Lecture Notes in Computer Science 10057

More information about this series at http://www.springer.com/series/7409

Andreas Holzinger · Alan Pope ·
Hugo Plácido da Silva (Eds.)

Physiological Computing Systems

International Conferences
PhyCS 2016, Lisbon, Portugal, July 27–28, 2016
PhyCS 2017, Madrid, Spain, July 27–28, 2017
PhyCS 2018, Seville, Spain, September 19–21, 2018
Revised and Extended Selected Papers

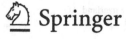
Springer

Editors
Andreas Holzinger ⓘ
Medical University of Graz
Graz, Austria

Alan Pope
NASA Langley Research Center
Hampton, VA, USA

Hugo Plácido da Silva ⓘ
IT - Instituto de Telecomunicações
Lisbon, Portugal

ISSN 0302-9743   ISSN 1611-3349   (electronic)
Lecture Notes in Computer Science
ISBN 978-3-030-27949-3   ISBN 978-3-030-27950-9   (eBook)
https://doi.org/10.1007/978-3-030-27950-9

LNCS Sublibrary: SL3 – Information Systems and Applications, incl. Internet/Web, and HCI

This Springer imprint is published by the registered company Springer Nature Switzerland AG
The registered company address is: Gewerbestrasse 11, 6330 Cham, Switzerland

Preface

Physiological data in its different dimensions, either bioelectrical, biomechanical, biochemical or biophysical, collected through specialized biomedical devices (video and image capture or other sources) is opening new boundaries in the field of human-computer interaction into what can be defined as Physiological Computing. The International Conference on Physiological Computing Systems (PhyCS) is a series of annual meetings of the physiological interaction and computing community, and serves as the main international forum for engineers, computer scientists, and health professionals, interested in outstanding research and development that bridges the gap between physiological data handling and human-computer interaction.

Given the topical nature of this subject, the present book includes extended and revised versions of a set of selected papers from the Third International Conference on Physiological Computing Systems (PhyCS 2016), 4th International Conference on Physiological Computing Systems (PhyCS 2017), and the 5th International Conference on Physiological Computing Systems (PhyCS 2018), which brought together people interested in creating novel interaction devices, adaptable interfaces, algorithms, and tools, through the study, planning, and design of interfaces between people and computers that are supported by multimodal biosignals.

This volume is a collection of the best papers, resulting in a final acceptance rate of approximately 20%, selected by the event chairs and their selection is based on a number of criteria that include the classifications and comments provided by the Program Committee members, the Session Chairs' assessment and also the Program Chairs' global view of all papers included in the technical program. The authors of selected papers were then invited to submit a revised and extended version of their papers having at least 30% innovative material.

The papers selected to be included in this book contribute to the understanding of relevant trends of current research on physiological computing systems, including brain-computer interfaces, virtual reality, psychophysiological load assessment in unconstrained scenarios, body tracking and movement pattern recognition, emotion recognition, machine learning applied to diabetes and hypertension, tangible biofeedback technologies, multimodal sensor data fusion, and deep learning for hand gesture recognition.

We would like to express our gratitude, first of all, to the contributing authors of the technical papers, whose work and dedication made it possible to put together an exciting program of high technical quality. We would also like to thank all the members of the international Program Committee and auxiliary reviewers, who provided a comprehensive set of thoughtful reviews, helping us with their expertise and

time. We would also like to thank the invited speakers for their invaluable contribution
and for sharing their vision in their talks. We are especially grateful to the INSTICC
Steering Committee whose invaluable work made this event possible.

September 2018   Andreas Holzinger
                                                                          Alan Pope
                                                                     Hugo Plácido Silva

Organization

Conference Co-chairs

Alan Pope   NASA, Retired, Distinguished Research Associate, USA

Hugo Plácido Silva   IT - Institute of Telecommunications, Portugal

Program Co-chairs

2016

Abraham Otero   Universidad San Pablo CEU, Spain

Stephen Fairclough   Liverpool John Moores University, UK

Andreas Holzinger   Medical University Graz, Austria

2017

Andreas Holzinger   Medical University Graz, Austria

2018

Juan-Manuel Belda-Lois   Instituto de Biomecánica de València, Spain

Chen Wang   Xinhua Net, China

Manuel Domínguez Morales   University of Seville, Spain

Program Committee

2016

Mohamed Abouelhoda   Nile University, Egypt

Jean-Marie Aerts   M3-BIORES, Katholieke Universitëit Leuven, Belgium

Jesús B. Alonso   Universidad de Las Palmas de Gran Canaria, Spain

Farid Amirouche   University of illinois at Chicago, USA

Luis Azevedo   Anditec, Portugal

Carryl Baldwin   George Mason University, USA

Panagiotis Bamidis   Aristotle University of Thessaloniki, Greece, and Leeds Institute of Medical Education, University of Leeds, UK

Adrian Barb   Penn State University, USA

Emiliano Barreto-Hernandez   Universidad Nacional de Colombia, Colombia

Bert-Jan van Beijnum   University of Twente, The Netherlands

Juan-Manuel Belda-Lois   Instituto de Biomecánica de València, Spain

Peter Bentley   UCL, UK

Kin-chuen Hui	The Chinese University of Hong Kong, SAR China
Ivan Ivanov	Technical University Sofia, Bulgaria
Sandeep Jha	Indian Institute of Technology Delhi, India
Bo Jin	MilliporeSigma, Merck KGaA, USA
Visakan Kadirkamanathan	The University of Sheffield, UK
Bozena Kaminska	Simon Fraser University, Canada
Bridget Kane	Karlstad University Business School, Sweden
Anastasia Kastania	Athens University of Economics and Business, Greece
Jonghwa Kim	University of Science and Technology, South Korea
Andrzej Kloczkowski	Ohio State University, USA
Stefanos Kollias	National Technical University of Athens, Greece
Shin'ichi Konomi	The University of Tokyo, Japan
Georgios Kontaxakis	Universidad Politecnica de Madrid, Spain
Ondrej Krejcar	University of Hradec Kralove, Czech Republic
Vaclav Kremen	Czech Technical University in Prague, Czech Republic
Dean Krusienski	Virginia Commonwealth University (VCU), USA
Vinod Kumar	IIT Roorkee, India
Iolanda Leite	INESC-id, Instituto Superior Técnico, Portugal
Lenka Lhotska	Czech Technical University in Prague, Czech Republic
Jiang Li	Old Dominion University, USA
Ying Li	IBM T. J. Watson Research Center, USA
Chun-Cheng Lin	National Chiao Tung University, Taiwan
Huei-Yung Lin	National Chung Cheng University, Taiwan
Giuseppe Liotta	University of Perugia, Italy
Benny Lo	Imperial College London, UK
Daniel Lopes	INESC ID Lisboa, Portugal
Martin Lopez-Nores	University of Vigo, Spain
Paulo Luzio de Melo	IDMEC-IST, MIT, USA
Mai Mabrouk	Misr University for Science and Technology, Egypt
Ratko Magjarevic	Faculty of Electrical Engineering and Computing, Croatia
Jarmo Malinen	Aalto University, Finland
Dan Mandru	Technical University of Cluj Napoca, Romania
Francesco Marcelloni	University of Pisa, Italy
Elena Marchiori	Radboud University, The Netherlands
Jan Mares	University of Chemistry and Technology, Czech Republic
G. Matsopoulos	School of Electrical and Computer Engineering, National Technical University of Athens, Greece
Gianluigi Me	Luiss University, Italy
Gerrit Meixner	Heilbronn University, Germany
Nuno Mendes	Instituto de Biologia Experimental e Tecnológica, Portugal
Silvano Mignanti	Sapienza University of Rome, Italy
Ji Ming	Queen's University Belfast, UK
Yehya Mohamad	Fraunhofer FIT, Germany

| Li Zhuo | Beijing University of Technology, China |
| André Züquete | IEETA, IT, Universidade de Aveiro, Portugal |

2017

Jean-Marie Aerts	M3-BIORES, Katholieke Universitëit Leuven, Belgium
Jesüs B. Alonso	Universidad de Las Palmas de Gran Canaria, Spain
Philip Azariadis	University of the Aegean, Greece
Luis Azevedo	Anditec, Portugal
Panagiotis Bamidis	Aristotle University of Thessaloniki, Greece, and Leeds Institute of Medical Education, University of Leeds, UK
Emiliano Barreto-Hernandez	Universidad Nacional de Colombia, Colombia
Bert-Jan van Beijnum	University of Twente, The Netherlands
Juan-Manuel Belda-Lois	Instituto de Biomecánica de València, Spain
Peter Bentley	UCL, UK
Dinesh Bhatia	North Eastern Hill University, India
Luciano Boquete	Alcala University, Spain
Alfred Bruckstein	Technion, Israel
Ahmet Çakir	ERGONOMIC Institute, Germany
Mónica Cameirão	Madeira Interactive Technologies Institute, Portugal
Eric Campo	LAAS CNRS, France
John Chuang	UC Berkeley, USA
Pietro Cipresso	IRCCS Istituto Auxologico Italiano, Italy
Miguel Coimbra	IT, University of Porto, Portugal
Jan Cornelis	VUB, Belgium
David Cornforth	University of Newcastle, Australia
Fernando Cruz	College of Technology of Setubal, Polytechnic Institute of Setubal, Portugal
Antoine Danchin	Institut Cochin INSERM U1016, CNRS UMR8104, Université Paris Descartes, France
Thomas Dandekar	University of Würzburg, Germany
George Dulikravich	Florida International University, USA
Gintautas Dzemyda	Vilnius University, Lithuania
Anastasios Economides	University of Macedonia, Greece
Christo El Morr	York University, Canada
George Eleftherakis	CITY College, International Faculty of the University of Sheffield, Greece
Mireya Fernández Chimeno	Universitat Politècnica de Catalunya, Spain
Fabrizio Ferre	University of Rome Tor Vergata, Italy
Leonardo Franco	Universidad de Málaga, Spain
Christoph Friedrich	University of Applied Sciences and Arts Dortmund, Germany
Ioannis Fudos	University of Ioannina, Greece
Juan Carlos Garcia	University of Alcala, Spain

Nuno Garcia	University of Beira Interior, Portugal
Max Garzon	The University of Memphis, USA
Aaron Golden	National University of Ireland Galway, Ireland
Daniel Gonçalves	INESC-ID, Instituto Superior Técnico, Portugal
David Greenhalgh	University of Strathclyde, UK
Clemens Heitzinger	Technical University Vienna (TU Vienna), Austria
Thomas Hinze	Friedrich Schiller University Jena, Germany
Chun-Hsi Huang	University of Connecticut, USA
Ivan Ivanov	Technical University Sofia, Bulgaria
Bart Jansen	Vrije Universiteit Brussel, Belgium
Sandeep Jha	Indian Institute of Technology Delhi, India
Bo Jin	MilliporeSigma, Merck KGaA, USA
Bozena Kaminska	Simon Fraser University, Canada
Bridget Kane	Karlstad University Business School, Sweden
Stefanos Kollias	National Technical University of Athens, Greece
Georgios Kontaxakis	Universidad Politecnica de Madrid, Spain
Ondrej Krejcar	University of Hradec Kralove, Czech Republic
Vaclav Kremen	Czech Technical University in Prague, Czech Republic
Dean Krusienski	Virginia Commonwealth University (VCU), USA
Vinod Kumar	IIT Roorkee, India
Lenka Lhotska	Czech Technical University in Prague, Czech Republic
Ying Li	IBM T. J. Watson Research Center, USA
Huei-Yung Lin	National Chung Cheng University, Taiwan
Giuseppe Liotta	University of Perugia, Italy
Benny Lo	Imperial College London, UK
Daniel Lopes	INESC ID Lisboa, Portugal
Martin Lopez-Nores	University of Vigo, Spain
Paulo Luzio de Melo	IDMEC-IST, MIT, USA
Mai Mabrouk	Misr University for Science and Technology, Egypt
Dennis Majoe	ETH Zurich, Switzerland
Jarmo Malinen	Aalto University, Finland
Dan Mandru	Technical University of Cluj Napoca, Romania
Francesco Marcelloni	University of Pisa, Italy
Jan Mares	University of Chemistry and Technology, Czech Republic
Jorge Martins	Instituto Superior Técnico, Portugal
Gerrit Meixner	Heilbronn University, Germany
Silvano Mignanti	Sapienza University of Rome, Italy
Ji Ming	Queen's University Belfast, UK
Miroslav Minovic	University of Belgrade, Serbia
Yehya Mohamad	Fraunhofer FIT, Germany
Mihaela Morega	University Politehnica of Bucharest, Romania
Kazuya Murao	Ritsumeikan University, Japan
Robert Newcomb	University of Maryland, USA
Domen Novak	University of Wyoming, USA

Ian Oakley   Ulsan National Institute of Science and Technology,
                              South Korea
Rui Pedro Paiva   University of Coimbra, Portugal
Krzysztof Pancerz   University of Rzeszow, Poland
Shahram Payandeh   Experimental Robotics and Graphics Laboratory,
                              Canada
Evan Peck   Bucknell University, USA
Gennaro Percannella   University of Salerno, Italy
Horacio Pérez-Sánchez   Catholic University of Murcia, Spain
Vitor Pires   Escola Superior de Tecnologia de Setübal,
                              Instituto Politécnico de Setübal, Portugal
Ales Prochazka   University of Chemistry and Technology,
                              Czech Republic
José Joaquín Rieta   Universidad Politécnica de Valencia, Spain
Luís Rocha   University of Minho, Portugal
Carsten Röcker   Ostwestfalen-Lippe aus, Fraunhofer IOSB-INA,
                              Germany
Marcos Rodrigues   Sheffield Hallam University, UK
Heather Ruskin   Dublin City University, Ireland
Wim Rutten   University of Twente, The Netherlands
Seonghan Ryu   Hannam University, South Korea
Maytham Safar   Kuwait University, Kuwait
George Sakellaropoulos   University of Patras, Greece
J. Salgado   University of Chile, Chile
Ovidio Salvetti   National Research Council of Italy - CNR, Italy
Andres Santos   Universidad Politécnica de Madrid, Spain
Henrique Santos   University of Minho, Portugal
Nilanjan Sarkar   Vanderbilt University, USA
Chutham Sawigun   Mahanakorn University of Technology, Thailand
Emanuele Schiavi   Universidad Rey Juan Carlos, Spain
Tanja Schultz   Cognitive Systems Lab (CSL), University of Bremen,
                              Germany
Tapio Seppänen   University of Oulu, Finland
Pavel Smrz   Brno University of Technology, Czech Republic
Alcimar Soares   Universidade Federal de Uberlândia, Brazil
Jiri Spilka   Czech Technical University in Prague, Czech Republic
Mu-Chun Su   National Central University, Taiwan
Miguel Tavares da Silva   Instituto Superior Técnico, Portugal
António Teixeira   University of Aveiro, Portugal
Carlos M. Travieso   University of Las Palmas de Gran Canaria, Spain
Alexander Tsouknidas   Aristotle University of Thessaloniki, Greece
Luis Valente   Universidade do Minho, Portugal
Rob van der Mei   CWI Amsterdam, The Netherlands
Alfredo Vellido   Universitat Politècnica de Catalunya, Spain
Justin Wan   University of Waterloo, Canada
Yuanyuan Wang   Fudan University, China

Junzo Watada	Universiti Teknologi PETRONAS, Malaysia
Quan Wen	University of Electronic Science and Technology of China, China
Didier Wolf	Research Centre for Automatic Control, CRAN CNRS UMR 7039, France
Vera Yashina	Dorodnicyn Computing Center of the Russian Academy of Sciences, Russia
Leming Zhou	University of Pittsburgh, USA
Li Zhuo	Beijing University of Technology, China
André Züquete	IEETA, IT, Universidade de Aveiro, Portugal

2018

Jean-Marie Aerts	M3-BIORES, Katholieke Universitëit Leuven, Belgium
Jesús B. Alonso	Universidad de Las Palmas de Gran Canaria, Spain
Carryl Baldwin	George Mason University, USA
Panagiotis Bamidis	Aristotle University of Thessaloniki, Greece, and Leeds Institute of Medical Education, University of Leeds, UK
Dinesh Bhatia	North Eastern Hill University, India
Ahmet Çakir	ERGONOMIC Institute, Germany
Mónica Cameirão	Madeira Interactive Technologies Institute, Portugal
Eric Campo	LAAS CNRS, France
Pierre Chalfoun	Ubisoft, Canada
John Chuang	UC Berkeley, USA
Miguel Coimbra	IT, University of Porto, Portugal
Jan Cornelis	VUB, Belgium
Manuel Domínguez Morales	University of Seville, Spain
George Dulikravich	Florida International University, USA
Gintautas Dzemyda	Vilnius University, Lithuania
Mireya Fernández Chimeno	Universitat Politècnica de Catalunya, Spain
Leonardo Franco	Universidad de Málaga, Spain
Claude Frasson	University of Montreal, Canada
Christoph Friedrich	University of Applied Sciences and Arts Dortmund, Germany
Ioannis Fudos	University of Ioannina, Greece
Juan Carlos Garcia	University of Alcala, Spain
Miguel García Gonzalez	Universitat Politècnica de Catalunya, Spain
Max Garzon	The University of Memphis, USA
Paulo Gil	Universidade Nova de Lisboa, Portugal
Kiel Gilleade	University of Illinois, USA
Daniel Gonçalves	INESC-ID, Instituto Superior Técnico, Portugal
David Greenhalgh	University of Strathclyde, UK
Thomas Hinze	Friedrich Schiller University Jena, Germany
Chun-Hsi Huang	University of Connecticut, USA

Ivan Ivanov   Technical University Sofia, Bulgaria
Sandeep Jha   Indian Institute of Technology Delhi, India
Bo Jin   MilliporeSigma, Merck KGaA, USA
Stefanos Kollias   National Technical University of Athens, Greece
Georgios Kontaxakis   Universidad Politecnica de Madrid, Spain
Ondrej Krejcar   University of Hradec Kralove, Czech Republic
Vaclav Kremen   Czech Technical University in Prague, Czech Republic
Dean Krusienski   Virginia Commonwealth University (VCU), USA
Chun-Cheng Lin   National Chiao Tung University, Taiwan
Giuseppe Liotta   University of Perugia, Italy
Benny Lo   Imperial College London, UK
Martin Lopez-Nores   University of Vigo, Spain
Jarmo Malinen   Aalto University, Finland
Dan Mandru   Technical University of Cluj Napoca, Romania
Jan Mares   University of Chemistry and Technology,
                              Czech Republic
Jorge Martins   Instituto Superior Técnico, Portugal
Gianluigi Me   Luiss University, Italy
Yehya Mohamad   Fraunhofer FIT, Germany
Pedro Monteiro   INESC-ID, IST - Universidade de Lisboa, Portugal
Umberto Morbiducci   Politecnico di Torino, Italy
Alexandru Morega   University Politehnica of Bucharest, Romania
Mihaela Morega   University Politehnica of Bucharest, Romania
Robert Newcomb   University of Maryland, USA
Domen Novak   University of Wyoming, USA
Helcio Orlande   POLI/COPPE Federal University of Rio de Janeiro,
                              Brazil
Rui Pedro Paiva   University of Coimbra, Portugal
Krzysztof Pancerz   University of Rzeszow, Poland
Shahram Payandeh   Experimental Robotics and Graphics Laboratory,
                              Canada
José Pazos-Arias   University of Vigo, Spain
Vitor Pires   Escola Superior de Tecnologia de Setúbal,
                              Instituto Politécnico de Setúbal, Portugal
José Joaquín Rieta   Universidad Politécnica de Valencia, Spain
Luís Rocha   University of Minho, Portugal
Simona Rombo   Dipartimento di Matematica e Informatica,
                              Università degli Studi di Palermo, Italy
Heather Ruskin   Dublin City University, Ireland
Seonghan Ryu   Hannam University, South Korea
Maytham Safar   Kuwait University, Kuwait
George Sakellaropoulos   University of Patras, Greece
J. Salgado   University of Chile, Chile
Ovidio Salvetti   National Research Council of Italy - CNR, Italy
Akio Sashima   AIST, Japan
Chutham Sawigun   Mahanakorn University of Technology, Thailand

Reinhold Scherer	University of Essex, UK
Emanuele Schiavi	Universidad Rey Juan Carlos, Spain
Thomas Schlitt	Novartis Institute of BioMedical Research, Switzerland
Tapio Seppänen	University of Oulu, Finland
Kulwinder Singh	University of South Florida, USA
Pavel Smrz	Brno University of Technology, Czech Republic
Mu-Chun Su	National Central University, Taiwan
Miguel Tavares da Silva	Instituto Superior Técnico, Portugal
António Teixeira	University of Aveiro, Portugal
Vitor Teodoro	Universidade Nova Lisboa, Portugal
William Toscano	NASA Ames, USA
Carlos M. Travieso	University of Las Palmas de Gran Canaria, Spain
Rob van der Mei	CWI Amsterdam, The Netherlands
Alfredo Vellido	Universitat Politècnica de Catalunya, Spain
Francisco Veredas	Universidad de Málaga, Spain
Susana Vinga	IDMEC, Portugal
Justin Wan	University of Waterloo, Canada
Chen Wang	Xinhua Net, China
Yuanyuan Wang	Fudan University, China
Quan Wen	University of Electronic Science and Technology of China, China
Didier Wolf	CRAN UMR CNRS 7039, Université de Lorraine, France
Erliang Zeng	University of Iowa, USA
Leming Zhou	University of Pittsburgh, USA

Additional Reviewers

2016

Michael Bauer	Heilbronn University, Germany
Sebastian Rauh	Heilbronn University, Germany

2017

Tiago Pereira	Universidade do Minho - Escola de Engenharia, Portugal

Invited Speakers

2016

Kevin Warwick	Coventry University, UK
Tanja Schultz	Cognitive Systems Lab (CSL), University of Bremen, Germany
Anastasios Economides	University of Macedonia, Greece

2017

Pablo Cesar   Centrum Wiskunde and Informatica, The Netherlands
Juan-Manuel Belda-Lois Instituto de Biomecánica de València, Spain

2018

Eduardo Rocon   Consejo Superior de Investigaciones Científicas, Spain
Lucas Noldus   Noldus Information Technology bv, The Netherlands
Georgios N. Yannakakis University of Malta, Malta
Norbert Streitz   Founder and Scientific Director, Smart Future
                        Initiative, Germany

Contents

Development and Assessment of a Self-paced BCI-VR Paradigm Using Multimodal Stimulation and Adaptive Performance

Athanasios Vourvopoulos[1,2,3](✉) , André Ferreira[1],
and Sergi Bermudez i Badia[1,2]

[1] Faculdade das Ciências Exatas e da Engenharia, Universidade da Madeira,
Campus Universitário da Penteada, 9020-105 Funchal, Portugal
[2] Madeira Interactive Technologies Institute, Polo Científico e
Tecnológico da Madeira, Caminho da Penteada, 9020-105 Funchal, Portugal
athanasios.vourvopoulos@m-iti.org
[3] University of Southern California, Los Angeles, CA, USA

Abstract. Motor-Imagery based Brain-Computer Interfaces (BCIs) can provide alternative communication pathways to neurologically impaired patients. The combination of BCIs and Virtual Reality (VR) can provide induced illusions of movement to patients with low-level of motor control during motor rehabilitation tasks. Unfortunately, current BCI systems lack reliability and good performance levels in comparison with other types of computer interfaces. To date, there is little evidence on how BCI-based motor training needs to be designed for transferring rehabilitation improvements to real life. Based on our previous work, we showcase the development and assessment of NeuRow, a novel multiplatform immersive VR environment that makes use of multimodal stimulation through vision, sound and vibrotactile feedback and delivered through a VR Head Mounted Display. In addition, we integrated the Adaptive Performance Engine (APE), a statistical approach to optimize user control in a self-paced BCI-VR paradigm. In this paper, we describe the development and pilot assessment of NeuRow as well as its integration and assessment with APE.

Keywords: Brain-Computer Interfaces · Motor imagery · Virtual reality · Adaptive performance · Neurorehabilitation

1 Introduction

Motor Imagery (MI) is the mental rehearsal of movement -without any muscle activation- and is a mental ability strongly related to the body or 'embodied' cognition [1]. MI appears to largely share the control mechanisms and neural substrates of actual movement both in action execution and action observation [2], providing a unique opportunity to study neural control of movement in either healthy people or patients [3, 4]. Since MI leads to the activation of overlapping brain areas with actual movement, and because sensory and motor cortices can dynamically reorganize [5, 6], MI can be an important strategy for motor learning and recovery. Hence, MI has important

© Springer Nature Switzerland AG 2019
A. Holzinger et al. (Eds.): PhyCS 2016–2018, LNCS 10057, pp. 1–22, 2019.
https://doi.org/10.1007/978-3-030-27950-9_1

benefits and is currently utilized as a technique in neurorehabilitation for people with neurological impairments [7].

MI offers an important basis for the development of brain-to-computer communication systems called Brain–Computer Interfaces (BCIs). BCIs are capable of establishing an alternative pathway between the brain and a computer or prosthetic devices [8] that could assist (assistive BCI) or rehabilitate physically (restorative BCI) disabled people and stroke survivors [9].

More recently, Virtual Reality (VR) feedback has also been used in MI BCI training, offering a more compelling experience to the user through 3D virtual environments [10, 11]. The fusion of BCI and VR (BCI-VR) allows a wide range of experiences where participants can control various aspects of their environment -either in an explicit or implicit manner-, by using mental imagery alone [12]. This direct brain-to-VR communication can induce illusions mostly relying on the sensorimotor contingencies between perception and action [13].

The idea of utilising BCIs in virtual rehabilitation (virtual reality and tele-medicine for neurorehabilitation), was fostered in order to complement current VR rehabilitation strategies [14, 15] where patients with low level of motor control –such as those suffering of flaccidity or increased levels of spasticity [16] - could not benefit due to low range of motion, pain, fatique, etc.

The main challenge in the use of BCIs, regardless of the BCI cost, lies in the lack of reliability and good performance at the system level that inexperienced users have [17] due to BCI "illiteracy" of users (inability of the user to produce vivid mental images of movement resulting in poor BCI performance) [18, 19]. Although previous studies have shown mixed results, the combination of haptic and visual feedback seems to increase performance [20, 21]. It has been shown that replacing the standard visual BCI feedback with vibrotactile feedback does not interfere with the EEG signal acquisition [22] and also does not impact negatively the classification performance [22, 23]. On the other hand, it has been shown to have a positive effect on visual workload measured in a multiple object tracking task (MOT) where the data revealed significant differences between visual or tactile feedback [24]. It has also been shown that with the use of haptic feedback, the user can pay more attention to the task instead of to the feedback [23], and in [25] users achieved higher scores in the vibrotactile feedback setting. Vibrotactile feedback has also been used in a hybrid BCI system [26], where MI with selective sensation (SS) were used in order to increase performance. On this system, equal vibration is applied to both wrists of the user and he/she has to imagine that the vibration to one of the sides is stronger than the other. SS combined with MI increased the overall performance of the system. In [25], it is also reported that the vibrotactile feedback applied on the user's hand significantly increases MI performance. In [27] the use of vibrotactile feedback directly applied to certain tendons is used to convey the illusion of movement to the user, and in conjunction with a virtual representation of the arm, significantly increased the accuracy of a BCI system. Further, recent findings with the use of virtual arms have shown that the combination of motor priming (physical rehearsal of a movement) preceding BCI-VR MI training can improve performance as well as the capacity to modulate and enhance sensorimotor brain activity rhythms, important in rehabilitation research [28].

In addition, there is an increased need for alternative motivational mechanisms and feedback approaches for BCI systems [29, 30]. Previous research in learning states that a poorly designed feedback can actually deteriorate motivation and impede successful learning [31]. On the other hand, providing extensive feedback to the user can lead to efficient and high quality learning [32]. Lotte et al. recommended a set of guidelines for a good instructional design in BCI training, in which (1) the user should only be presented with the correct classified action for enhancing the feeling of competence; (2) provide a simplified and intuitive task; (3) meaningful and self-explanatory task; (4) challenging but achievable, with feedback on progress of achievement; and finally (5) in an engaging 3D virtual environment [30].

To date, and to the best of our knowledge, there is not a holistic approach in BCI MI training that combines the advantages of different feedback modalities (immersive VR environment, vibrotactile feedback), training approaches (motor priming preceding MI) and motivational mechanisms (game-like tasks). Further, in order to be able to harness the benefits of BCI in neurorehabilitation, two questions need to be addressed: (a) how can we increase user performance in BCI MI training, and (b) how can we maximize the activation of the brain areas responsible for actual movement. Answering these questions will enable the appearance of novel BCI paradigms that will allow us to promote more efficiently reorganization of sensorimotor cortices of motor impaired patients (such as for instance stroke), which ultimately can lead to higher levels of recovery.

The purpose of this paper is twofold. First we describe the development and pilot assessment of NeuRow [33], a novel VR environment for MI training. Secondly, we present the integration with and assessment of the Adaptive Performance Engine (APE) [34]. The combination of APE with NeuRow is an attempt to optimize user control in a self-paced BCI-VR paradigm. NeuRow makes use of multimodal feedback (auditory, haptic and visual) in a VR environment delivered through an immersive Head Mounted Display (HMD), integrated in a BCI MI training task (left|right hand motor imagery). Current results are presented through two studies. (1) Development and assessment of the NeuRow VR setup in terms of performance and feedback, and (2) assessment of use performance in NeuRow integrated with APE in terms of sense of control.

2 Development and Assessment of the VR Training Paradigm

In this chapter, we describe the design, development and early assessment of NeuRow including the preliminary results.

2.1 Experimental Setup

The experimental setup was composed by a desktop computer (OS: Windows 8.1, CPU: Intel® Core™ i5-2400 at 3.10 GHz, RAM: 4 GB DDR3 1600 MHz, Graphics: AMD Radeon HD 6700), running the acquisition software, the BCI-VR task, HMD, EEG system, and the vibrotactile module.

EEG Acquisition. The BCI system for the first study consisted of 8 active electrodes equipped with a low-noise biosignal amplifier and a 16-bit A/D converter at 256 Hz (g.MOBIlab+ biosignal amplifier, g.tec, Graz, Austria). The spatial distribution of the electrodes followed the 10–20 system configuration [35] with the following electrodes over the somatosensory and motor areas: Frontal-Central (FC5, FC6), Central (C1, C2, C3, C4), and Central-Parietal (CP5, CP6) (see Fig. 1a). The BCI system was connected via bluetooth to the dedicated desktop computer for the EEG signal acquisition. EEG data acquisition and processing was performed through the OpenVibe platform [36] combined with the Reh@Panel (RehabNet Control Panel) [37] via the VRPN protocol [38] to control the virtual environment. The Reh@Panel is a free tool that acts as a middleware between multiple interfaces and virtual environments.

Feedback Presentation. For delivering feedback to the user, the Oculus Rift DK1 HMD was used (Oculus VR, Irvine, California, USA). The HMD is made of one 7″ 1280 × 800 60 Hz LCD display (64 × 800 resolution per eye), one aspheric acrylic lens per eye, 110° Field of View (FOV), internal tracking through a gyroscope, accelerometer, and magnetometer, with a tracking frequency of 1000 Hz (Fig. 1b).

Vibrotactile Feedback. A custom vibrotactile feedback module was developed with out-of-the-box components including an Arduino Mega 2560 board and vibrating motors. The vibrating motors (10 mm diameter, 2.7 mm thick) performed at 11000 RPM at 5 V and were mounted on cylindrical tubes that acted as grasping objects for inducing the illusion of movement during the BCI task (Fig. 1c). In our setup, a pair of carton-based tubes with 12 cm of length and 3 cm diameter were used. Finally, 3D printed cases were produced to accommodate the vibrating motors inside the tubes (see Fig. 2). All hardware and software blueprints are made available free online.

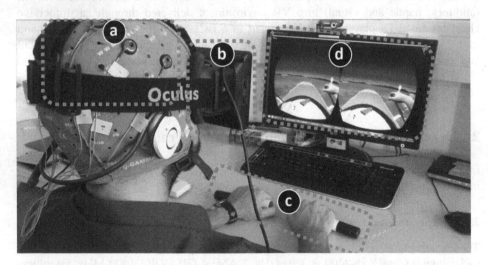

Fig. 1. Experimental setup (a) EEG cap with 8 active electrodes, (b) HMD, (c) vibrotactile modules, (d) BCI feedback, adapted from [32].

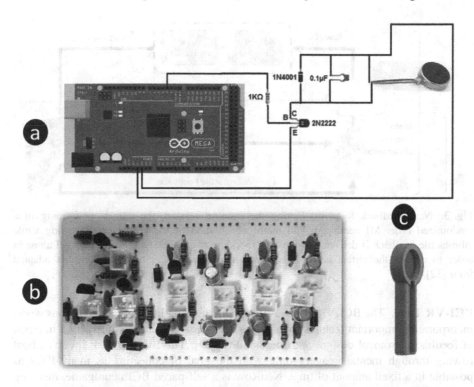

Fig. 2. (a) Arduino board schematic including the necessary electronic components (for one motor), (b) custom Arduino shield, (c) 3D printed casing for motors. Code and schematics can be downloaded from: http://neurorehabilitation.m-iti.org/bci/neurow/vibrotactile-module/.

2.2 BCI Task Design

BCI-VR Training Protocol. The training protocol was designed and adapted based on the Graz-BCI paradigm [39], substituting the standard feedback presented (directional arrows) by multimodal VR feedback. The first step of the training consisted on the acquisition of the raw EEG data to train a linear discriminant classifier to distinguish Right and Left imagined hand movements. Throughout the training session, the user performs mental imagery of the corresponding hand (based on the presented stimuli). For each hand, the user is stimulated visually (VR action observation), auditorily, and haptically through the vibration on the corresponding hand (Fig. 3a). The training session was configured to acquire data in 24 blocks (epochs) per class (Right or Left hand imagery) in a randomized order. Following the training, data are used to compute a Common Spatial Patterns (CSP) filter, a spatial filter that maximizes the difference between the signals of the two classes. Finally, the raw EEG and the spatial filter are used to train a Linear Discriminant Analysis (LDA) classifier.

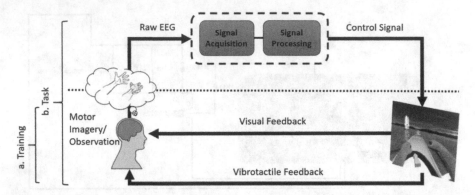

Fig. 3. Neurofeedback loop. (a) During the training session, the user is performing in a randomized order MI combined with motor observation of the virtual hands rowing while vibrotactile feedback is delivered to the corresponding hand. (b) The user relies on MI alone in order to control the virtual hands in a closed-loop system after training. Figure is adapted from [32].

BCI-VR Task. The BCI-VR task was designed based on literature and previous work, incorporating important features for a successful brain-to-computer interaction in terms of feedback, protocol design, and accessibility [29]. The BCI-VR task involves boat rowing through mental imagery only with the goal of collecting as many flags as possible in a fixed amount of time. NeuRow is a self-paced BCI neurogame, meaning that is not event related, and the user controls the timing of rowing actions like he/she would do in real-life (Fig. 3b). NeuRow is a multiplatform virtual environment developed in Unity game engine (Unity Technologies, San Francisco, California, USA). Finally, NeuRow is optimized for different platforms, however with different features (Table 1. NeuRow features for the different supported platforms Table 1). Namely:

- *Desktop:* The standalone version for PC, supports high quality graphics for an immersive VR experience with the support of the Oculus Rift DK1 headset and the HTC Vive, the Leap Motion hand controller (Motion control, San Francisco, California, USA) available for optional motor-priming before the MI BCI session. Finally, vibrotactile feedback is supported by using custom-made hardware for controlling through USB up to 6 vibration motors (Fig. 2). Data logging is supported for boat trajectory, target location, score and time.
- *Mobile:* The mobile version is built for Android OS devices, receiving data via the RehabNet UDP protocol through the Reh@panel. For phones, the VR feature is utilized for VR glasses (e.g. Google VR) by applying lens correction for each eye, and using the phone gyroscope and magnetometer for head tracking, offering an immersive experience similar to the Oculus DK1 HMD.
- *Web Browser:* The web version uses the Unity web player (compatible through Internet Explorer, Firefox or Opera), does not support the networking, HMD and haptic components due to security restrictions. Instead, the web NeuRow acquires data through emulated keyboard events generated by the Reh@panel.

Table 1. NeuRow features for the different supported platforms. Adapted from [32].

Features/platform	Desktop	Android	Web
Logging	✓	X	X
VR	✓ (Oculus DK, HTC Vive)	✓ (Google VR)	X
Hand tracking	✓ (Leap Motion)	X	X
Networking	✓	✓	X
Platform independent	X	X	✓
Vibrotactile feedback	✓ (Arduino)	X	X

The in-game interface is simple, with two high fidelity virtual arms to rotate the oars, time indication, score and navigational aids (Fig. 4). NeuRow can be customized with different settings, depending on the experimental setup, BCI paradigm and running platform. Through the settings, one can choose if the session is part of the MI training or self-paced online control of the boat. During training, the navigational arrow and the targets are removed to focus the user only on the multimodal MI BCI-VR task. During self-paced mode, the behavior of the boat can be changed by setting the heading speed, turn speed and cut-off angle. The cut-off angle is the allowed angle that the boat can be off-course with respect to the target flag before stopping. This serves as a protection mechanism to help the player not to deviate in excess from the target.

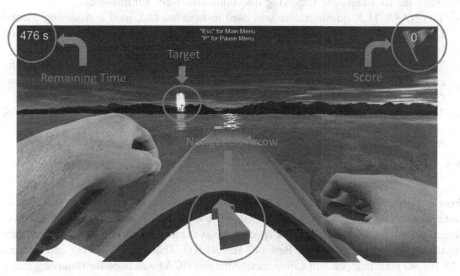

Fig. 4. In-game interface. An arrow indicates the direction of the target and also the distance by changing its color (red for far blending up to green for close). Top Left: Remaining time for the end of the session. Middle: A flag with a ray acts as the game targets, Top Right: Game scoring, counting the number of targets. Adapted from [32]. (Color figure online)

2.3 Participants

A voluntary sample of 13 users (mean age of 28 ± 5 years old) was recruited for the pilot study, based on their motivation to participate in the study. All participants were male and right handed with no previous known neurological disorder, nor previous experience in BCIs. Participants were either university students or academic staff. Finally, all participants provided their written informed consent before participating in the study.

2.4 Questionnaires

Before each BCI training session, demographics and user data were gathered through the following questionnaires:

- The Vividness of Movement Imagery Questionnaire-2 (VMIQ2) was used to assess the capability of the participant to perform an imagined movement (Kinesthetic Imagery) [40]. Kinesthetic Imagery (KI) questions were combined with mental chronometry by measuring the response time in perceptual-motor tasks with the help of a timer.
- For assessing gaming experience we used the Gamer Dedication (GD) questionnaire, a 15 factor classification questionnaire in which participants are asked whether they "strongly disagree," or "strongly agree" with a series of statements about their gaming habits [41].
- After the BCI task, the following questionnaires were administered:
- The NASA TLX questionnaire was used to measure task load considering Mental Demand, Physical Demand, Temporal Demand, Performance, Effort and Frustration [42].
- The core modules of the Game Experience Questionnaire (GEQ) were used at the end of the BCI session. GEQ assesses game experience using Immersion, Flow, Competence, Positive and Negative Affect, Tension, and Challenge [43].
- The System Usability Scale (SUS) is a ten-item scale giving a global view of subjective assessments of usability [44].

2.5 EEG Data

Power Spectral Density (PSD). EEG signals were processed in Matlab (MathWorks Inc., Massachusetts, US) with the EEGLAB toolbox [45] for extracting the Power Spectral Density (PSD). The power spectrum was extracted for the following frequency rhythms: Alpha (8 Hz–12 Hz), Beta (12 Hz–30 Hz), Theta (4 Hz–7 Hz), and Gamma (25 Hz–90 Hz). Independent Component Analysis (ICA) was used for removing major artefacts related with power-line noise, eye blinking, ECG and EMG activity. For the current analysis, and because we were only measuring from sensory-motor areas, data were averaged for all the channels for each experimental condition.

Engagement Index. The Engagement Index (EI) is a metric proposed at NASA Langley for evaluating operator engagement in automated tasks, was validated through a bio-cybernetic system for Adaptive Automation [46], and is widely used in EEG studies for assessing engagement [47]. We therefore computed engagement index from the EEG power spectrum according to the EI formula (Eq. 1), where α = Alpha band, β = Beta band and θ = Theta band:

$$EI = \beta/(\alpha + \theta) \tag{1}$$

2.6   Preliminary Results

In the following section, we analyzed NeuRow's BCI task performance in terms of classifier score during training, user acceptance as assessed by the SUS, GEX and TLX questionnaires, and finally the relationship between game behavior and user experience through the questionnaires and also the EEG activity.

Performance. Comparing the performance score with previous studies which used LDA classifiers in two class (left, right hand) MI, we are able to gain insights concerning the effectiveness of our BCI-VR paradigm in terms of user control [48–51]. As illustrated in Fig. 5, the comparison places NeuRow as the fourth highest with a mean performance of 70.7% out of 12 studies. Moreover, of those studies that used exactly the same feature extraction technique of band power (BP) and CSP [17], NeuRow scores the highest. Finally, of those studies that used VR as a training environment [28], again NeuRow scores first.

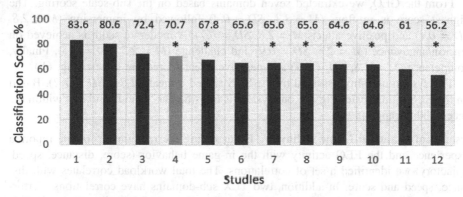

Fig. 5. Ranked accuracy of performance in pure MI based BCI studies using two classes (left and right hand imagery) with respect to LDA classification [47–50]. The asterisk (*) over 4,5,7,8,9,10 and 12 [16, 27] indicates studies which use the same feature extraction method (BP with CSP). The data of this study corresponds to the 4th best. Adapted from [32].

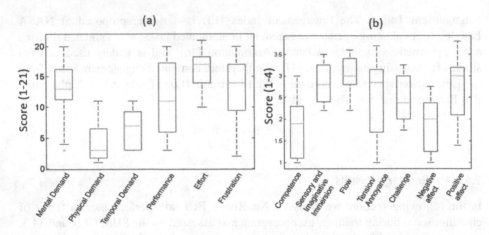

Fig. 6. (a) TLX scores between 1–20 for mental demand, physical demand, temporal demand, performance, effort and frustration. (b) Scores for the GEQ core questionnaire domains.

User Acceptance. To assess different aspects of the user experience during online control of NeuRow, the mental workload, gaming experience and system usability were assessed after the task.

For workload, the NASA-TLX mean score was relatively high at 66.8/100 ($SD = 14.5$). As it is illustrated in Fig. 6a, the two lowest scores are those for physical ($M = 4.4$, $SD = 3.4$) and temporal ($M = 6.5$, $SD = 3$) demand. The highest score is on effort ($M = 16.4$, $SD = 5.2$) followed closely by frustration ($M = 13.3$, $SD = 5.2$) and mental demand ($M = 12.8$, $SD = 5$). Performance lies in the middle ($M = 11.4$, $SD = 6.2$).

From the GEQ, we extracted seven domains based on the sub-scale scoring. The highest score is in flow ($M = 3.1$, $SD = 0.4$) followed by immersion ($M = 2.8$, $SD = 0.4$) and positive affect ($M = 2.8$, $SD = 0.7$). A moderate score is achieved on tension/annoyance ($M = 2.5$, $SD = 0.9$) and challenge ($M = 2.5$, $SD = 0.5$). Finally, competence ($M = 1.8$, $SD = 0.7$) and negative affect scored the lowest (Fig. 6b).

The system usability assessed by the SUS scored a mean of 74 ($SD = 7.2$). Based on the SUS rating scale (Fig. 7), our system is classified as "Good" and it is within the acceptability range [52].

User-Profile and In-Game Behavior. By assessing the relationship of the reported experience and the EEG activity with the in-game behavior (score, distance, speed, trajectory) we identified a set of correlations. The total workload correlates with distance, speed and score. In addition, two TLX sub-domains have correlations. Performance is significantly correlated with distance and speed, as well as frustration is significantly correlated with distance, speed and score. Furthermore, mental chronometry (the response time in perceptual-motor tasks), significantly correlates with distance, speed and score. Finally, from the extracted EEG bands and the resulting Engagement Index, we can see that Alpha and Theta bands are reversely correlated with distance and speed. Finally, Engagement Index is interestingly correlated with all in-game metrics. In particular, distance, speed, score and trajectory smoothness.

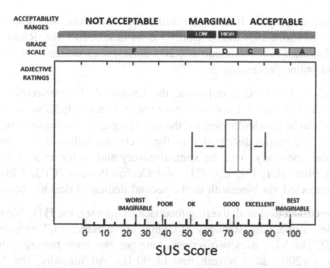

Fig. 7. SUS results for all users. Acceptability scales are displayed on top (not acceptable, marginal and acceptable), followed by the grade scale (A to F) and the adjective rating (0–100). Adapted from [32].

Overall, we identified an imbalance between theoretical training performance (LDA) and actual quality of the online performance (game score and control). In current MI-BCI interaction users undergo long, tiresome and complex periods of training so that EEG classification score can reach acceptable performance rates. On the following chapter, we propose to reverse the problem and make MI-BCI interaction adaptive to the user, so that we can guarantee a satisfactory performance rates by softening decisions – making them probabilistic and non-time-constrained – depending on our confidence on the user's EEG data.

3 Augmenting Control Through Adaptive Performance

Following the design and development stage of NeuRow, as a next step, we conducted a complementary assessment by incorporating the APE module together with the Reh@Panel. APE aims at adapting the BCI interaction to each user in order to maximize the level of control on their actions, whatever their performance level is. Our objective is evaluating the improvements in performance and perceived sense of control -at the user level instead of the classifier output- with the APE. For this, we integrated a state-of-the-art HMD for increased immersion and an ultraportable wireless EEG system.

3.1 Experimental Setup

For this second study, a dedicated desktop computer was used for delivering the multimodal feedback: the VR environment, the vibrotactile module and the HMD (OS: Windows 10 Pro, CPU: Intel® Core™ i7-6700 at 3.40 GHz, RAM: 8GM DD3

1600 MHz, Graphics: AMD Radeon R9 390 Series). Additionally, a second desktop (OS: Windows 10 Pro, CPU: Intel® Core™ i5-4440 at 3.10 GHz, RAM: 8GM DD3 1600 MHz, Graphics: AMD Radeon R7 200 Series) was utilized for the EEG data acquisition and online processing.

EEG Acquisition. For EEG acquisition, the Enobio 8 (Neuroelectrics, Barcelona, Spain) system had been used. Enobio, is a wearable, wireless EEG sensor with 8 EEG channels and a triaxial accelerometer, for the recording and visualization of 24 bit EEG data at 500 Hz. The spatial distribution of the electrodes followed the same electrode placement as the first study, over the somatosensory and motor areas: Frontal-Central (FC5, FC6), Central (C1, C2, C3, C4), and Central-Parietal (CP5, CP6). The BCI system was connected via bluetooth to the second dedicated desktop computer.

Feedback Presentation. For delivering feedback to the user, the HTC Vive HMD was used (HTC, New Taipei City, Republic of China; Valve, Kirkland, Washington, United States) (Fig. 8). The Vive uses two screens, one per eye, each having a display resolution of 108 × 1200 and a refresh rate of 90 Hz. Additionally, the Vive uses a gyroscope, accelerometer and laser position sensors, and operates in a 4.6 × 4.6 m (15-by-15-ft) tracking space by using two "Lighthouse" base stations that track the user's movement with sub-millimeter precision. The Lighthouse system uses photosensors by sweeping structured light lasers within a space.

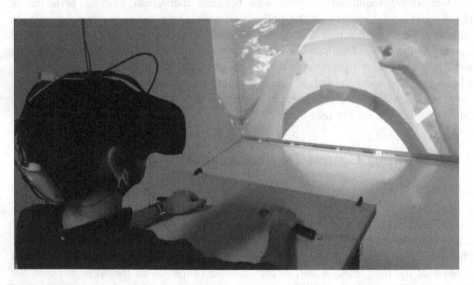

Fig. 8. NeuRow setup including the HTC Vive HMD and Enobio 8 EEG headset (projected feedback is for illustration purposes only).

3.2   BCI Protocol

For both the training and the BCI task, an identical protocol and setup to the previous experiment were used. During training the NeuRow feedback had been displayed for left|right motor observation and motor imagery of the rowing task, delivering also vibrotactile feedback. Following training, two conditions were delivered in random order: (1) standard output of the LDA classifier, and (2) the APE (see Fig. 9).

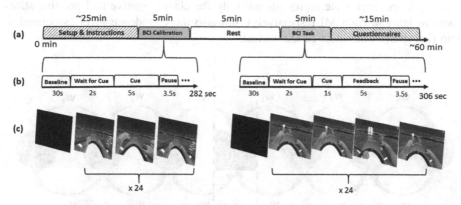

Fig. 9. BCI protocol for training and online control.

3.3 The Adaptive Performance Engine

The Adaptive Performance Engine (APE) is composed by 2 main components: (a) a Bayesian Inference Layer (BIL) (b) a Finite State Machine (FSM). The BIL was used in order to formulate the input into a model, where we translate the continuous BCI classification data into probability. BIL was chosen since is a simple computational approach and more efficient as compared to other supervised learning techniques such as artificial neural networks. As for decision making, we made use of an FSM because of its efficiency and non-linear properties. More concretely:

Bayesian Inference Layer. BIL was design to complement the standard Linear discriminant analysis (LDA) classifier that results from MI BCI training, and is used to compute the likelihood of the classifier output for each class (left vs. right motor-imagery). This is done by modeling the data belonging to each class as a Gaussian distribution, where μ and σ indicate their mean and standard deviation values $(MI_i(\mu, \sigma), i = [left, right])$. We then compute the Likelihood of a specific LDA output belonging to each MI class with:

$$P(i|LDAoutput) = \frac{MI_i(LDA\ output, \mu_i, \sigma_i) * P_i}{\sum_j MI_j(LDA\ output, \mu_j, \sigma_j)} \tag{2}$$

Where P_i indicates the prior probability of action i (0.5 for left vs. right MI). μ and σ are updated at each iteration, taking into account all previous history of the user for the given i MI action. $LDAoutput$ indicates the output value of the LDA classifier.

Finite State Machine. Following the BIL, the likelihood of each MI classification forwarded into a FSM. The role of the FSM is to transform binary MI classifications – such as left vs. right as given by the LDA – into evidence-based states (S_i). FSM is composed of 7 states, a neutral (S_0) and three for each MI class ($S_{1/-1}$, $S_{2/-2}$, $S_{3/-3}$). Each state has a transition threshold associated with it (w_1, w_2, w_3), and can only transition to one of the nearest neighbors or stay in the same state (see Fig. 10). As input, the FSM uses the difference of the posterior probabilities of left and right MI from Eq. 2 and each state represents not only the class (negative and positive states represent left and right MI respectively), but also the confidence level associated to them (being $S_{3/-3}$ the most certain states).

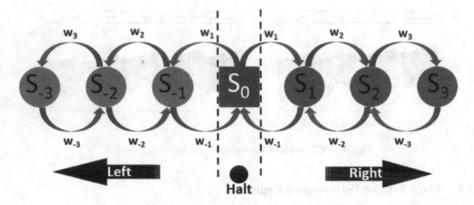

Fig. 10. State transition diagram. Adapted from [33].

Previous results with the APE compared with other classifier performance datasets, have shown an increase in performance up to 20% combined with LDA in a two class MI paradigm [34]. This study aims at measuring its impact in users' perceived performance complementing our previous machine learning assessment.

3.4 Participants

For assessing the APE, a sample of 8 users (mean age of 27 ± 3.5 years old) was recruited, based on their motivation. All participants were male and right handed with no previous known neurological disorder. Four of the users had little prior experience with MI-based BCI. All participants were university students of the University of Madeira and provided their written informed consent before participating in the study.

3.5 Questionnaires and EEG Data

Before each session, the Movement Imagery Questionnaire—Revised second version (MIQ-RS)) [53] was admitted to each participant. MIQ-RS is an 18-item questionnaire for mental imagery comprised of nine visual imagery and nine kinesthetic imagery items, each of which involves the movement of an arm, leg or the entire body. To complete each item, four steps are required: (1) The starting position for each movement is described, and the participant is initiating that position, (2) The movement is then described and the participant physically performs the movement, (3) The participant retakes the starting position, and images the movement without physically performing the movement, (4) Finally, the participant rates the ease or difficulty of imaging the movement on a 7-point scale anchored by 1 = very easy to picture/feel and 7 = very difficult to picture/feel. Following MIQ-RS, the Vividness of Movement Imagery Questionnaire-2 (VMIQ2) (Roberts et al. 2008) was used including the visual and kinesthetic parts of the questionnaire.

After each session, the NASA TLX questionnaire was used to measure task load considering Mental Demand, Physical Demand, Temporal Demand, Performance, Effort and Frustration [42].

Finally, on each condition, the raw EEG data were logged in order to extract the different EEG bands and the Engagement Index derived from these bands as explained in Sect. 2.5.

3.6   Results

For quantifying the quality of control between the two conditions, we analyzed the in-game data (trajectory, score), perceived experience through the SOPI and TLX questionnaires, and finally, the EEG bands modulation including the Engagement Index.

Quality of Control. In terms of control, Fig. 11 illustrates the in-game boat trajectories resulting from the Raw LDA control (blue) compared with the APE decision mechanism (orange) for the same task, subject, and with the in-game targets on the same positions. The trajectory with APE is steadier than the Raw LDA control, displaying a smoother trajectory. It is also visible in the APE trial that users could perform equally both left and right turns, while the Raw LDA trajectory is generally dominated by one dominant hemisphere, resulting in frequent rotation in one direction.

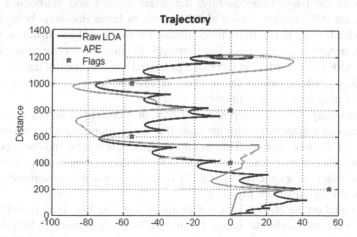

Fig. 11. Example in-game boat trajectory during raw LDA classification output vs APE output for subject 1. (Color figure online)

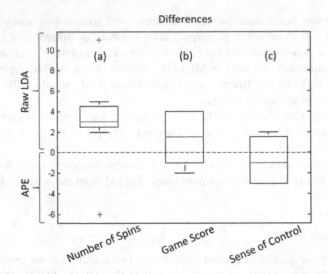

Fig. 12. In-game data and self-report of control. (a) Number of boat spins (180° rotation), (b) game score in terms of flags captured, (c) reported sense of control

The improvement in control is also apparent by the number of sudden trajectory changes or "spins" present during navigation, being considerably higher for Raw LDA than for APE (see Fig. 12a). When comparing the scores for both conditions, we observe that Raw LDA captures more in-game targets than APE. However, the lower performance for APE could be related to the fact that it is a statistical system that adds a third state to the LDA output, allowing for indecisions during noisy data (see Fig. 12b). Instead, the Raw LDA forces the user rowing left or right, making the boat always move towards the flags. Consequently, the added control and confidence on each decision by the APE system -which also translates to fewer decisions being made by the system- leads to more inactivity time, making the user travel less distance, therefore achieving less targets for the same time interval. Finally, the increased accuracy per decision of APE is reflected in an increased perceived sense of control during APE (see Fig. 12c). Nevertheless, neither the in-game scores nor the reported sense of control differ significantly between conditions.

When designing APE, we hypothesized that an increased sense of control could provide increased engagement with the task. If a user is more engaged, he/she may try harder and for a longer period. This is important for users who require repeated MI training for rehabilitation purposes. Our assessment of engagement through the engagement index as extracted by the EEG data reveals a non-significant higher engagement during APE (see Fig. 13).

Finally, based on the NASA TLX sub-domains (see Fig. 14), users report increased effort and a higher workload index for the APE configuration. Additionally, the reported performance is lower and the levels of frustration are increased. This contrast with the increased sense of control and engagement during APE. This may indicate that the increased control that APE affords has as consequence higher mental, physical and temporal demands on users. Hence, making the APE setup a preferred option for users who require continuous training with a MI BCI system.

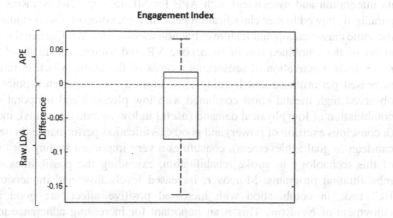

Fig. 13. Difference in Engagement index as extracted by the EEG bands in Eq. 1.

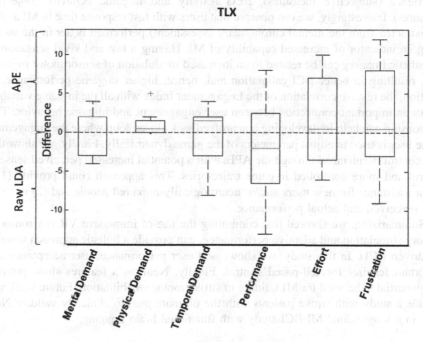

Fig. 14. NASA TLX sub-domains.

4   Conclusions

In this paper, we describe the development and pilot assessment of NeuRow as well as its integration and assessment with APE for MI training. The NeuRow BCI training paradigm showed higher classification performance, compared with studies which used the same classification and feature extraction methods for MI. Current data illustrate the effect of the combined use of immersive VR and vibrotactile feedback, resulting in more distinct activation of sensorimotor areas of the brain, which in turn can lead to increased performance and learning [54]. From a user experience point of view, we observed high mental effort combined with low physical and temporal demand. The combination of low physical demand (useful in low mobility patients), increased effort (a conscious exertion of power) and good classification performance (better control that can lean in goal achievement), constitutes a very important finding for the integration of this technology in stroke rehabilitation, extending the possibilities of ICT-based rehabilitation programs. Moreover, increased levels flow and immersion during the BCI task, in combination with increased positive affect, are good indicators of enjoyment of NeuRow. This is an important for increasing adherence to the therapy through motivating and engaging mechanisms. Furthermore, we showed that people with increased workload will perform worse by comparing the data between user experience (subjective measures), EEG activity and in-game behavior (objective measures). Interestingly, we can observe that users with fast response time in MI ability (as extracted from the mental chronometry assessment) performed better in the game, being an indicator of increased capability of MI. Having a fast and vivid sensation of kinesthetic imagery can be related to an increased modulation of sensorimotor rhythms [55], resulting in better BCI calibration and, hence, higher in-game performance. In addition, the reverse correlation of the Engagement Index with all the in-game variables shows an important connection between user engagement and in-game behavior. This relationship can help in developing a neurofeedback closed loop where the engagement of the user is used to adjust parameters of the game dynamically. Finally, we show that user control is enhanced through the APE, with a potential increased perceived sense of control and more controlled in-game trajectories. This approach could provide (1) a major assistance for new users and/or neurologically impaired people and (2) increase both perceived and actual performance.

Summarizing, we showed that combining the use of immersive VR environment, sensory stimulation and adaptive performance, can provide a holistic approach towards MI driven BCIs. In this study, we showcased user performance, user acceptance and important features for self-paced control. Finally, NeuRow's features show promise and potential to be used for MI training in stroke motor rehabilitation. Future work will include a study with stroke patients with the ultimate goal to clinically validate Neu-Row in a longitudinal MI-BCI study with functional brain imaging.

Acknowledgements. This work was supported by the European Commission through the RehabNet project - Neuroscience Based Interactive Systems for Motor Rehabilitation - EC (303891 RehabNet FP7-PEOPLE-2011-CIG), by the MACBIOIDI project financed by the EC through the INTERREG program (MAC/1.1.b/098), by the Fundação para a Ciência e Tecnologia (Portuguese Foundation for Science and Technology) through SFRH/BD/97117/2013, and LARSyS (Laboratório de Robótica e Sistemas em Engenharia e Ciência) through UID/EEA/50009/2013.

References

1. Hanakawa, T.: Organizing motor imageries. Neurosci. Res. **1**, 56–63 (2015)
2. Eaves, D.L., Haythornthwaite, L., Vogt, S.: Motor imagery during action observation modulates automatic imitation effects in rhythmical actions. Front. Hum. Neurosci. **8**, 28 (2014)
3. Neuper, C., Scherer, R., Wriessnegger, S., Pfurtscheller, G.: Motor imagery and action observation: modulation of sensorimotor brain rhythms during mental control of a brain–computer interface. Clin. Neurophysiol. **120**, 239–247 (2009)
4. Mulder, T.: Motor imagery and action observation: cognitive tools for rehabilitation. J. Neural Transm. **114**, 1265–1278 (2007)
5. Lledo, P.-M., Alonso, M., Grubb, M.S.: Adult neurogenesis and functional plasticity in neuronal circuits. Nat. Rev. Neurosci. **7**, 179–193 (2006)
6. Rossini, P.M., Calautti, C., Pauri, F., Baron, J.-C.: Post-stroke plastic reorganisation in the adult brain. Lancet Neurol. **2**, 493–502 (2003)
7. Dickstein, R., et al.: Effects of integrated motor imagery practice on gait of individuals with chronic stroke: a half-crossover randomized study. Arch. Phys. Med. Rehabil. **94**, 2119–2125 (2013)
8. Wolpaw, J.R., Birbaumer, N., McFarland, D.J., Pfurtscheller, G., Vaughan, T.M.: Brain-Computer Interfaces for communication and control. Clin. Neurophysiol. Off. J. Int. Fed. Clin. Neurophysiol. **113**, 767–791 (2002)
9. Dobkin, B.H.: Brain-computer interface technology as a tool to augment plasticity and outcomes for neurological rehabilitation. J. Physiol. **579**, 637–642 (2007)
10. Lotte, F., et al.: Combining BCI with virtual reality: towards new applications and improved BCI. In: Allison, B., Dunne, S., Leeb, R., Del, R., Millán, J., Nijholt, A. (eds.) Towards Practical Brain-Computer Interface. Springer, Heidelberg (2013). https://doi.org/10.1007/978-3-642-29746-5_10
11. Vourvopoulos, A., Niforatos, E., Hlinka, M., Škola, F., Liarokapis, F.: Investigating the effect of user profile during training for BCI-based games. In: 2017 9th International Conference on Virtual Worlds and Games for Serious Applications (VS-Games), pp. 117–124 (2017)
12. Friedman, D.: Brain-computer interfacing and virtual reality. In: Nakatsu, R., Rauterberg, M., Ciancarini, P. (eds.) Handbook of Digital Games and Entertainment Technologies, pp. 1–22. Springer, Singapore (2015). https://doi.org/10.1007/978-981-4560-52-8_2-1
13. Slater, M.: Place illusion and plausibility can lead to realistic behaviour in immersive virtual environments Philos. Trans. R. Soc. Lond. B Biol. Sci. **364**, 3549–3557 (2009)
14. Bermudez i Badia, S., Cameirao, M.S.: The Neurorehabilitation Training Toolkit (NTT): a novel worldwide accessible motor training approach for at-home rehabilitation after stroke. Stroke Res. Treat. **2012** (2012). https://doi.org/10.1155/2012/802157
15. Lange, B., et al.: Designing informed game-based rehabilitation tasks leveraging advances in virtual reality. Disabil. Rehabil. **34**, 1863–1870 (2012).
16. Trompetto, C., et al.: Pathophysiology of spasticity: implications for neurorehabilitation. BioMed Res. Int. **2014** (2014). https://doi.org/10.1155/2014/354906

17. Vourvopoulos, A., Bermúdez i Badia, S.: Usability and cost-effectiveness in brain-computer interaction: is it user throughput or technology related? In: Proceedings of the 7th Augmented Human International Conference, Geneva, Switzerland. ACM (2016)
18. Allison, B.Z., Neuper, C.: Could anyone use a BCI? In: Tan, D.S., Nijholt, A. (eds.) Brain-Computer Interfaces, pp. 35–54. Springer, London (2010). https://doi.org/10.1007/978-1-84996-272-8_3
19. Vidaurre, C., Blankertz, B.: Towards a cure for BCI illiteracy. Brain Topogr. **23**, 194–198 (2009)
20. Gomez-Rodriguez, M., Peters, J., Hill, J., Schölkopf, B., Gharabaghi, A., Grosse-Wentrup, M.: Closing the sensorimotor loop: haptic feedback facilitates decoding of motor imagery. J. Neural Eng. **8**, 036005 (2011)
21. Hinterberger, T., et al.: A multimodal brain-based feedback and communication system. Exp. Brain Res. **154**, 521–526 (2004)
22. Leeb, R., Gwak, K., Kim, D.-S., del R Millán, J.: Freeing the visual channel by exploiting vibrotactile BCI feedback. In: Conference Proceedings: Annual International Conference of the IEEE Engineering in Medicine and Biology Society. IEEE Engineering in Medicine and Biology Society Annual Conference 2013, pp. 3093–3096 (2013)
23. Cincotti, F., et al.: Vibrotactile feedback for brain-computer interface operation. Comput. Intell. Neurosci. **2007**, e48937 (2007)
24. Gwak, K., Leeb, R., Millan, J.D.R., Kim, D.-S.: Quantification and reduction of visual load during BCI operation. In: 2014 IEEE International Conference on Systems, Man and Cybernetics (SMC), pp. 2795–2800 (2014)
25. Jeunet, C., Vi, C., Spelmezan, D., N'Kaoua, B., Lotte, F., Subramanian, S.: Continuous tactile feedback for motor-imagery based brain-computer interaction in a multitasking context. In: Abascal, J., Barbosa, S., Fetter, M., Gross, T., Palanque, P., Winckler, M. (eds.) INTERACT 2015. LNCS, vol. 9296, pp. 488–505. Springer, Cham (2015). https://doi.org/10.1007/978-3-319-22701-6_36
26. Yao, L., Meng, J., Zhang, D., Sheng, X., Zhu, X.: Combining motor imagery with selective sensation toward a hybrid-modality BCI. IEEE Trans. Biomed. Eng. **61**, 2304–2312 (2014)
27. Leonardis, D., Frisoli, A., Solazzi, M., Bergamasco, M.: Illusory perception of arm movement induced by visuo-proprioceptive sensory stimulation and controlled by motor imagery. In: 2012 IEEE Haptics Symposium (HAPTICS), pp. 421–424 (2012)
28. Vourvopoulos, A., Bermúdez i Badia, S.: Motor priming in virtual reality can augment motor-imagery training efficacy in restorative brain-computer interaction: a within-subject analysis. J. NeuroEng. Rehabil. **13**, 69 (2016)
29. Lotte, F.: On the need for alternative feedback training approaches for BCI. Presented at the Berlin Brain-Computer Interface Workshop September (2012)
30. Lotte, F., Larrue, F., Mühl, C.: Flaws in current human training protocols for spontaneous Brain-Computer Interfaces: lessons learned from instructional design. Front. Hum. Neurosci. **7**, 568 (2013)
31. Shute, V.J.: Focus on formative feedback. Rev. Educ. Res. **78**, 153–189 (2008)
32. Hattie, J., Timperley, H.: The power of feedback. Rev. Educ. Res. **77**, 81–112 (2007)
33. Vourvopoulos, A., Ferreira, A., Bermúdez i Badia, S.: NeuRow: an immersive VR environment for motor-imagery training with the use of Brain-Computer Interfaces and vibrotactile feedback. Presented at the PhyCS 2016 - 3rd International Conference on Physiological Computing Systems Lisbon, July 2016
34. Ferreira, A., Vourvopoulos, A., Bermúdez i Badia, S.: Optimizing performance of non-expert users in brain-computer interaction by means of an adaptive performance engine. In: Guo, Y., Friston, K., Aldo, F., Hill, S., Peng, H. (eds.) BIH 2015. LNCS (LNAI), vol. 9250, pp. 202–211. Springer, Cham (2015). https://doi.org/10.1007/978-3-319-23344-4_20

35. Klem, G.H., Lüders, H.O., Jasper, H.H., Elger, C.: The ten-twenty electrode system of the International Federation. The International Federation of Clinical Neurophysiology. Electroencephalogr. Clin. Neurophysiol. Suppl. **52**, 3–6 (1999)
36. Renard, Y., et al.: OpenViBE: an open-source software platform to design, test, and use Brain-Computer Interfaces in real and virtual environments. Presence Teleoperators Virtual Environ. **19**, 35–53 (2010)
37. Vourvopoulos, A., Faria, A.L., Cameirao, M.S., Bermudez i Badia, S.: RehabNet: a distributed architecture for motor and cognitive neuro-rehabilitation. In: 2013 IEEE 15th International Conference on e-Health Networking, Applications Services (Healthcom), pp. 454–459 (2013)
38. Taylor II, R.M., Hudson, T.C., Seeger, A., Weber, H., Juliano, J., Helser, A.T.: VRPN: a device-independent, network-transparent VR peripheral system. In: Proceedings of the ACM Symposium on Virtual Reality Software and Technology, pp. 55–61. ACM, New York (2001)
39. Pfurtscheller, G., et al.: Graz-BCI: state of the art and clinical applications. IEEE Trans. Neural. Syst. Rehabil. Eng. Publ. IEEE Eng. Med. Biol. Soc. **11**, 177–180 (2003)
40. Roberts, R., Callow, N., Hardy, L., Markland, D., Bringer, J.: Movement imagery ability: development and assessment of a revised version of the vividness of movement imagery questionnaire. J. Sport Exerc. Psychol. **30**, 200–221 (2008)
41. Adams, E., Ip, B.: From casual to core: a statistical mechanism for studying gamer dedication. http://www.gamasutra.com/view/feature/131397/from_casual_to_core_a_statistical_.php
42. Hart, S.G., Staveland, L.E.: Development of NASA-TLX (task load index): results of empirical and theoretical research. In: Hancock, P.A., Meshkati, N. (eds.) Advances in Psychology, pp. 139–183. North-Holland, Amsterdam (1988)
43. IJsselsteijn, W., Poels, K., de Kort, Y.A.: The Game Experience Questionnaire: development of a self-report measure to assess player experiences of digital games. TU Eindh,. Eindhoven, Netherlands (2008)
44. Brooke, J.: SUS-A quick and dirty usability scale. Usability Eval. Ind. **189**, 194 (1996)
45. Delorme, A., Makeig, S.: EEGLAB: an open source toolbox for analysis of single-trial EEG dynamics including independent component analysis. J. Neurosci. Methods **134**, 9–21 (2004)
46. Pope, A.T., Bogart, E.H., Bartolome, D.S.: Biocybernetic system evaluates indices of operator engagement in automated task. Biol. Psychol. **40**, 187–195 (1995)
47. Berka, C., et al.: EEG correlates of task engagement and mental workload in vigilance, learning, and memory tasks. Aviat. Space Environ. Med. **78**, B231–B244 (2007)
48. Boostani, R., Moradi, M.H.: A new approach in the BCI research based on fractal dimension as feature and Adaboost as classifier. J. Neural Eng. **1**, 212–217 (2004)
49. Garcia, G.N., Ebrahimi, T., Vesin, J.: Support vector EEG classification in the Fourier and time-frequency correlation domains. In: First International IEEE EMBS Conference on Neural Engineering. Conference Proceedings, pp. 591–594 (2003)
50. Obermaier, B., Guger, C., Neuper, C., Pfurtscheller, G.: Hidden Markov models for online classification of single trial EEG data. Pattern Recogn. Lett. **22**, 1299–1309 (2001)
51. Solhjoo, S., Moradi, M.: Mental task recognition: a comparison between some of classification methods. In: BIOSIGNAL 2004 International EURASIP Conference, pp. 24–26 (2004)
52. Bangor, A., Kortum, P., Miller, J.: Determining what individual SUS scores mean: adding an adjective rating scale. J Usability Stud. **4**, 114–123 (2009)
53. Gregg, M., Hall, C., Butler, A.: The MIQ-RS: a suitable option for examining movement imagery ability. Evid. Based Complement. Altern. Med. ECAM. **7**, 249–257 (2010)

54. Sigrist, R., Rauter, G., Riener, R., Wolf, P.: Augmented visual, auditory, haptic, and multimodal feedback in motor learning: a review. Psychon. Bull. Rev. **20**, 21–53 (2013)
55. Neuper, C., Scherer, R., Reiner, M., Pfurtscheller, G.: Imagery of motor actions: differential effects of kinesthetic and visual-motor mode of imagery in single-trial EEG. Brain Res. Cogn. Brain Res. **25**, 668–677 (2005)

Bio-behavioral Modeling of Workload and Performance

Jean-François Gagnon[1(✉)], Olivier Gagnon[2], Daniel Lafond[1],
Mark Parent[3], and Sébastien Tremblay[3]

[1] Thales Research and Technology, Thales Canada, Québec, Canada
{jean-francois.gagnon,
daniel.lafond}@ca.thalesgroup.com
[2] Department of Electrical and Computer Engineering,
Université Laval, Québec, Canada
olivier.gagnon.7@ulaval.ca
[3] School of Psychology, Université Laval, Québec, Canada
{mark.parent,sebastien.tremblay}@psy.ulaval.ca

Abstract. Research on adaptive systems based on human psychophysiological assessments has been growing rapidly over the last decade. One fundamental component of such a system is human state assessment, on which the adaptation depends, at least partly. This is critical as the confidence of operators in such system will be determined to some extent by the accuracy of the models responsible for the assessment. This chapter presents work carried out in order to better understand the relationship between bio-behavioral data, psychological state, and operational performance of the operators. Modeling physiological parameters and performance was performed through a manipulation of three factors. The first factor was the size of smoothing window for performance. The second factor was the performance decrement threshold for labelling functional and sub-functional states. Finally, the third factor was the mode of classification being either prospective or descriptive. We used two types of classifiers, a linear and a non-linear classifier, and compared performance. Insights emerging from this work support that the use of multiple sources of bio-behavioral data, combined in a non-linear fashion, increases the psychometric qualities of state classifiers. This suggests that if such systems are to be used in safety-critical systems, they should be implemented using a wide variety of sensors to increase classification accuracies of performance.

Keywords: Operator functional state · Psychophysiological modeling ·
Machine learning · Data processing

1 Introduction

The development of low cost and mobile devices capable of sensing human bio-behavioral activities has enabled a series of research efforts aiming to use such data for the assessment of operator functional state (OFS) in various contexts. OFS refers to "The multidimensional pattern of human psychophysiological condition that mediates performance in relation to physiological and psychological costs" [1]. Assessment of

A. Holzinger et al. (Eds.): PhyCS 2016–2018, LNCS 10057, pp. 23–38, 2019.
https://doi.org/10.1007/978-3-030-27950-9_2

OFS has great value, especially in safety critical systems where information about the state of operators could support decision makers or closed loop automated systems [2].

Significant progress in the development of models of OFS has been made, but it still faces several challenges before such models are used in the field, especially in safety-critical applications. Indeed, transitioning models to uncontrolled conditions has been identified as an important challenge by many [3, 4]. Specifically, two issues need to be addressed. The first issue concerns the constraints associated with the data, both in terms of quality and availability. The second issue is at the other end of the spectrum and concerns the formalization of the concept of OFS itself. This paper addresses these issues.

1.1 Data

In field operations, several constraints will impede the use of sensors or degrade the quality of the sampled data. It is not always possible to equip with head-worn gear, or the task may be ambulatory by nature which may introduce motion artefacts in the signals. Although benefits associated with the use of central nervous system sensors in the modeling of OFS and similar concepts were demonstrated [5, 6], some contexts will only allow for the collection of peripheral nervous system measures. Despite promising results that show that the removal of motion artefacts from the signals might be possible [7], there is a value in investigating the possibility to model OFS using only behavioral and peripheral nervous system sensors. But are they sufficient? Is there really OFS information in the data collected by these sensors? Indeed, the vast majority of studies that model OFS in near real-time rely at least if not only on central nervous system sensors.

Previous work has shown that perceptual attention tasks elicited a small but significant increase in breathing rate [8]. Also, in applied settings, such as office-like situations, breathing rate has shown to be positively associated with stress [9].

Heart rate variability (HRV) is the (ir)regularity of consecutive heartbeats, and has been widely associated with the balance between sympathetic and parasympathetic systems. Among others, HRV was associated with mental overload in a simulated piloting task [5] and stress in musical performance [10].

Eye-related activity may also provide information associated with OFS. Eye-related attributes should however not require a priori knowledge about the visual scene to facilitate use of the model in new contexts. Such attributes include eye velocity, pattern of saccadic and fixation activity [11], blink frequency and blink duration.

Altogether, such attributes have shown to be sensitive to levels of workload, but divergent [12]. One potential approach to increase specificity is to combine attributes through machine learning techniques in order to discover multi-modal classification rules.

1.2 OFS Ground Truth

But what exactly is this information about the operator that such models attempt to provide? Gaillard [13] argued that the goal of OFS assessment "is to detect significant deviations from the optimal bio behavioral state that may indicate an enhanced risk for performance degradation". This conceptualization disentangles performance from OFS by introducing the notion of enhanced risk, which is reasonable since performance greatly depends on contextual factors. Indeed, the concept of performance is arguably further away from the bio-behavioral state than the level of workload or fatigue. It is a multi-determined concept that involves a complex combination of psycho-physiological state, task difficulty, and other contextual factors.

Because of this, one of the most studied components of OFS is mental workload [14, 15], which refers to the portion of operator information processing capacity or resources that is actually required to meet system demands. From a theoretical standpoint, the assessment of mental workload is critical since excessive demand on cognitive resources may result in performance degradation [16]. Still, the relationship between mental workload and performance is not straightforward as other factors come into play, such as level of expertise, fatigue, and motivation. Because the relationship between mental workload and performance is not direct, we might be missing the target. Are the predicted levels of workload really associated with enhanced risk of performance degradation?

This raises the question of how to obtain a valid and reliable ground truth of "enhanced risk for performance degradation". One way to achieve this might be to collect data on standardized fundamental tasks and maximize control of contextual factors. In this context, observed performance degradations should mostly be due to individual as opposed to contextual factors and may therefore be used as a ground truth for OFS. Nevertheless, there are still pending issues we discuss and address here.

1.3 Objectives

The main objectives of this study are (1) to demonstrate the feasibility of modeling OFS without the use of central nervous system sensors and (2) to evaluate various operationalization of OFS ground truth and evaluate how OFS models fare in comparison to models of mental workload. Three specific research questions are addressed.

First, performance and physiology may vary on asynchronous time scales. Indeed, a performance decrement can happen very fast, within seconds, whereas some physiological responses may have a slower onset. Therefore, is the OFS better conceptualized (and classified) as a punctual or a longer term general state?

Second, it is unclear whether physiological responses cause performance decrements, or if it is the other way around [17]. Are the physiological signals able to predict performance decrements (i.e., prospective mode) or are they limited to describing an ongoing state? If the performance decrement causes a physiological response, it may be hard to predict decrements in advance. Conversely, if physiological patterns lead to performance decrements, it may be reasonable to have some level of predictability.

Finally, to be reliably detectable, a physiological response must have some level of amplitude. It is unclear however if there is a relationship between the amplitude of the performance decrement and the physiological response. Is there a performance decrement threshold that can be associated with physiological patterns regardless of the task? In other words, what is the magnitude of change necessary in performance to be reflected in physiological response, if any? This paper reports a systematic assessment of these issues.

2 Method

This study investigates the aforementioned questions using an experimental design that manipulates task difficulty in order to foster performance decrements. Participants perform the tasks while peripheral bio-behavioral data is collected. Then, a series of models was developed to map the relationship between bio-behavioral data and performance. For each model, a new set of parameters was manipulated for the operationalization of performance. Models are tested on new participants in order to assess cross-subject generalization. This section details the key elements of the method, including data collection, parameter selection, and modeling procedure.

2.1 Experiment

Participants. Seventeen volunteers - 9 males, mean age (sd) = 24.58 (3.74) - participated in the experiment. They were recruited on the university campus and received a financial compensation for their participation. Inclusion criteria were having normal or corrected vision and no known health issues.

Design. The experimental design involved two tasks: visual search and N-Back. Each participant completed eight consecutive experimental sessions separated by five-minute breaks to avoid carry over effects of physiological response. Each task comprised two conditions, easy and hard. This was done to ensure variability in performance data of the participants. These conditions were counterbalanced across participants and played twice. Total duration of the experimental sessions including practice sessions and breaks was approximately 90 min. Prior to the experimental sessions, participants were trained on each of the two tasks.

Visual Search. Visual search is a computerized task that requires the participants to identify a target letter among a series of distractors (Fig. 1). The task requires visually scanning the screen to search for the target letter. The participants select the target by clicking on the letter. Participants performed 60 trials in each experimental session resulting in 240 trials overall. Task difficulty is manipulated by varying the complexity of the rule of the target letter. In the easy condition, the target is a vowel. In the hard condition, the target is an unrotated vowel. Response times are recorded and represent the measure of performance.

N-Back. The N-Back is a computerized task that requires participants to identify a target letter among a series of distractors presented sequentially in time (one every 2 s). The participants are presented a series of letters and must tell whether the actual letter is the same (target) or a different one (distractor) from the N previous letter. Participants must answer with the keyboard (i.e., "M" = same, "Z" = different). Participants performed 60 trials in each experimental session resulting in 240 trials overall. See (Fig. 2) for a schematic representation of the task. Difficulty is operationalized by varying the number of elements to retain, manipulate, and update in memory (i.e., N = 1 [easy] and N = 2 [hard]). Response times are recorded and represent the measure of performance. Accuracy was also recorded; however, we used response times as the principal measure of performance for comparison purposes with the visual search task.

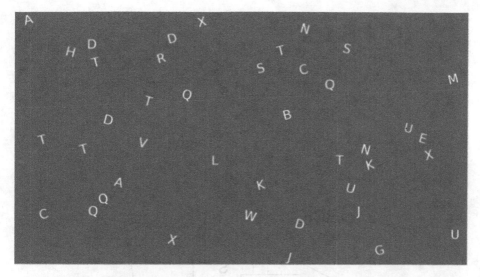

Fig. 1. Visual search is an attentional task that involves an active visual scan of the environment for a specific target (e.g., unrotated vowel [U]) among distractors (e.g., consonant and rotated vowels). Extracted from [18].

Sensing. During the completion of these tasks, participants were equipped with two devices for bio-behavioral sensing. The Zephyr Bio Harness 3 was used for electro-cardiography (ECG) and respiratory induced plethysmography (RIP). ECG was sampled at 250 Hz, and RIP was sampled at 18 Hz. Data were wirelessly transmitted to the logging device through Bluetooth. The ASL Mobile Eye system was used for eye-tracking. It sampled the position and the dimension of the pupil of the right eye at approximately 30 Hz.

Sampled signals were then validated in terms of quality. All data were compared to theoretical boundaries and were investigated further if different from the expected range. Some levels of invalid data were tolerated (up to 20% over a moving window of 10 s) to reflect operational conditions. This resulted in approximately 8% of the data removed for model training, validation, and testing.

Attributes. From the remaining validated signals, a series of attributes were calculated. These attributes are associated with the behavior of the eyes, cardiac activity or respiratory activity.

Eye-related attributes included velocity, proportion of fixations, proportion of involuntary fixations, proportion of saccades, blink frequency, and blink duration [19]. Fixations and saccades were computed using a velocity-based algorithm [20]. Areas of interest were not used to avoid task specific attributes.

Several implementations of HRV measures exist and are typically categorized as being either in the temporal, frequency, or non-linear domains [21]. Since the frequency and temporal domains allow for precise analyses of the variability and was previously associated with mental effort, we adopted these two types. The standard-deviation of heart inter-beat intervals (SDRR) was used for the temporal domain HRV.

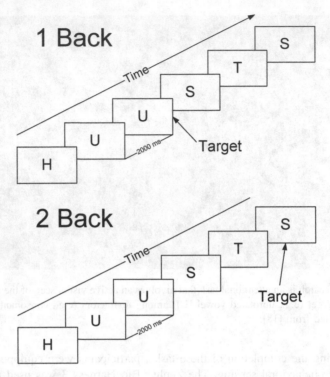

Fig. 2. The N-Back task is a working memory task in which the participants must preserve, manipulate and update information in active memory. Extracted from [18].

Frequency attributes were computed by estimating power spectral density of high (.15–.4 Hz), low (.05–.15 Hz), very low (.03–.05), and ultra low (.03–.0) frequency of inter-beat intervals. The LF/HF attribute was also calculated. Attributes associated with HRV were extracted using the default values of the RHRV package [22]. The frequency bands were extracted over a short window of five minutes and a very short window of two minutes.

In the present study, breathing rate and breathing amplitude were used as the attributes for respiratory activity.

Since the signals were originally sampled at asynchronous rates, we interpolated the values of the attributes with the last valid value between two consecutive samples. The last valid value was used to replicate the functional constraint of the device used for wireless data collection and integration. In fact, all processing is feasible in real-time to acknowledge for operational requirements. All the attributes were then sampled down to 1 Hz. The resulting data set was composed of roughly 28,000 observations of 41 attributes. From these 41 attributes, 24 ($\sim 58\%$) were obtained from the eye, 15 ($\sim 37\%$) from the heart and 2 ($\sim 5\%$) from respiratory activity.

2.2   Ground Truth Parameters

Decontextualized dynamic performance (DDP) was adapted from previous research and consists of a dynamic standardization of the median response times over the last N seconds [23]. The median response times are standardized so that the resulting score is comparable across tasks. DDP represents the formalization of OFS and allows the direct comparison of multiple tasks in terms of performance.

Aligned with the objectives of the paper, three parameters associated with the calculation (and prediction) of the DDP were manipulated (these parameters are reported in Table 1):

1. Length in seconds of the median response time window. Two windows were compared: 10 vs. 70 s. The shortest window reflects a "punctual" state whereas the longest one represents a "general" state.
2. Threshold of the z score at which the sub functional level is specified. Three levels were tested: 0, −1 and −1.5. In Gagnon [23], this parameter was estimated with Yen's method, but its impact was not systematically assessed.
3. Finally, two types of classification modes were compared: Descriptive of actual state (bio-signals and performance metrics come from the same time window) versus prospective (bio-signals come from a first time window, and performance is assessed using the subsequent time-window).

Table 1. OFS parameters. Extracted from [18].

Sub functional threshold (z score)	Window	
	Punctual (10 s)	General (70 s)
0	Descriptive vs. Prospective	Descriptive vs. Prospective
−1	Descriptive vs. Prospective	Descriptive vs. Prospective
−1.5	Descriptive vs. Prospective	Descriptive vs. Prospective

The manipulation of these parameters results in 12 versions of OFS ground truth which will be systematically assessed in the results section.

Mental workload, as operationalized by task difficulty (easy vs. hard) was used as an additional ground truth. This ground truth is used to assess the additional difficulty associated with classification of OFS when compared to intermediate psychological states such as mental workload.

2.3 Modeling

In previous work, many classes of models have been used, including support vector machines, decision trees, and linear discriminant analysis, but none have been granted with superior performances [23]. Because of this, we restrained the classifiers to two types: stochastic gradient boosting machine (GBM) and generalized linear model (GLM). Ensemble methods such as GBM have been used with success in similar contexts [24]. We compare their performance with GLM, a classic modeling framework that is also known to be resilient to overfitting.

GBM model training was performed using a cross validation procedure implemented in the R caret package [25]. The procedure involved leaving out the data of one participant at a time for training. Data were shuffled prior to input.

The procedure was performed for 4620 (2 X 154 X 3 X 5) iterations: manipulated parameters were interaction depth (2), number of trees (154), shrinkage (3), and minimal observations in node (5).

The threshold used for labelling the data generated imbalanced classes. For instance, the −1 and −1.5 Z score threshold generates sub-functional vs. functional classes comprising ∼16% vs. 84% and ∼7% vs. 93% of samples, respectively. In order to minimize complications associated with class imbalance, we performed a SMOTE procedure [26] and classifiers were evaluated using balanced accuracy. This statistic measures classifier accuracy while correcting for class imbalance. It therefore represents a good impartial measure when comparing several scenarios with different class distributions.

For each ground truth (i.e., combination of OFS time window, sub-functional threshold, and mode, and mental workload levels), the best set of parameters was used to train a final model with the data of the 15 training participants. Results report statistics on the testing sample. The test set was divided into eight data bins for each of which balanced accuracy values, sensitivity, and specificity were calculated.

In addition a classifier was trained per participant in order to quantify the loss of accuracy of a generalized model in comparison with a subject-specific model.

3   Results

Before the development of the psychophysiological models, we first validated that the experimental conditions did have a significant impact on performance of the participants. Analyses revealed that responses times were statistically different between low and high workload conditions for both N-Back t(16) = 8.29, p < .001 and visual search t(16) = 10.63, p < .001. The distributions are represented in Figs. 3 and 4.

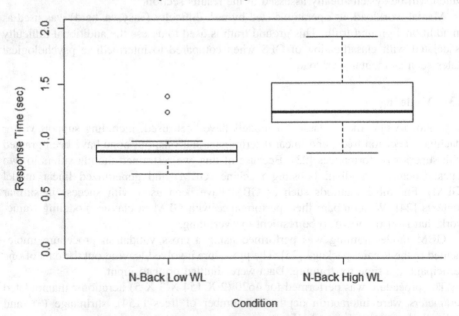

Fig. 3. Distribution of response times for the N-Back task by condition. Extracted from [18].

Results showed that balanced accuracy was significantly higher for the best mental workload classifier compared to the best OFS classifier t(15) = 4.85, p < .001. Indeed, the best average balanced accuracy values on the test set was of .77 (.05) for mental workload whereas it was of .66 (.04) for OFS. Moreover, for the best combination of parameters, both mental workload t(7) = 14.58, p < .001 and OFS t(7) = 11.29, p < .001 predictive accuracy was significantly superior to chance.

A repeated measures analysis of variance (ANOVA) was carried out to test the effect of classifiers (GBM vs. GLM), time frame (punctual vs. general), mode (descriptive vs. prospective), and threshold (−1.5, −1, 0) on balanced accuracy, specificity, and sensitivity. Statistics are reported in Tables 2, 3, and 4 for balanced accuracy, sensitivity and specificity respectively. Data for sensitivity and specificity are reported in Figs. 5 and 6 respectively.

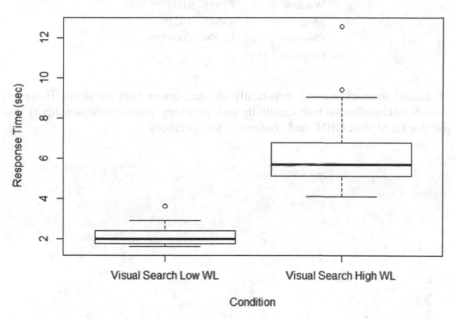

Fig. 4. Distribution of response times for the Visual Search task by condition. Extracted from [18].

Table 2. ANOVA - Effect of threshold, window, mode, and classifier on balanced accuracy. Extracted from [18].

	df	F	p
Threshold	2	1.1745	0.3112
Window	1	27.5743	<.001***
Mode	1	3.8706	0.0506
Classifier	1	0.2908	0.5903
Residuals	186		

Table 3. ANOVA - Effect of threshold, window, mode, and classifier on sensitivity. Extracted from [18].

	df	F	p
Threshold	2	3.9429	0.0210*
Window	1	3.2754	0.0719
Mode	1	3.349	0.0688
Classifier	1	5.9328	0.0158*
Residuals	186		

Table 4. ANOVA - Effect of threshold, window, mode, and classifier on specificity. Extracted from [18].

	df	F	p
Threshold	2	5.2295	0.0061**
Window	1	7.2587	0.0077**
Mode	1	0.4965	0.4819
Classifier	1	17.4499	<.001***
Residuals	186		

Balanced accuracy was not statistically different across OFS classifiers. However, classifiers had an effect on both sensitivity and specificity. Indeed, mean sensitivity was higher for GLM than GBM, and conversely for specificity.

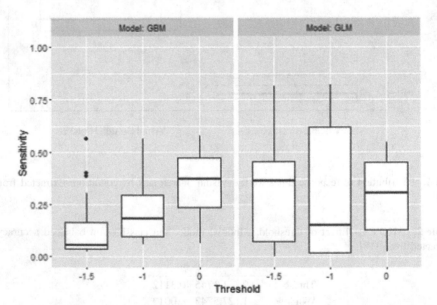

Fig. 5. Sensitivity by classifier (left: GBM, right: GLM) and threshold on test data. Extracted from [18].

The effect of time window on balanced accuracy was statistically significant. Indeed, observed balanced accuracy on test set was higher for punctual window (M = .59, SD = .07) than general window (M = .54, SD = .07). The time window also had an effect on specificity, but not sensitivity. Indeed, specificity was lower when OFS was conceptualized with a general window than when compared to a punctual window.

There was no effect of threshold on balanced accuracy, but its impact was significant on both sensitivity and specificity. Lower thresholds were on average associated with higher specificity, but lower sensitivity.

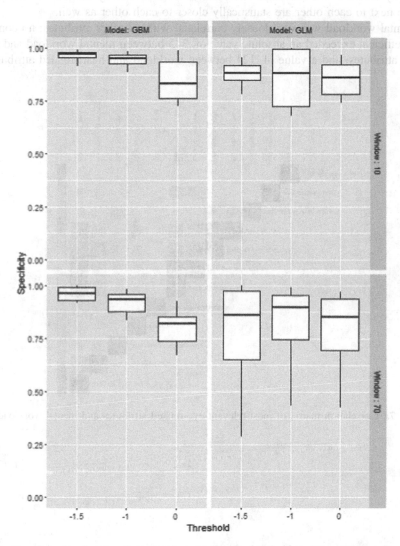

Fig. 6. Specificity by classifier (left: GBM, right: GLM), threshold, and time window (top: 10 s, bottom: 70 s) on test data. Extracted from [18].

Finally, the effect of the classification mode (descriptive vs. prospective) on balanced accuracy was marginally significant. Indeed, balanced accuracy in descriptive mode (M = .58, SD = .07) was almost higher than in the prospective mode (M = .56, SD = .07). There was no effect on specificity and sensitivity.

A series of linear correlational analyses were also carried out to assess the relationship between attributes and mental workload. Figure 7 shows the correlation matrix between eye-related attributes and mental workload whereas Fig. 8 shows the matrix for heart and respiration related attributes. All attributes were not represented for simplicity reasons. The attributes were clustered hierarchically so that two attributes that are next to each other are statistically closer to each other as well.

Mental workload was very loosely correlated with all other attributes: no correlation coefficient exceeded an absolute value of .345 between mental workload and eye-related attributes, and a value of .124 between workload and heart-related attributes.

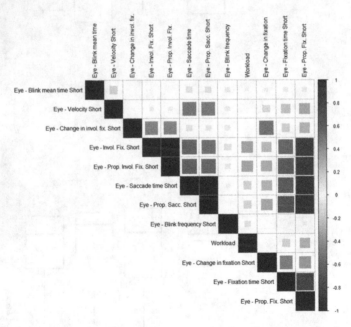

Fig. 7. Correlation matrix of most relevant eye-related attributes and mental workload.

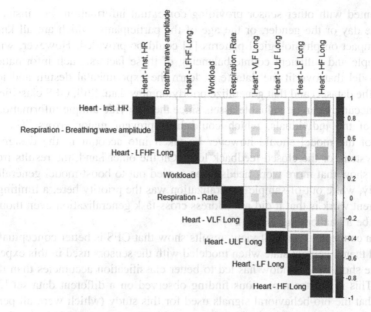

Fig. 8. Correlation matrix of most relevant heart and respiration-related attributes and mental workload.

4   Discussion

This work concerned the modeling of the link between bio-behavioral state of individuals and more specifically, the likelihood of performance decrements (i.e., OFS), which should be avoided in safety-critical applications. Model accuracy when classifying performance vs. mental workload, and we assessed the impact of key parameters of OFS conceptualization. This is critical as these parameters have a great impact on the ground truth metric, which supports supervised learning. Specifically, this study investigated if OFS is better conceptualized as a punctual or a general state, as a small or a large variation of performance, and whether a prospective approach can lead to results comparable to the descriptive mode.

Results show that the link between the bio-behavioral measures of individuals and performance is less strong than the link between measures and intermediate variables such as level of mental workload. This is exhibited by higher classifier performance when discriminating workload levels compared to OFS levels (functional vs. subfunctional). This result expected as it was hypothesized that performance is more dependent of contextual factors not captured in bio-behavioral signals than mental workload. Moreover, because results show that it is possible to classify workload relatively well, we are confident that the collected data does in fact carry valid information about the state of the operator.

Results also show that OFS was classified above chance level, but that more information, probably contextual, is needed to achieve high levels of accuracy. This suggests that if such models are to be used in operational contexts, they should be complemented with other sensor providing contextual information. For instance, the time of the day or the gender, or the age of the participants, which are all known to have an impact on physiological patterns [1] could be provided. However, without a larger sample and sufficient counterbalancing of these factors, such information will lead to model that overfit the data (e.g., learn the experimental design and idiosyncrasies in the dataset) and that generalize poorly on new data. Still, OFS classifiers with moderate accuracy can be valuable assets since they provide unique information about the state of the individuals, which could help prevent major errors. The limited accuracy of the model should however be taken into account in the design of the warning system, or the closed feedback loop. On the other hand, the results from this work also show that more work needs to be carried out to boost model generalization. Specifically, while out-of-sample generalization was the priority here, a limiting factor of the current work is that it did not address cross-task generalization even though it is known to be a challenging issue [27].

From a conceptual point of view, results show that OFS is better conceptualized as a punctual than a general state when modeled with the sensors used in this experiment. Indeed, the short time window has led to better classification accuracies than the long window. This replicates a previous finding observed on a different data set [22] and suggests that the bio-behavioral signals used for this study (which were all peripheral sensors) are capturing physiological dynamics that operate on relatively short time scales.

Interestingly, there was no effect of threshold on balanced accuracy. However this parameter, as well as time window and classifier type, had significant impacts on specificity and sensitivity. This is very important, especially in the context of safety critical systems, since you may want to boost one of these metrics over the other. As such, the present findings provide useful insights about parameter tradeoffs and how to prioritize true-positives or true-negatives without compromising balanced accuracy.

Weak linear relationship between mental workload and attributes, and the significant difference observed across classifiers support the use of non-linear models for classifying psychophysiological states. Indeed, as it was shown before, physiological data sources are complementary, rather than redundant [12], and may also yield more information when combined in non-linear fashion, suggesting complex physiological manifestation of psychological states.

Acknowledgments. This research was supported by a Mitacs internship awarded to Mark Parent, funded by NSERC and Thales Canada. The authors would also like to thank Margot Beugniot for her participation in data collection.

References

1. Carter, R., Cheuvront, S.N., Sawka, M.N.: Operator Functional State Assessment (l'évaluation de l'aptitude opérationnelle de l'opérateur humain). Army research institute (2004)

2. Bracken, B.K., Palmon, N., Romero, V., Pfautz, J., Cooke, N.J.: A prototype toolkit for sensing and modeling individual and team state. In: Proceedings of the Human Factors and Ergonomics Society Annual Meeting, vol. 58, pp. 949–953 (2014). https://doi.org/10.1177/1541931214581199

3. Durkee, K.T., Pappada, S.M., Ortiz, A.E., Feeney, J.J., Galster, S.M.: System decision framework for augmenting human performance using real-time workload classifiers. Presented at the 2015 IEEE International Multi-Disciplinary Conference on Cognitive Methods in Situation Awareness and Decision Support (CogSIMA), Orlando, FL (2015)

4. Yin, Z., Zhang, J.: Operator functional state classification using least-square support vector machine based recursive feature elimination technique. Comput. Methods Programs Biomed. 113, 101–115 (2014). https://doi.org/10.1016/j.cmpb.2013.09.007

5. Durantin, G., Gagnon, J.-F., Tremblay, S., Dehais, F.: Using near infrared spectroscopy and heart rate variability to detect mental overload. Behav. Brain Res. 259, 16–23 (2014). https://doi.org/10.1016/j.bbr.2013.10.042

6. Hogervorst, M.A., Brouwer, A.-M., van Erp, J.B.F.: Combining and comparing EEG, peripheral physiology and eye-related measures for the assessment of mental workload. Front. Neurosci. 8 (2014). https://doi.org/10.3389/fnins.2014.00322

7. Tobon, D.V., Falk, T., Maier, M.: MS-QI: a modulation spectrum-based ECG quality index for telehealth applications. IEEE Trans. Biomed. Eng. 99, 1 (2014)

8. Overbeek, T.J., van Boxtel, A., Westerink, J.H.: Respiratory sinus arrhythmia responses to cognitive tasks: effects of task factors and RSA indices. Biol. Psychol. 99, 1–14 (2014)

9. Wijsman, J., Grundlehner, B., Liu, H., Penders, J., Hermens, H.: Wearable physiological sensors reflect mental stress state in office-like situations. In: 2013 Humaine Association Conference on Affective Computing and Intelligent Interaction (ACII), pp. 600–605 (2013). https://doi.org/10.1109/acii.2013.105

10. Williamon, A., Aufegger, L., Wasley, D., Looney, D., Mandic, D.P.: Complexity of physiological responses decreases in high-stress musical performance. J. R. Soc. Interface 10 (2013). https://doi.org/10.1098/rsif.2013.0719

11. Régis, N., et al.: Formal detection of attentional tunneling in human operator-automation interactions. IEEE Trans. Hum. Mach. Syst. 44(3), 326–336 (2014)

12. Matthews, G., Reinerman-Jones, L.E., Barber, D.J., Abich, J.: The psychometrics of mental workload multiple measures are sensitive but divergent. Hum. Factors J. Hum. Factors Ergon. Soc. 57, 125–143 (2015). https://doi.org/10.1177/0018720814539505

13. Gaillard, A.W.: Fatigue assessment and performance protection. NATO Sci. Ser. Sub Ser. I Life Behav. Sci. 355, 24–35 (2003)

14. Eggemeier, F.T., Wilson, G.F., Kramer, A.F., Damos, D.L.: Workload Assessment in Multi-Task Environments. Multiple-Task Performance, pp. 207–216 (1991)

15. Wilson, G.F., Russell, C.A.: Real-time assessment of mental workload using psychophysiological measures and artificial neural networks. Hum. Factors 45, 635–643 (2003)

16. Nourbakhsh, N., Wang, Y., Chen, F.: GSR and blink features for cognitive load classification. In: Kotzé, P., Marsden, G., Lindgaard, G., Wesson, J., Winckler, M. (eds.) Human-Computer Interaction–INTERACT. LNCS, vol. 8117, pp. 159–166. Springer, Heidelberg (2013). https://doi.org/10.1007/978-3-642-40483-2_11

17. Brouwer, A.-M., Zander, T.O., van Erp, J.B.F., Korteling, J.E., Bronkhorst, A.W.: Using neurophysiological signals that reflect cognitive or affective state: six recommendations to avoid common pitfalls. Front. Neurosci. 9 (2015). https://doi.org/10.3389/fnins.2015.00136

18. Gagnon, J.-F., Gagnon, O., Lafond, D., Parent, M., Tremblay, S.: A systematic assessment of operational metrics for modeling operator functional state: In: Proceedings of the 3rd International Conference on Physiological Computing Systems, pp. 15–23 SCITEPRESS - Science and Technology Publications, Lisbon, Portugal (2016). https://doi.org/10.5220/0005921600150023

19. Poole, A., Ball, L.J.: Eye tracking in human-computer interaction and usability research: current status and future prospects. In: Encyclopedia of Human-Computer Interaction, pp. 211–219 (2005). https://doi.org/10.4018/978-1-59140-562-7

20. Salvucci, D.D., Goldberg, J.H.: Identifying fixations and saccades in eye-tracking protocols. In: Proceedings of the 2000 Symposium on Eye Tracking Research & Applications, pp. 71–78. ACM (2000)

21. Boonnithi, S., Phongsuphap, S.: Comparison of heart rate variability measures for mental stress detection. Comput. Cardiol. **2011**, 85–88 (2011)

22. Rodríguez-Liñares, L., Vila, X., Mendez, A., Lado, M., Olivieri, D.: RHRV: an R-based software package for heart rate variability analysis of ECG recordings. In: 3rd Iberian Conference in Systems and Information Technologies (CISTI 2008), Vigo, Spain (2008)

23. Gagnon, O., Lafond, D., Gagnon, J-F., Parizeau, M.: Comparing methods for assessing operator functional state. In: Proceedings of the 2016 IEEE International Inter-Disciplinary Conference on Cognitive Methods in Situation Awareness and Decision Support (CogSIMA), San Diego, CA, USA, 21–25 March 2016

24. Oh, H., et al.: A composite cognitive workload assessment system in pilots under various task demands using ensemble learning. In: Schmorrow, Dylan D., Fidopiastis, Cali M. (eds.) AC 2015. LNCS (LNAI), vol. 9183, pp. 91–100. Springer, Cham (2015). https://doi.org/10.1007/978-3-319-20816-9_10

25. Kuhn, M.: caret: classification and regression training. Astrophys. Source Code Libr. **1**, 05003 (2015)

26. Torgo, L.: Data Mining with R, Learning with Case Studies. Chapman and Hall/CRC (2010). http://www.dcc.fc.up.pt/~ltorgo/DataMiningWithR

27. Wang, Z., Hope, R.M., Wang, Z., Ji, Q., Gray, W.D.: Cross-subject workload classification with a hierarchical Bayes model. NeuroImage Neuroergon. Hum. Brain Action Work **59**, 64–69 (2012). https://doi.org/10.1016/j.neuroimage.2011.07.094

Simple and Robust Automatic Detection and Recognition of Human Movement Patterns in Tasks of Different Complexity

Lisa Gutzeit[1](✉), Marc Otto[1], and Elsa Andrea Kirchner[1,2]

[1] Robotics Research Group, University of Bremen, Robert-Hooke-Str.1,
28359 Bremen, Germany
lisa.gutzeit@uni-bremen.de
[2] Robotics Innovation Center, German Research Center for Artificial
Intelligence (DFKI), Robert-Hooke-Str.1, 28359 Bremen, Germany
http://www.informatik.uni-bremen.de/robotik

Abstract. In many different research areas it is important to understand human behavior, e.g., in robotic learning or human-computer
interaction. To learn new robotic behavior from human demonstrations,
human movements need to be recognized to select which sequences should
be transferred to a robotic system and which are already available to the
system and therefore do not need to be learned. In interaction tasks,
the current state of a human can be used by the system to react to the
human in an appropriate way. Thus, the behavior of the human needs to
be analyzed. To apply the identification and recognition of human behavior in different applications, it is of high interest that the used methods
work autonomously with minimum user interference. This paper focuses
on the analysis of human manipulation behavior in tasks of different
complexity while keeping manual efforts low. By identifying characteristic movement patterns in the movement, human behaviors are decom-
posed into elementary building blocks using a fully automatic segmentation algorithm. With a simple k-Nearest Neighbor classification these
identified movement sequences are assigned to known movement classes.
To evaluate the presented approach, pick-and-place, ball-throwing, and
lever-pulling movements were recorded with a motion tracking system. It
is shown that the proposed method outperforms the widely used Hidden
Markov Model-based classification. Especially in case of a small number of labeled training examples, which considerably minimizes manual
efforts, our approach still has a high accuracy. For simple lever-pulling
movements already one training example per class sufficed to achieve a
classification accuracy of above 95%.

Keywords: Human movement analysis · Behavior segmentation ·
Behavior recognition · Manipulation · Motion tracking

© Springer Nature Switzerland AG 2019
A. Holzinger et al. (Eds.): PhyCS 2016–2018, LNCS 10057, pp. 39–57, 2019.
https://doi.org/10.1007/978-3-030-27950-9_3

1   Introduction

In the future, novel approaches in industry, production, personal services, health care, or medical applications, require a close collaboration of humans with robotic systems. To facilitate the requirements of these new approaches, not only the robotic systems must be equipped with enlarged mechanisms and skills that allow intuitive and safe interaction, but also the human intention, behavior and habits have to be better understood [11]. To allow this, novel methods to analyze human behavior are needed, which can easily be applied in different applications.

Understanding human behaviors is one important factor to successfully achieve intuitive human-computer interaction. For example, based on the knowledge of the current state of the human, systems can interact with humans in an appropriate manner. To obtain this knowledge, it is necessary to identify the representative parts of the human behavior and to assign the identified behaviors into categories which induce different reactions of the system. Only if the state of the human and the context which is described by this state are known, the system can follow the working steps that are required in this situation or can support the human if desired.

If robots become part of our everyday life in the future, it becomes important that also non-experts can teach a robotic system new skills. Robotic learning from demonstration is an active research area in robotics that promises to be a powerful tool to reach this goal, see for example [8,13,15,16]. With learning from demonstration approaches, human demonstrations of a task can be transferred to a robotic system and generalized to solve different but similar tasks [8]. This allows also non-experts to demonstrate the system a way to solve a certain task without knowledge about robot control techniques. However, transferring a complex behavior to a system can be very time-consuming or even impossible. In order to learn also complex behaviors, the demonstration should be segmented into its main building blocks to be learned more efficiently [18]. By grouping segments that belong to the same behavior and by recognizing these behaviors, it can be determined which segments are needed to be learned for a certain situation. Beyond that, movements can be identified that can already be executed by the system and thus do not need to be learned.

Behavioral studies indicate that also humans learn complex behavior incrementally, as can be seen, e.g., in a study on infants [2]. The hypothesis is that complex behaviors are learned based on simple individual building blocks that are chunked together to a more complex behavior [7]. The idea in this work is to identify building blocks of human manipulation demonstrations so that they can be learned by the robotic system. In this way the system can learn a repertoire of behavior building blocks based on human demonstration which can easily be combined to different complex manipulation movements. To detect building blocks of human demonstrations, characteristic movement patterns have to be identified. In manipulation behaviors, bell-shaped velocity profiles have been found to be a suitable pattern [14]. In this work, a velocity-based behavior segmentation algorithm, introduced in previous work as velocity-based Multiple

Change-point Inference (vMCI) [18], is used to segment recorded human manipulation movements. The applied algorithm detects movement sequences that show a bell-shaped velocity profile and are therefore assumed to be building blocks of human behavior. Furthermore, the vMCI algorithm identifies movement building blocks automatically without need for parameter tuning despite noise in the data [18].

The identified building blocks of human movements have also to be classified according to the actual behavior they belong to. By assigning suitable annotations to the recognized movement classes, the selection as well as the detection of the required behavior becomes intuitive and easy to use in different interaction scenarios. For supervised movement classification approaches the training data needs to be manually labeled. To keep the manual input low, it is desirable that the classification works with small sets of training data. We propose to classify detected building blocks by using simple k-Nearest Neighbor (k-NN) classification which satisfies this condition.

In this paper, our previous work presented in [9] is recapped and extended with an additional experiment and evaluation. Beside the application of our methods on pick-and-place and ball-throwing movements, the proposed methods are additionally applied to segment and recognize lever-pulling movements in a third experiment. The paper is organized as follows: In Sect. 2, different state-of-the-art approaches for segmentation and recognition of human movements are summarized. Our approach is described in Sect. 3. Afterwards in Sect. 4, the approach is evaluated on real human manipulation movements in tasks of different complexity. All results are compared to Hidden Markov Model (HMM)-based approaches which are widely used in the literature to represent and recognize movements. At the end of this paper, a conclusion is given.

2   Related Work

Depending on the modality to record human movements, there are a lot of different methods to recognize human behaviors. In many applications, human actions are recognized in videos, e.g., to find tackles in soccer games, to support elderly in their homes or for gesture recognition in video games [17]. Human action classification is just as important as detecting the human itself in video-based action recognition. Algorithms like Support Vector Machines, or their probabilistic variant the Relevance Vector Machines, Hidden Markov Models, k-Nearest Neighbors or Dynamic Time Warping-based classification are used to classify the observed actions. A more detailed overview is given in [17].

If the human behavior is not observed in a video but using motion tracking, e.g., with markers placed on the body, the segmentation of the recorded movements is next to the classification of high interest. For example in [4], human arm movements were tracked and segmented into so-called movement primitives at time points where the angular velocity of a certain number of degrees of freedom crosses zero. After a PCA-based dimensionality reduction, the identified movements were clustered using k-Means. Even though this approach promises to identify the primitive units of human movements, it requires the selection of thresholds to determine the segment borders. This is very sensitive to noise in the input data which results in over-segmentation of the data and requires adaption of the parameters for different applications. Gong et al., on the other hand, propose Kernelized Temporal Cut to segment full body motions, which is based on Hilbert space embedding of distributions [5]. In their work, different actions are recognized using Dynamic Manifold Warping as similarity measure. In contrast to the analysis of full body motions, we focus on the identification and recognition of manipulation movements which show special patterns in the velocity which should be considered for segmentation.

Beyond that, HMM-based approaches are often used in the literature, both for movement segmentation as well as for movement recognition. For example, Kulic et al. stochastically determine motion segments which are then represented using HMMs [12]. The derived segments are incrementally clustered using a tree structure and the Kullback-Leibler distance as segment distance measure. In a similar fashion, Gräve and Behnke represent probabilistically derived segments with HMMs, where segments that belong to the same movement are simultaneously classified into the same class if they can be represented by the same HMM [6]. Besides these approaches, solely training-based movement classification with HMMs is widely used, e.g. in [1,19]. Because HMMs are expected to perform not well when few training data is available, we propose to use k-NN instead and compare it with the HMM approach.

3 Methods

This section describes a velocity-based movement segmentation algorithm which automatically identifies building blocks in human manipulation movements without the need of parameter tuning. In the second part of this section, an approach to recognize different known movement segments in an observed behavior is described.

3.1 Segmentation of Human Movement into Building Blocks

The purpose of this work it to find sequences in human manipulation movements that correspond to elementary building blocks which are characterized by bell-shaped velocity profiles as shown in [14]. Therefore, a segmentation algorithm is needed that identifies these building blocks. A second important property of the algorithm is the ability to handle variations in the movements. Human movement shows a lot of variations both during the execution by different persons as well as by the same person. For this reason, it is important that the algorithm for human movement segmentation finds sequences that correspond to the same behavior despite differences in their execution. Furthermore, the algorithms should be applicable to different tasks with low efforts. This can be accomplished with an algorithm that does not require parameter tuning if different types of movements are analyzed.

In previous work, we introduced the velocity-based Multiple Change-point Inference (vMCI) algorithm which tackles these issues [18]. The algorithm detects building blocks in human manipulation movements fully automatic. It is an probabilistic method, which can handle variations in the movement and the direct parameters of the data model are inferred from the data. It is based on the Multiple Change-point Inference (MCI) algorithm [3] in which segments are found in time series data using Bayesian Inference. Each segment $y_{i+1:j}$, starting at time point i and ending at j, is represented with a linear regression model (LRM) with q predefined basis functions ϕ_k:

$$y_{i+1:j} = \sum_{k=1}^{q} \beta_k \phi_k + \varepsilon, \tag{1}$$

where ε models the noise that is assumed in the data and $\beta = (\beta_1, ..., \beta_q)$ are the model parameters [18]. It is assumed that a new segment starts if the underlying LRM changes. This modeling of the observed data allows to handle technical noise in the data as well as variation in the execution of the same movement. To determine the segments online, the segmentation points are modeled via a Markov process in order that an online Viterbi algorithm can be used to determine their positions [3].

We expanded the MCI algorithm in our previous work to detect movement sequences that correspond to building blocks characterized by a bell-shaped velocity profile [18]. To accomplish this, the LRM of Eq. 1 is split to model the velocity of the hand independent from its position with different basis functions, where the basis function for the velocity dimension is chosen in a way that it has a bell-shaped profile. In detail this means that the velocity y^v of the observed data sequence is modeled by

$$y^v = \alpha_1 \phi_v + \alpha_2 + \varepsilon, \tag{2}$$

with weights $\alpha = (\alpha_1, \alpha_2)$ and noise ε [18]. The model has two basis functions. First, the bell-shaped velocity curve is modeled using a single radial basis function [18]:

$$\phi_v(x_t) = \exp\left\{-\frac{(c - x_t)^2}{r^2}\right\}. \tag{3}$$

If half of the segment length is chosen for the width parameter r, the basis function can cover the whole segment. The center c is determined automatically by the algorithm and regulates the alignment to velocity curves with peaks at different positions. Additionally, the basis function 1 weighted with α_2 accounts for velocities unequal to zero at start or end of the segment. As in the original MCI method, an online Viterbi algorithm can be used to detect the segment borders.

Figure 1 shows an exemplary result of the segmentation of artificial data using the vMCI algorithm. At the top, a one-dimensional simulated movement can be seen. The lower figure shows the corresponding velocity. To simulate two different behavior segments, the movement is slowed down at time point 0.4. For

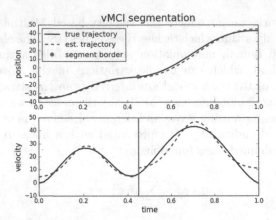

Fig. 1. Artificial movement consisting of two sequences with a bell-shaped velocity. The vMCI segmentation successfully detected the transition point. Extracted from [9].

the position dimension, the algorithm fits LRMs to the data according to Eq. 1 with pre-defined basis functions. In this case, autoregressive basis functions are chosen. The velocity dimension is simultaneously fit with a LRM as introduced in Eq. 2. The algorithm automatically selects the models which best fits parts of the data. In this case, it is most likely that the data arises from two different underlying models. This results in a single segmentation point which matches the true segmentation point within an acceptable margin. In contrast to other segmentation algorithms, for example a segmentation based on the detection of local minima, vMCI is very robust against noise in the data, as shown in [18]. Furthermore, the method is not sensitive to the choice of its hyper-parameters [18], hence, no parameter tuning is needed if it is applied to different data.

3.2 Recognition of Human Movement

There are many different possibilities to classify human movements, as reviewed in Sect. 2. The goal in this work is to choose a simple and robust classification method. To make the algorithm easily applicable on different manipulation data, minimal need for parameter tuning is of high interest. Furthermore, manual efforts can be minimized if the algorithm reliably classifies movement segments even if only a small training set is available. For this reasons we use a k-NN classifier for movement recognition. It has only one parameter, k, and is able to classify manipulation movements with a high accuracy given a small training set, as shown in our experiments.

Feature Extraction. Movement trajectories of markers placed at certain positions on the demonstrator are used in this work as features for the classification. The movements are recorded in Cartesian coordinates which results in different time series if the same movement is executed at a different position. Thus, the data is transposed into a coordinate system which is not global but relative to the human demonstrator. The position of the back is used as reference point (see Fig. 2a) at the first time point of a segment, i.e. the data is transformed into a coordinate system centered at this point. Additionally, variances in the execution of the same movement are reduced by normalizing each movement segment to zero mean.

To successfully classify movement segments, additional features may be relevant. In manipulation movements where objects are involved, the positions of the objects as well as their spatial relation to the demonstrator are important features to distinguish between movement classes. Thus, the distance of the human hand to the manipulated object as well as the object speed are used in the pick-and-place experiment described in Sect. 4.2 to classify manipulation segments into distinct movements. Depending on the recognition task additional features, like the rotation of the hand to distinguish between different grasping positions, can be relevant.

Movement Classification. Due to its simplicity, we propose to use a k-NN classifier to distinguish between different movements. In the k-NN classification, an observed movement sequence is assigned to the movement class, which is the most common among its k closest neighbors of the training examples. To determine the closest neighbors, we use the standard Euclidean distance metric. All segments are interpolated to the mean segment length in order to account for segments of unequal length. Alternatively, dynamic time warping (DTW) could be used as a distance measure. However, in a preliminary analysis of k-NN classification on manipulation behaviors the presented approach outperformed a DTW-based k-NN. The number of neighbors k is set to 1. That means just the closest neighbor is considered for classification which leads to a good accuracy in case of small number of training examples. A bigger k could result in more classification errors due to the very low number of examples of each class.

4   Experiments

The proposed segmentation and classification methods are evaluated in this section on real human manipulation movements tracked using a motion capturing system. The experimental setup including the evaluation technique used in three different experiments are described in Sect. 4.1. Afterwards, the application and evaluation of the presented approaches on several demonstrations of three different manipulation movements are described. The evaluation on a pick-and-place and ball-throwing tasks were already part of our previous publication [9] and are recapped here. Additionally, we evaluated the approaches on a lever-pulling task in Sect. 4.4. For all experiments it is shown that the vMCI algorithm correctly detects segments in the recorded demonstrations which correspond to behavior building blocks with a bell-shaped velocity pattern. Furthermore, the classification with k-NN using small number of training data is evaluated and compared to the results with an HMM-based classification.

4.1 Experimental Setup

The demonstrations of all manipulation movements were tracked using a marker-based motion tracking system. The 3D positions of visual markers placed on the subject were measured with 7 motion capture cameras at a frequency of 500 Hz. In a pre-processing step this data was down-sampled to 25 Hz. The positions of the markers can be seen in Figs. 2 and 3. Three markers were placed on the back of the demonstrator to determine the position of the back and its orientation. This was used to transform the recorded data into the coordinate system relative to the back, as described in Sect. 3.2. To track the movement of the manipulating arm, markers were placed at the shoulder, the elbow, and the back of

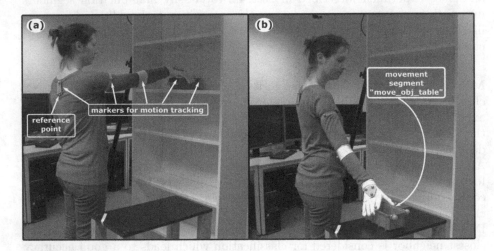

Fig. 2. Snapshots of the pick-and-place task analyzed in this work. The images show the grasping of the object from the shelf (a) which is then placed on a table standing on the right hand side (b) which corresponds to the movement segment move_obj_table. Extracted from [9].

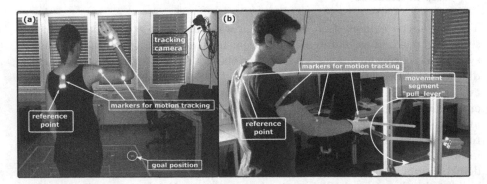

Fig. 3. Snapshot of the ball-throwing (a), extracted from [9], and the lever-pulling task (b).

the hand. The orientation of the hand was determined by placing three markers instead of one on it. Grasping movements in the pick-and-place demonstrations were recorded using additional markers which were placed at thumb, index, and middle finger. Furthermore, two more markers were placed on the manipulated object in this experiment to determine its position and orientation. However, the tasks in our experiments required only basic manipulation movements, e.g., approaching the object or moving the object. Thus, just the position of the hand and the manipulated object were used for segmentation and recognition. However, the orientations are needed if the demonstrated movements should be transferred in a further step to a robotic system using learning from demonstration techniques [8].

Movement building blocks were identified in the demonstrations using the vMCI algorithm described in Sect. 3.1. The segmentation algorithm was applied on the position and the velocity of the recorded hand movements. As proposed in [18], the recorded positions of each demonstration were pre-processed to a zero mean and such that the variance of the first order differences of each dimension is equal to one.

To evaluate the proposed classification method, the resulting movement segments were manually labeled into one of the movement classes defined for each experiment. However, some of the obtained segments could not be assigned to one of these classes because they contain only parts of the movement. This could result from errors in the segmentation as well as from demonstrations where a movement was slowed down before the movement class ends. A case would be when the subject thought about the exact position to grasp the object. An example can be seen in the top plot of Fig. 4. The concatenation of the first two detected segments belong to the class approach_forward. Nonetheless, the vMCI algorithm detected two segments, both with a bell-shaped velocity curve, because the subject slowed down the movement right before reaching the object. These incomplete movement segments were discarded for the evaluation of the classification approach. Furthermore, some of the identified movement segments did not belong to one of the pre-defined movement classes of the experiment. Usually, these nonassignable segments belonged to small extra movements, that were not part of the main movement task and thus were not considered in the defined movement classes. These movement segments were as well not used for the evaluation of the classification.

Before classification, the original recorded marker positions of each obtained segment were pre-processed as described in Sect. 3.2. Depending on the manipulation task, additional features were calculated. As proposed in Sect. 3.2, the obtained segments were classified using the 1-NN algorithm. For each of the two experiments, the accuracy of the 1-NN classification was evaluated using a stratified 2-fold cross-validation with a fixed number of examples per class in the training data. The training set sizes were varied from 1 example per class to 20 examples per class and the remaining data was used for testing. Since we want to show the performance of the classification with small training set sizes, the maximal number of training examples per class was kept low. For each number of examples per class in the training data, the cross-validation was performed with 100 iterations.

For comparison, the data was also classified using a HMM-based approach, which is a standard representation method for movements in the literature, see Sect. 2. In the HMM-based classification, one single HMM was trained for each movement class. To classify a test segment, the probability of the segment to be generated by each of the trained HMMs was calculated. The label of the most likely underlying HMM was assigned to the segment. The number of states in the HMMs was determined with a stratified 2-fold cross-validation repeated 50 times with equally sized training and test sets. As a result, we trained each HMM with one hidden state. The accuracy of the HMM-based classification with 1 hidden state per trained HMM was evaluated like the 1-NN classification with a stratified 2-fold cross-validation with fixed numbers of training examples for each class.

4.2   Segmentation and Recognition of Pick-and-Place Movements

In the first experiment, the presented approach was evaluated on pick-and-place movements. The task of the human demonstrator, partly shown in Fig. 2, was to grasp a box from a shelf, move it to a table standing on the right side of the subject, and move the box back to the shelf. After placing the box on the table or the shelf, the subject should move the arm into a rest position in which it loosely hangs down. This task resulted in 6 different main movement classes: approach_forward, move_obj_table, move_to_rest_right, approach_right, move_obj_shelf, and move_to_rest_down. Short periods of time in which the demonstrator did not move his arm were assigned to the class idle.

The pick-and-place task was performed by three different subjects, repeated 6 times by each. Two of these subjects performed the task again with 4 repetitions while their movements were recorded with slightly different camera positions and a different global coordinate system. This resulted in different positions of the person and the manipulating object in the scene which should be handled by the presented movement segmentation and recognition methods. A total of 26 different demonstrations from different subjects and with varying coordinate systems were available to evaluate the proposed approaches.

Results. The demonstrations of the pick-and-place task could be successfully segmented into movement parts with a bell-shaped velocity profile using the vMCI algorithm. Three examples of the segmentation results can be seen in Fig. 4. The resulting movement segments were manually labeled into one of the 7 movement classes described above. This resulted in 155 labeled movement segments with different occurrences of each class, as summarized in Table 1.

As described in Sect. 4.1, next to the positions of the markers attached on the subject, the distance from the hand to the object and the object velocity were calculated as additional features in this experiment. An example result of the classification using 1-NN is shown in Fig. 5. For this example demonstration of the pick-and-place task, all segments have been labeled with the correct annotation using a training set with 5 examples for each class.

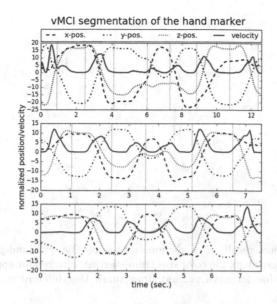

vMCI segmentation of the hand marker

Fig. 4. Segmentation results of three different demonstrations of the pick-and-place task. The x-, y- and z-position of the hand are visualized with black lines. The blue line corresponds to its velocity and the red vertical lines are the segment borders determined by the vMCI algorithm. Extracted from [9].

Table 1. Occurences of each class in the recorded pick-and-place data [9].

Movement class	num. examples
approach_forward	20
move_obj_table	26
move_to_rest_right	25
approach_right	23
move_obj_shelf	26
move_to_rest_down	24
idle	11

The results of the cross-validation using 1-NN and HMM-based classification are shown in Fig. 6. Because the data contains 7 different classes, an accuracy of 14.3% can be achieved by guessing. The 1-NN classification clearly outperforms the HMM-based classification using training sets with occurrences of each class smaller or equal to 20. Already with 1 example per class an accuracy of nearly 80% can be achieved using 1-NN. With 10 examples per class, the accuracy is 97.5% and with 20 examples per class 99.2%. In contrast, 14 examples per class are needed in the HMM-based classification to achieve an accuracy of 90% in this evaluation. With not more than 10 examples per class, the accuracy of the HMM-based classification is considerably below the achieved accuracy using 1-NN.

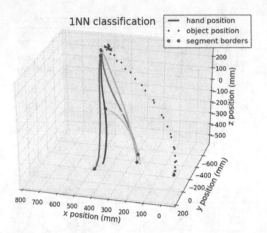

Fig. 5. Classification result of a demonstration of the pick-and-place task with 1-NN. Different colors along the color spectrum starting with red for `approach_forward` and ending with blue for `move_to_rest_down` mark the different movement classes. Extracted from [9].

These results show that with the proposed 1-NN classification, manipulation movements can be assigned to known movement classes with a very small number of training examples. This means that with minimal need for manual training data labeling and no parameter tuning, very good classification results can be achieved using the proposed approach. Furthermore, the 1-NN classification considerably outperforms the widely used HMM-based classification in case that only a small number of training examples is available.

4.3   Segmentation and Recognition of Ball-Throwing Movements

The vMCI segmentation and the 1-NN classification were evaluated in a second experiment on ball-throwing demonstrations. Compared to the pick-and-place experiment, this task is more challenging because no fixed objects are involved resulting in more possibilities of movement execution. The task of the subject was to throw a ball to a goal position on the ground located approximately 1.5 m away. The numerous possibilities to throw the ball were limited by the restriction that the ball should be thrown from above, i.e. the hand has a position higher than the shoulder before the ball leaves the hand, see Fig. 3a. Nonetheless, the recorded throws show high variations in the demonstrations compared to the pick-and-place task. This could stem from different experiences in ball-throwing of the different subjects and training effects.

Before and after the throw, the subject had to move into a rest position, in which the arm loosely hangs down. The individual movement parts of each throw could be divided into four different main classes: `strike_out`, `throw`, `swing_out` and `idle`. In contrast to the pick-and-place task, only the movement of the arm was tracked in this task and not the position of the involved object, the ball. This is because in this experiment, the spatial distance of the ball to the demonstrator plays only a minor role and the movement of the arm has a much higher relevance to distinguish between movement classes. Furthermore, it was not recorded if the goal position was actually hit by the ball.

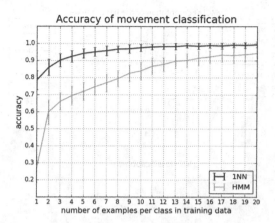

Fig. 6. Comparison of the accuracy of the classification of pick-and-place movement segments using 1-NN and HMM-based classification. Extracted from [9].

The ball-throwing task was demonstrated by 10 different subjects, each performing 24 throws.

Results. In a previous evaluation of the vMCI method on ball-throwing movements, it was already shown that the algorithm is able to identify the individual throws based on the position and velocity of the hand [18]. This result was confirmed by the evaluation of the demonstrations conducted for this work. A representative example of the segmentation result is shown in Fig. 7(a). Segment borders were correctly identified at positions were bell-shaped curves of the velocity profile end.

The resulting segments of all 240 ball-throw demonstration were manually assigned to one of the four movement classes to evaluate the classification. Again, each class had a different occurrence in the available data, as summarized in Table 2.

Table 2. Occurrences of each class in the ball-throwing data [9].

Movement class	num. examples
strike_out	221
throw	227
swing_out	339
idle	208

The positions of the markers attached to the subject, see Fig. 3a, were used as features for the movement classification in this experiment. Figure 7(b) shows an example classification result using 1-NN and 5 examples per class in the

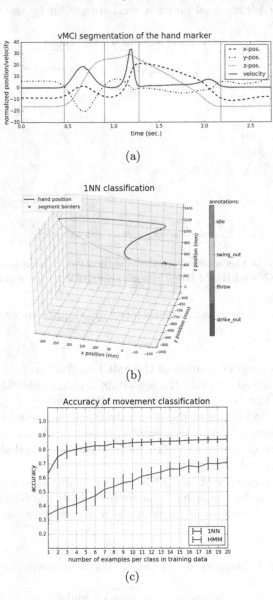

(a)

(b)

(c)

Fig. 7. Segmentation (a) and classification (b) result of one demonstration of the ball-throwing task. The presented methods successfully identified the segment borders and recognized the different movement classes. (c) Comparison of the accuracy of the classification of ball-throwing segments of all demonstrations using 1-NN and HMM-based classification. Extracted from [9].

training data. The 5 movement segments were correctly classified into one of the predefined classes.

The results of the cross-validation comparing 1-NN with HMM-based classification are visualized in Fig. 7(c). Like in the pick-and-place experiment, 1-NN outperforms HMM-based classification in the case of small training data sets. This experiment contains considerably more demonstrated movements and higher variance along demonstrations compared to the pick-and-place task. In here, the difference between classification algorithms is more contrasting. With one example per class in the training data, an accuracy of 62.9% using 1-NN can be achieved and only 33.8% by using HMM-based classification. This experiment contains 4 different classes, i.e. an accuracy of 25% can be achieved by guessing. Using 1-NN, a classification accuracy of 80% is accomplished using 4 examples per class during training. In contrast to this, this accuracy is not reached using HMM-based classification in this evaluation. For comparison, the evaluation was additionally conducted using 100 examples per class during training. This resulted in an accuracy of 91.5% using 1-NN, and 77.8% using HMM-based classification. This shows that even if more training data is available, the 1-NN classification outperforms the HMM-based approach.

4.4   Segmentation and Recognition of Lever-Pulling Movements

In a third experiment, the presented methods were evaluated on lever-pulling demonstrations. The task of the subject was to pull a lever down. The lever was fixed to a table and thus movement execution was in comparison to the other two experiments strongly predetermined, see Fig. 3b. At the beginning of each demonstration the subject was in a rest position with the arm hanging down at the side of the body. Next, the subject reached for the lever with the right arm and pulled down the lever. Finally, the subject turned the arm back to the rest position (arm hanging down). After returning to the rest position, the lever had to be pulled up again, which was done with the left arm and had not been recorded by motion tracking. We chose this very simple behavior to show that for simple movements only very few demonstrations are needed for classification.

The individual movement parts of each movement could be divided into 4 different main classes: `idle`, `approach_forward`, `move_lever`, `move_to_rest`. As for the ball-throwing experiment, only the movement of the arm was tracked and not the position of the involved object, the lever. This is because in this experiment, the spatial distance of the lever to the demonstrators hand is fixed and plays no role. Only the movement of the arm can be used to distinguish between movement classes.

The lever-pulling task was demonstrated by two different subjects, performing 32 and 36 pulls, respectively.

Results. In this task the velocity of the movements did not always show smooth bell-shaped curves like in the previous experiments. This is because the positions of the hand was more predetermined. The subjects could not move their hand free, resulting in some cases in a slowed down movement with a more noisy velocity profile. This effect may be minimized by more demonstration trails generating a training effect on the subjects. Nonetheless, the vMCI algorithm successfully segmented the trajectories of the lever-pulling demonstrations without any adaptions of (hyper-)parameters or an additional preprocessing of the data. An example of the segmentation results can be seen in Fig. 8(a). The resulting

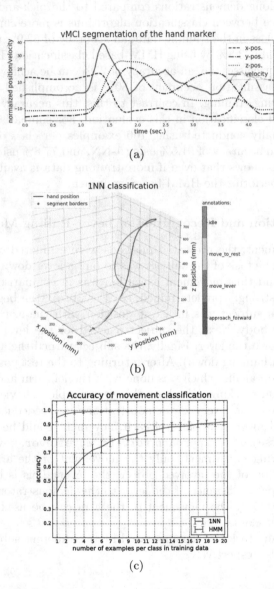

(a)

(b)

(c)

Fig. 8. Segmentation (a) and classification (b) result of one demonstration of the lever-pulling task. (c) Comparison of the accuracy of the classification of lever-pulling segments of all demonstrations using 1-NN and HMM-based classification.

movement segments were manually labeled into one of the 4 movement classes that are present in the lever-pulling task. The occurrences of each class can be found in Table 3.

Table 3. Occurences of each class in the lever-pulling data.

Movement class	num. examples
move_lever	62
approach_forward	76
move_to_rest	72
idle	72

The positions of the markers attached to the subject, see Fig. 3b, were used as features for the automatic movement classification. Figure 8(b) shows an example classification result using 1-NN and only one example per class in the training data. The 4 movement segments were correctly classified into one of the predefined classes.

The results of the cross-validation comparing 1-NN with HMM-based classification are visualized in Fig. 8(c). As in the other two experiments, 1-NN outperforms HMM-based classification in the case of small training data sets. In this experiment, which contains simpler movements compared to the ball-throwing and the pick-and-place examples, the difference between the classification algorithms is very vivid in the area of very few training examples. Indeed, very high accuracy can already be achieved with one training example for each class, i.e., 95.3% using 1-NN but only 42.1% by using HMM-based classification. Using 1-NN, a classification accuracy of 99.0% is accomplished using 4 examples per class during training. In contrast to this, this accuracy is not reached using HMM-based classification in this evaluation.

This experiment shows that even if very few training data is available, training is possible resulting in a high accuracy using 1-NN classification in case that the movements are very simple.

5   Conclusions

We presented in this paper an approach to segment and classify human manipulation behavior. The segmentation was done using the unsupervised vMCI segmentation, formerly introduced in [18], which identifies building blocks of manipulation movements based on the velocity profile of the hand. For classification, we applied a simple 1-NN classifier using the Euclidean distance measure. Both algorithms were applied on pick-and-place, ball-throwing and lever-pulling movements. All these manipulation movements of different complexity could be successfully segmented and classified without the need of manual adaptions of the algorithms like, e.g., parameter tuning. Although a supervised classification method like 1-NN always needs manually labeled training data, we showed that the recognition of the movements can be done using a small set of training data, which considerably minimizes manual efforts. For the lever-pulling task, which is the simplest of the considered movements, a high classification accuracy could be achieved with just one training example per class. In comparison to widely used HMM-based movement classification, the accuracy was a considerably higher with small training sets in all experiments. Furthermore, the good classification results were achieved without any sophisticated feature selection methods.

For the development of embedded multimodal interfaces [10], simple approaches as the one presented here allow to use miniaturized processing units with relatively low processing power and energy consumption. This is, e.g., relevant in robotics, since the integration of interfaces into a robotic system is limited. But also wearable assisting devices have limitations regarding size, energy and computing power. For these applications not only accurate but also simple methods are needed. With the evaluation of our approaches we show that both, accuracy and simplicity, can be accomplished.

For future work, an integrated algorithm for segmentation and classification should be considered. Especially when extra segments are generated, e.g., caused by not fluently executed movements, an integrated algorithm where segmentation and classification influence each other becomes relevant. Such segments could be merged by identifying that only their concatenation can be assigned to one of the known movement classes.

In addition, manual effort needed for classification should be further minimized by recognizing the movement segments using an unsupervised approach. Annotations, like `move_object`, which are needed in many applications, e.g. to select segments that should be imitated by a robot, are ideally done without manual interference. These movement annotations can, e.g., be derived by analyzing features of the movement arising from different modalities. Psychological data, such as eye-tracking or electroencephalographic-data, could be used for this.

References

1. Aarno, D., Kragic, D.: Motion intention recognition in robot assisted applications. Robot. Auton. Syst. **56**, 692–705 (2008)
2. Adi-Japha, E., Karni, A., Parnes, A., Loewenschuss, I., Vakil, E.: A shift in task routines during the learning of a motor skill: Group-averaged data may mask critical phases in the individuals' acquisition of skilled performance. J. Exp. Psychol. Learn. Mem. Cogn. **24**, 1544–1551 (2008)
3. Fearnhead, P., Liu, Z.: On-line inference for multiple change point models. J. Roy. Stat. Soc. Ser. B (Stat. Methodol.) **69**, 589–605 (2007)
4. Fod, A., Matrić, M., Jenkins, O.: Automated derivation of primitives for movement classification. Auton. Robots **12**, 39–54 (2002)
5. Gong, D., Medioni, G., Zhao, X.: Structured time series analysis for human action segmentation and recognition. IEEE Trans. Pattern Anal. Mach. Intell. **36**(7), 1414–1427 (2013). http://doi.org/4B458234-5E6D-453D-B6A0-C9F3A51683BB. http://www.ncbi.nlm.nih.gov/pubmed/24344075

6. Gräve, K., Behnke, S.: Incremental action recognition and generalizing motion generation based on goal-directed features. In: 2012 IEEE/RSJ International Conference on Intelligent Robots and Systems (IROS), pp. 751–757 (2012). http://ieeexplore.ieee.org/xpls/abs_all.jsp?arnumber=6386116

7. Graybiel, A.: The basal ganglia and chunking of action repertoires. Neurobiol. Learn. Mem. **70**, 119–136 (1998)

8. Gutzeit, L., Fabisch, A., Otto, M., Metzen, J.H., Hansen, J., Kirchner, F., Kirchner, E.A.: The besman learning platform for automated robot skill learning. Front. Robot. AI **5**, 43 (2018). https://doi.org/10.3389/frobt.2018.00043. https://www.frontiersin.org/article/10.3389/frobt.2018.00043

9. Gutzeit, L., Kirchner, E.A.: Automatic detection and recognition of human movement patterns in manipulation tasks. In: Proceedings of the 3rd International Conference on Physiological Computing Systems (2016)

10. Kirchner, E.A., Fairclough, S., Kirchner, F.: Embedded multimodal interfaces in robotics: Applications, future trends and societal implications. In: Oviatt, S., Schuller, B., Cohen, P., Sonntag, D. (eds.) Handbook of Multimodal-Multisensor Interfaces, vol. 3, Chap. IX, p. n.A. ACM Books, Morgan Claypool (2017)

11. Kirchner, E.A., de Gea Fernandez, J., Kampmann, P., Schröer, M., Metzen, J.H., Kirchner, F.: Intuitive interaction with robots – technical approaches and challenges. In: Drechsler, R., Kühne, U. (eds.) Formal Modeling and Verification of Cyber-Physical Systems, pp. 224–248. Springer, Wiesbaden (2015). https://doi.org/10.1007/978-3-658-09994-7_8

12. Kulić, D., Ott, C., Lee, D., Ishikawa, J., Nakamura, Y.: Incremental learning of full body motion primitives and their sequencing through human motion observation. Int. J. Robot. Res. **31**(3), 330–345 (2012)

13. Metzen, J.H., Fabisch, A., Senger, L., Gea Fernández, J., Kirchner, E.A.: Towards learning of generic skills for robotic manipulation. KI - Künstliche Intelligenz **28**(1), 15–20 (2013). https://doi.org/10.1007/s13218-013-0280-1

14. Morasso, P.: Spatial control of arm movements. Exp. Brain Res. **42**, 223–227 (1981)

15. Mülling, K., Kober, J., Koemer, O., Peters, J.: Learning to select and generalize striking movements in robot table tennis. Int. J. Robot. Res. **32**, 263–279 (2013)

16. Pastor, P., Hoffmann, H., Asfour, T., Schaal, S.: Learning and generalization of motor skills by learning from demonstration. In: 2009 IEEE International Conference on Robotics and Automation, pp. 763–768. IEEE, May 2009. https://doi.org/10.1109/ROBOT.2009.5152385. http://ieeexplore.ieee.org/lpdocs/epic03/wrapper.htm?arnumber=5152385

17. Poppe, R.: A survey on vision-based human action recognition. Image Vis. Comput. **28**(6), 976–990 (2010). https://doi.org/10.1016/j.imavis.2009.11.014. http://linkinghub.elsevier.com/retrieve/pii/S0262885609002704

18. Senger, L., Schröer, M., Metzen, J.H., Kirchner, E.A.: Velocity-based multiple change-point inference for unsupervised segmentation of human movement behavior. In: Proccedings of the 22th International Conference on Pattern Recognition (ICPR2014), pp. 4564–4569 (2014). https://doi.org/10.1109/ICPR.2014.781

19. Stefanov, N., Peer, A., Buss, M.: Online intention recognition in computer-assisted teleoperation systems. In: Kappers, A.M.L., van Erp, J.B.F., Bergmann Tiest, W.M., van der Helm, F.C.T. (eds.) EuroHaptics 2010. LNCS, vol. 6191, pp. 233–239. Springer, Heidelberg (2010). https://doi.org/10.1007/978-3-642-14064-8_34

From Body Tracking Interaction in Floor Projection Displays to Elderly Cardiorespiratory Training Through Exergaming

Afonso Gonçalves[1,2]($\boxtimes$) (iD), Filipa Nóbrega[2], Mónica Cameirão[1,2] (iD),
John E. Muñoz[1,2] (iD), Élvio Gouveia[1,3] (iD),
and Sergi Bermudez i Badia[1,2] (iD)

[1] Madeira Interactive Technologies Institute, Funchal, Portugal
{afonso.goncalves,monica.cameirao,john.cardona,
sergi.bermudez}@m-iti.org
[2] Faculdade de Ciências Exatas e da Engenharia, Universidade da Madeira,
Funchal, Portugal
[3] Faculdade de Ciências Sociais, Universidade da Madeira, Funchal, Portugal
erubiog@uma.pt

Abstract. The opportunity to develop new natural user interfaces has come
forward due to the recent development of inexpensive full body tracking sensors, which has made this technology accessible to millions of users. In this
paper, we present a comparative study between two natural user interfaces, and a
cardiorespiratory training exergame developed based on the study results. The
focus was on studying interfaces that could easily be used by an elderly population for interaction with floor projection displays. One interface uses both feet
position to control a cursor and feet distance to trigger activation. In the alternative interface, the cursor is controlled by forearm ray casting into the projection floor and interaction is activated by hand pose. These modes of
interaction were tested with 19 elderly participants in a point-and-click and a
drag-and-drop task using a between-subjects experimental design. The usability,
perceived workload and performance indicators were measured for each interface. Results show a clear preference towards the feet-controlled interface and a
marginally better performance for this method. The results from the study served
as a guide to the design of a cardiorespiratory fitness exergame for the elderly.
The game "Grape Stomping" uses ground projection and mapping to display
real-size winery elements. These virtual elements are used to simulate, in a
playful way, the process of grape maceration through repeated stomping.
A playtest session with nine elderly users was completed and its insights are
presented in addition to the description of the game.

Keywords: Large display interface · Floor projection · Elderly ·
Exergames natural user interface · Kinect

© Springer Nature Switzerland AG 2019
A. Holzinger et al. (Eds.): PhyCS 2016–2018, LNCS 10057, pp. 58–77, 2019.
https://doi.org/10.1007/978-3-030-27950-9_4

1 Introduction

Developed countries' populations are becoming increasingly older, with estimates that one-third of the European citizens will be over 65 years old by 2060 [1]. With the aging process, visual perception is commonly negatively affected [2] and the effects of sedentary lifestyles become more prominent. A computer system that could lighten such problems using large dimension displays and motion tracking interfaces could prove advantageous. More concretely, applications targeting engagement and physical fitness would provide extensive health benefits in older adults [3].

Meanwhile, the release of low-cost body tracking sensors for gaming consoles has made it possible for gesture detection to be present in millions of homes. Sensors like the Kinect V1, of which more than 24 million units were sold by Feb. 2014 [4], and Kinect V2, having 3.9 million units bundled and sold along with Xbox One consoles by Jan. 2014 [5]. The popular access to this technology opens the way for more *user natural* ways of interacting with computing systems. Natural user interfaces (NUI), where users act with and feel like *naturals*, aim at reflecting user skills and taking full advantage of their capacities to fit their task and context demands from the moment they start interacting [6]. In addition to the body tracking sensors' unique interface capabilities, they also provide exciting possibilities for automatic monitoring of health-related problems through kinematic data analysis. For example, automated systems for assessing fitness indicators in elderly [7, 8], automatic exercise rehabilitation guidance [9], or diagnosis and monitoring of Parkinson's disease [10].

The coupling of body tracking depth sensors, such as Kinect, and projectors enable systems to not only track the user movements relative to the sensor but also to map virtual content on the projection surfaces. In a well-calibrated system, where the transformation between the sensor and projector is known, this allows for immersive augmented reality experiences, such as the capability of augmenting a whole room with interactive projections [11].

In this paper, we present a comparative study of two interaction modalities for floor projections, and, based on the results of the comparison an exergame developed for cardiorespiratory training of the elderly. In the study, we combined floor projection mapping with whole body tracking to provide two modalities of body gesture NUIs in controlling a cursor. One modality is based on feet position over the display while the other uses forearm orientation (pointing). We assessed the interfaces with an abstraction of two common interaction tasks, the point-and-click and drag-and-drop, on an elderly population sample. The differentiation was done by evaluating the systems in terms of usability, perceived workload, and performance. The insights provided by the study results served as a preliminary step in the development of a senior exergame for cardiorespiratory fitness training. The game is projected on the ground and makes use of one-to-one mapping to project real-size winery elements. These virtual elements are used to mimic, in a fun and playful way, the process of grape maceration through stomping.

This work is an initial and important step in the development of content for a mobile autonomous robotic system designed to assist elderly in keeping an active lifestyle through adaptable exergames. The platform, equipped with a micro projector and depth sensor will be able to identify users and provide custom exergames through live projection mapping, or spatial augmented reality. While the results from this experiment guided the exergame interaction design, they will also help in the future development of a gesture interface for such mobile platform.

This paper is an extended version of the conference paper "Evaluating Body Tracking Interaction in Floor Projection Displays with an Elderly Population" [12], presented at the 3rd International Conference on Physiological Computing Systems PhyCS 2016. While it maintains the same structure and most of the original paper content, Sect. 6 was added as it represents work that was in progress at the time of the publication and a direct consequence of the original study results.

2   Related Work

While gesture-based interaction is not a requirement for an NUI, it is an evident candidate for the development of such an interface.

An area where several in-air gesture interfaces have been proposed is in pan-and-zoom navigation control. In [13] the authors investigated the impact three interaction variables had in task completion time and navigation overshoots when interacting with a wall-sized display. The variables were: uni- vs. bi-manual, linear vs. circular movements, and number of spatial dimensions for gesture guidance (in zooming). Panning was controlled by ray casting the dominant hand into the screen and activated by device clicking. Results showed that performance was significantly better when participants controlled the system bimanually (non-dominant hand zooming), with linear control and 1D guidance (mouse scroll wheel for zooming). An NUI for controlling virtual globes is introduced in [14]. The system uses a Kinect sensor to provide pan, zoom, rotation and street view navigation commands to Google Earth. The system presents an interesting possibility for an NUI as in-air gestures follow the same logic as common multi-touch gestures. Hand poses (open/close) are used to activate commands while the relative position of the hands is used to control the virtual globe. For street view control, it makes use of gestures that mimic the human walk, swinging arms makes the point-of-view move forward while twisting the shoulders rotates it. The use of metaphors that make computer controls relate to other known controls is not uncommon. In [15], two different approaches for interfacing with Bing Maps were tested for their usability, presence, and immersion. Using a Wiimote, the authors built a navigation interface inspired in the motorcycle metaphor. A handlebar like motion controlled turning and right-hand tilting acted as throttle. Additionally to the metaphor, altitude over the map was controlled by left-hand tilting. The alternative approach used the Kinect to provide control and feedback inspired in the bird metaphor. Raising the arms asymmetrically enables turning, both arms equally raised or lowered from a neutral position control altitude and moving the hands forward makes the user advance; the controls are enhanced by providing feedback in form of a bird/airplane avatar. Descriptive statistic results showed high levels of usability and presence for both systems, with higher values for the latter. The use of the torso angle to control an avatar in a virtual reality city and how this control method affected the user understanding of size proportions in the virtual world was investigated in [16]. The system uses forward/backward leaning and shoulder turning to move and turn in the respective direction. It was tested on participants chosen for their knowledge in urban planning and building design, and compared to the common first-person-shooter mouse/ keyboard interface. The results show that the system navigation was perceived as both easier and less demanding than the mouse/keyboard, and that it gave a better under-standing of proportions in the modeled world.

Beyond navigation interface, gesture NUIs have been studied in the context of controlling computerized medical systems. This is particularly important in the surgery room where doctors must maintain a sterile field while interacting with medical computers. In [17], the authors present their Kinect based system for touchless radi-ology imaging control. It replaces the mouse/keyboard commands with hand tracking controls where the right-hand controls the cursor and the left hand is used for clicking. The activation of the system was done by standing in front of the Kinect and waving. Tested for its qualitative rating with radiologists, 69% considered that the system would be useful in interventional radiology. The majority also found it easy to moderately difficult to accomplish the tasks. Similarly, in [18] the authors introduced a solution for interaction with these systems using inertial sensors instead. Here, the activation of the gesture detection was made by using a physical switch or voice commands.

Several exploratory research studies have been made to find the common gestures that naïve users would naturally perform. In [19] the authors found, by running an experiment in a Wizard of Oz set-up, that participants would adopt the point-and-click mouse metaphor when asked to perform tasks in a large display. In [20], participants were asked to propose gestures for common TV functions. The gesture agreement was assessed for each command and a set of guidelines proposed. Contrary to what was shown in [13] for pan and zoom gesture, here one hand gesturing was preferred. Hand posture naturally emerged as a way of communicating intention for gesture interaction.

When designing an NUI that supports in-air gestures one must be aware of the "live mic" issue. As the system is always listening, if not mitigated, this can lead to false positive errors [6]. Effective ways of countering the "live mic" problem are to reserve specific actions for interaction or reserve clutching mechanism that will disengage the gesture interpretation. The review made by Golod et al. [21] suggests a *gesture phrase* sequence of gestures to define one command, where the first phase is the activation. The activation serves as the segmentation cue to separate casual from command ges-tures. Some example guidelines are the definition of activation zones or dwell-based interactions. In [22], from a Wizard of Oz design, the authors tried to identify gestures for pan, zoom, rotate and tilt control. More importantly, by doing so they identified the natural clutching gestures for direct analog input, a subtle change from open-hand to semi open. Similarly, the system proposed in [23] used the hand palm facing the screen for activating cursor control. [24] proposed two activation techniques: holding a remote trigger, and activation through gaze estimation. These two activating techniques plus the control (trigger gesture of showing the palms to the screen) were tested for their hedonic and pragmatic qualities. Results showed that both the trigger gesture and remote trigger scored neutral on their hedonic and pragmatic scales. However, gaze activation scored high on both scales, achieving a "desired" rating.

Although much less common than vertical displays, interactive floors and floor projected interfaces possess unique features. In [25] the authors describe an interactive floor prototype, controlled by body movement and mobile phones, which was set-up on a large public library hall. This arrangement enabled them not only to take advantage of the open space, filled by the large projected interface but also from its public function of promoting social interaction. These types of interfaces were proposed as an alternative to interactive tabletops [26], useful for not being as spatially restraining as the latter. In their study, the authors also explored the preferred methods of activation for buttons in these floors, being feet *tap* their final choice of design.

Even though the literature on NUI is extensive, our review shows that most research has been made with exploratory or pilot designs and could be advanced with validation studies. Furthermore, while most studies target the general population, usually their samples are not representative of the elderly portion and thus ignore their specific limitations and needs. To generally address their visual perception impairments and support their needs of physical activity and engagement we focused our research on large interactive floors. To better understand how this population can interact with such an interface we proposed the following question:

- When designing an NUI to be used by an elderly population in floor projection displays what interaction is best?

This was narrowed down by limiting the answers to two types of interface control: arm ray casting, commonly studied for vertical displays, and a touch screen like control, where the user activates interaction through stepping on the virtual elements. Considering the goals of an interface, we chose three elements to be rated: usability, workload, and performance. As one method would provide clear mapping at the expense of increased physical activity (stepping), the other would free the user from such movements while requiring him to mentally project their arm into the floor. Therefore, we hypothesized that differences for each of the three evaluation elements would exist when considering the two NUIs proposed. To test this hypothesis, the two proposed modes of interface control were developed and tested on an elderly population sample for two types of tasks. We expected that raycasting would provide better results as it is more widely used for interaction with large displays and requires little physical effort by the user.

Next, we engaged in the development of an exergame for cardiorespiratory fitness training for the elderly. The design of exergames to promote physical activity in senior adults has been characterized for the lack of focused game design methodologies which can include appropriate content, real needs of the senior population and adapted interfaces for a natural interaction [27, 28]. To overcome these limitations, several investigations point at the need of including older adults in early design stages and to constantly evaluate playable prototypes to include real field data in the exergame design process [29]. For instance, Gerling and colleagues carried out a study showing how the frail elderly population may not be suitable for playing Wii games since the interface and the navigation through menu structures produce inadequate feedback [30]. Thus, the design of exergames oriented to cover individual fitness levels and user needs is essential to deliver positive user experiences that maximize the health benefits of training with this technology. A study with 170 senior adults also showed how a good knowledge of game preferences and motivations as well as an active participation of the target population within the design of novel games might produce more satisfactory experiences, which will facilitate a long-term adoption of this technology, one of the cornerstones for elderly exergaming [31]. Consequently, we adopted user-centered design methodologies to design, develop and partially evaluate interaction techniques in an exergame based on floor-projection to promote physical activity in a group of senior adults. By using these game design techniques, we aimed to: (a) provide a use case scenario for exercise promotion to integrate the previously studied interaction techniques, and (b) create better exergame experiences based on field tests to facilitate acceptance of such a technology.

The main contributions of this manuscript lies in the description of methods and results to: (a) evaluate body tracking interaction in floor projection with a group of active senior adults, aimed at elucidate the best interaction technique based in usability, workload and task performance measurements (Sects. 3 and 4); and (b) the integration of such results for the design and evaluation of a novel spatial augmenting reality exergame (Sect. 6).

3 Methods for Evaluating Body Tracking Interaction in Floor Projection Displays with an Elderly Population

The first experiment aimed at understanding the differences in terms of usability, workload levels, and task performance between two interaction modes in floor projections: forearm ray casting and feet interaction. This was evaluated using two different tasks: the point-and-click and the drag-and-drop.

3.1 Modes of Interacting

Two modes of interacting with the computer were developed based on the kinematic information provided by a Kinect V2 sensor and a display projection on the ground. In the first, henceforth named "*feet*", the cursor position is controlled by the average position of both feet on the floor plane; activation upon the virtual elements by the cursor is performed by placing the feet less than 20 cm apart. For the second mode of interaction, named "*arm*", the forearm position and orientation is treated as a vector (from elbow to wrist) and raycasted onto the floor plane, the cast controls the position of the cursor (as schematized in Fig. 1), while activation is done by closing the hand. Due to low reliability of the Kinect V2 sensor in detecting the closed hand pose, during the experiment this automatic detection was replaced by the visual detection done by the researcher in a Wizard of Oz like experiment.

3.2 Experimental Tasks' Description

The interfaces were tested in two different tasks to give a broader insight into what kind of interactions with computers our two systems would impact. A task to mimic the traditional point-and-click and another for the common drag-and-drop.

In both tasks, the participant controls a circular cursor (ø 17 cm) with 1 s activation duration, meaning that the activation gesture (feet together or hand closed) must be sustained for 1 s for the cursor to interact with the virtual element it is positioned on.

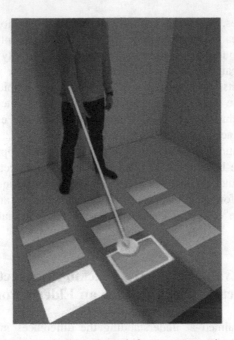

Fig. 1. Controlling the cursor position through forearm ray casting, extracted from [12].

This activation is represented on the cursor itself, which changes color in a circular way proportionally to the duration of the gesture.

Point-and-Click Task. In the point-and-click task, a set of 9 rectangles (40 cm × 25 cm) are projected in the floor, on a 3 by 3 configuration, separated 12 cm laterally and 8 cm vertically as shown in Fig. 2. Out of the 9 rectangles, 8 are distractors (blue) and one is the target (green). Every time the target is selected it trades places with a distractor chosen on a random sequence (the same random sequence was used for all participants). The purpose of the task is to activate the target repeatedly while avoiding activating the distractors. Performance is recorded in this task as a list of events and their time tags, the possible events being: target click (correct click); background click (neutral click); and distractor click (incorrect click). In this task, maintaining the activation pose while moving the cursor from inside a rectangle to outside, or vice versa, resets the activation timer.

Live feedback is given by drawing different colored frames around the rectangles. An orange frame is drawn around the rectangle over which the cursor is located. Upon activation, the frame changes color to red if the rectangle was a distractor or green if it was the target. This frame remains until the cursor is moved off the rectangle.

Drag-and-Drop Task. In the drag-and-drop task, 4 rectangles (40 cm × 25 cm) are projected on the ground, spaced 70 cm horizontally and 40 cm vertically, 3 of which are blue distractors and one is the target (green). In the center, a movable yellow rectangle (30 cm × 19 cm) is initially shown, as presented in Fig. 3. The participant can "*grab*" the yellow rectangle by activating it. Once it has been "*grabbed*", it can be

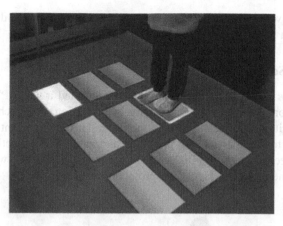

Fig. 2. Point-and-click task being performed with the *"feet"* interface, extracted from [12]. (Color figure online)

dropped by activating it again (joining the feet or closing the hand, depending on the mode of interaction). The purpose of the task is to "*grab*" the yellow rectangle and "*drop*" it onto the target repeatedly. Every time this is done successfully, the yellow rectangle is reset to the center and the target changes places with one of the distractors in a random sequence (the sequence was kept constant across all participants). Performance is recorded as a list of events and their time tags, the possible events for this task are: grab yellow (correct grab); attempt to grab anything else (neutral grab); drop yellow on target (correct drop); drop yellow on background (neutral drop); and drop yellow on distractors (incorrect drop). Maintaining the activation pose while moving the cursor from a rectangle to outside, or vice versa, resets the activation timer. Likewise, a set of colored frames are used to give live feedback to the users. An orange frame highlights any rectangle under the cursor. Once activated, the frame of the yellow object changes to green indicating that is being dragged by the cursor. Dropping

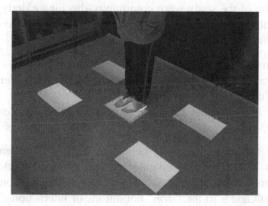

Fig. 3. The drag-and-drop task being performed with the *"feet"* interface, extracted from [12]. (Color figure online)

it on a distractor will create a red frame around the distractor, and dropping it on a target will show a green frame around it.

3.3 Technical Setup

The hardware was set up in a dimly illuminated room and a white PVC canvas was placed on the floor to enhance the reflectivity of projection. A Hitachi CP-AW100N projector was positioned vertically to face the floor. This arrangement enabled a high contrast of the virtual elements being projected and an area of projection greater than what our tasks needed (150 cm × 90 cm). A Microsoft Kinect V2 was placed horizontally next to the projector, facing the projection area (Fig. 4).

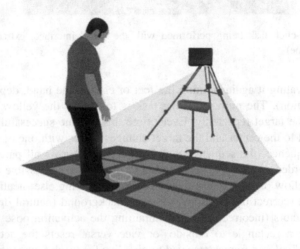

Fig. 4. Experimental setup diagram, extracted from [12].

3.4 Sample

The target population of the study were community-dwelling elderly. A self-selecting sample of this population was recruited at Funchal's Santo António civic center with the following inclusion criteria:

1. Being more than 60 years old;
2. Do not present cognitive impairments (assessed by the Mini-Mental State Examination Test [32]);
3. Do not present low physical functioning (assessed by the Composite Physical Function scale [33]).

The experiment took place over the course of 2 days. Nineteen participants (16 females; ages: M = 70.2 SD = 5.3) volunteered and provided written informed consent. The participants were randomly allocated to one of the two conditions, 10 being assigned to the "*feet*" and 9 to the "*arm*" conditions of interaction.

3.5 Experimental Protocol

The experiment followed a between-subjects design. The participants were asked to answer questionnaires regarding identification, demographical information, and level of computer use experience. They were evaluated with the Composite Physical Function Scale and Mini-Mental State Examination Test. During each individual participant trial, the point-and-click task was explained and shown being performed through example according to the participant experimental condition. This was followed by a training period and then by a 2 min' session while performance metrics were recorded. Lastly, participants were asked to fill the System Usability Scale (SUS) [34] and NASA-TLX (TLX) [35] questionnaires. After it, the same procedure was followed for the drag-and-drop task.

3.6 Analysis

For each participant data consisted of SUS score and TLX index (both measured from 0 to 100), and task-related performance, as described in Subsect. 3.2. Normality of the data distributions was assessed using the Kolmogorov-Smirnov test for measurements concerning performance. The variables that showed a normal distribution are highlighted in Tables 1 and 2. For the pairs (between conditions) of measurements that fitted the assumption of normality, parametric t-tests were used When significant differences in the pairs variances were present, shown by the Levene's test, equal variances were not assumed. All the others pairs were tested with Mann-Whitney's U test. Differences in the SUS and TLX scores (ordinal variables) between conditions were also tested with Mann-Whitney's U test. All statistical testing was done using 2-tailed testing at α .05 with the IBM software SPSS Statistics 22.

4 Results in Evaluating Body Tracking Interaction in Floor Projection Displays with an Elderly Population

4.1 Point-and-Click Task

For the "*feet*" condition in the point-and-click task, the descriptive statistics are presented in Table 1. We can observe very low values of incorrect clicks, and high median scores for the SUS, which is considered to be a good value when over 68. The descriptive statistics for the "*arm*" condition are also presented in Table 1. Higher values of neutral and incorrect clicks are visible compared to the previous condition. Similarly, it can be seen a decrease in the median of the SUS usability score and an increase of the TLX workload index.

Results revealed significant higher System Usability Scale scores for the participants interfacing with their feet compared to the participants interfacing with their dominant arm, U = 18.5, p < .05, with effect size r = −.4997. The Task Load Index scores were not significantly different for both interfaces, U = 24.5, p > .05 (Fig. 5). The number of correct and neutral clicks was not significantly different for both interfaces, U = 40.5 and U = 29.0, p > .05, respectively. However, it was found that there was a lower number of incorrect clicks for the participants interfacing with their feet compared to the participants interfacing with the arm, $U = 15.0$, $p < .05$, $r = -.5863$ (Fig. 6).

Table 1. Descriptive statistics of the measurements for the point-and-click task, extracted from [12].

Variable	"Feet" interface		"Arm" interface	
	Median	Interquartile range	Median	Interquartile range
SUS	91.25	21.25	72.50	25.00
TLX	23.75	27.71	40.83	18.33
Correct	29.50	10	28.00[a]	15
Neutral	1.00	2	4.00[a]	7
Incorrect	0.00	1	2.00[a]	3

[a]Normally distributed

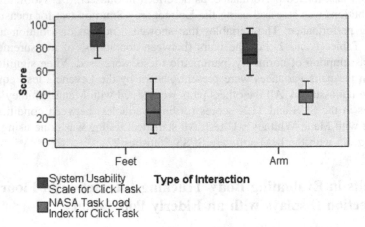

Fig. 5. System Usability Scale and Nasa-Task Load Index scores for the point-and-click task, extracted from [12].

4.2 Drag-and-Drop Task

The descriptive statistics for the "feet" condition, in the drag-and-drop task are presented in Table 2, where we can observe low values of incorrect drops and no neutral drops (accidental drops). The values of usability are very high and workload moderately low. In the "arm" condition of the drag-and-drop task we can see, in Table 2, a marginally good value for the SUS usability score, barely over 68. The TLX workload has relative medium levels and neutral drops (accidental) are present.

The results indicated again a significantly higher System Usability Scale score and lower Task Load Index score for the Feet interaction condition, with $U = 9$ and $U = 17$, $p < .05$, effect size $r = -.6777$ and $r = -.5247$ respectively (Fig. 7). There were no significant differences in correct grabs, neutral grabs, and correct drops,

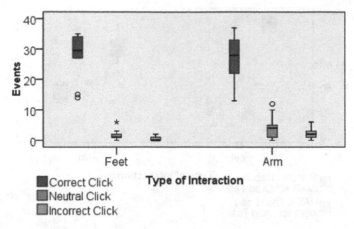

Fig. 6. Participants' performance on the point-and-click task (circles represent outliers and stars extreme outliers), extracted from [12].

Table 2. Descriptive statistics of the measurements for the drag-and-drop task, extracted from [12].

Variable	"Feet" interface		"Arm" interface	
	Median	Interquartile range	Median	Interquartile range
SUS	93.75	16.25	41.67	21.25
TLX	22.50	16.46	11.00[a]	22.50
Correct	14.50[a]	8	10.00[a]	9
Neutral	13.50[a]	4	10.00[a]	9
Incorrect	14.00[a]	7	1.00[a]	10

[a]Normally distributed

$t(17) = .565$, $t(17) = .863$ and $t(17) = 1.336$, $p > .05$, respectively. Neutral drops were significantly higher in the "arm" interaction condition, $U = 10$, $p < .05$, $r = -.7595$ and there were no significant differences between the number of incorrect drops, $U = 44.5$, $p > .05$ (Fig. 8).

5 Discussion Regarding the Evaluation of Body Tracking Interaction in Floor Projection Displays with an Elderly Population

For both the point-and-click and drag-and-drop tasks we identified a significant impact on system usability, being the "*feet*" interaction method preferable in both cases. The "*feet*" modality achieved high levels of usability, scores over 90, while the "*arm*" had levels of usability around 71, very close to the standard lower limit of good, 68. In the case of perceived workload indexes, for the point-and-click there were no significant differences found between the conditions. For drag-and-drop, the "*feet*" interface was

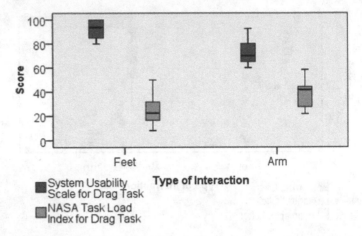

Fig. 7. System Usability Scale and Nasa-Task Load Index scores for the drag-and-drop task, extracted from [12].

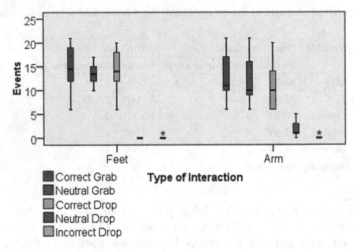

Fig. 8. Participants' performance on the drag-and-drop task, extracted from [12].

significantly less demanding for the participants. In both conditions, workload indexes for the "*feet*" were around 23 while for the "*arm*" the values were around 41. Although interfaces similar to our "*arm*" method have been the focus of previous research [13, 23] and shown to be a method that participants naturally display [19, 20, 22], in our experiment we found sufficient evidence that an alternative way of interacting with projected floor elements is preferred by elder people. This preference by the participants for the "*feet*" interface might be linked to the simpler mapping of the cursor control provided, which is known to have a lowering effect on cognitive load [16, 36]. In terms of performance, for the point-and-click task very low numbers of neutral and incorrect clicks (although significantly higher for the "*arm*") and a comparable number of correct clicks were observed. Similar results were found in the drag-and-drop task, with low numbers of neutral and incorrect drops for both methods and analogous values of correct grabs, neutral grabs, and correct drops. Still, the *"feet"* interface was again better, with the number of neutral drops being significantly lower than in the *"arm"* interface. Albeit these differences, the remaining performance indicators were shown not to be significantly different. Therefore, caution is advised in the interpretation of these results as proof of a clear performance advantage provided by any of the interfaces.

From the observed results, we can summarize a take-home message. When elderly interact with floor projection, a direct activation of the virtual elements with the feet is preferred for both usability and performance. In contrast, pointing and hand pose are considered less usable and more cumbersome.

6   Design of "Grape Stomping": A Cardiorespiratory Training Exergame for the Elderly

This section focuses on describing the "Grape Stomping" exergame, a cardiorespiratory training game using floor projection and feet interaction developed based on the observations from the previous section. The story and aesthetics were rooted in the traditional winemaking activities of the Douro region, an important activity for the development of the Portuguese economy, being the Douro Region the most famous and traditional region for wine production [37]. One of the most characteristic activities around the wine culture in Portugal is the grape stomping. The grapes are placed in large tanks, people tread knee-deep in grapes, arms linked as they stomp and dance on the grapes underfoot following the beats of the traditional folk music. This activity was recreated using a real-size floor projection of an ancient Portuguese winery, see Fig. 9. In this virtual world, there are two main elements: a row of three open-top tanks that can hold grapes and be used to stomp them, and a conveyor belt that continuously bring grapes into the play area. The tanks have two small footprints which are used to provide feedback over the position of the user and correct stepping height. Background sound with a folk music accompanies the interaction and sound effects were added to the stomping and tank filling events. GUI elements in the exergame include a countdown visualizer as well as individual counters for each tank showing the number of times it has been successfully filled.

The grape stomping activity was chosen taking two foundations in consideration, that general repeated stepping is the recommended exercise for cardiorespiratory fitness assessment [38, 39], and our interaction study results take-home message. In order to facilitate the interaction with the exergame, we used projection mapping technology which allows the augmentation of real-world spaces using simple projections instead of special displays [40]. With this technology, users are able to physically stomp the virtual grapes placed in the tanks projected on the floor in real scale. This game mechanic was directly inspired by the results (and product of the developed technology) presented in Sect. 4. Specifically, the direct mapping of the grape stepping action was inspired on the Point-and-Click task using the *feet* modality, while for the upper limb mechanics we avoided direct mapping and opted instead for gesture motion-based interaction.

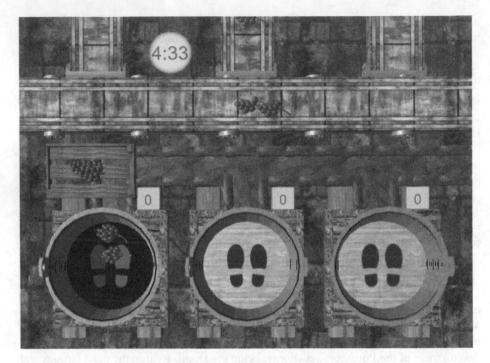

Fig. 9. A screenshot of the grape stomping exergame.

The goal of the exergame is to stomp on the grapes inside the tanks, pulled from the conveyor belt into the tank by small virtual baskets through repeated arm extension/flexion. The stomping process requires users to raise the knees to a pre-defined height when there are grapes in a tank, producing the grape juice. After filling up one of the tanks, users are free to move to the neighboring tanks to continue the exercise. The experience ends once the pre-established training time finalizes, presenting the total score in form of liters of wine produced, number of steps performed and number of grape bunches pulled.

An exergame playtest session was conducted in a local senior gymnasium in Madeira, Portugal, see Fig. 10. Nine older adults (8 females; ages M = 62.3, SD = 6.2) participated and two exercise instructors in the senior gymnasium were interviewed. From their feedback, we can enclose the main insights in the following items:

- Social aspect: senior elders enjoy playing exergames mainly for two reasons: they like to win competitions and they find here an opportunity to socialize (skills and experiences). Multiplayer playability is a key factor to improve technology adoption.
- In-time feedback: the lack of past experiences with gaming technologies obstructs a fluid interaction. Improving the quality and frequency of the feedback provided in the videogame facilitates the understanding of what to do, how to do and when to do it.

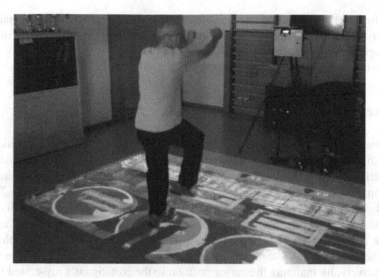

Fig. 10. "Grape Stomping" playtest at a local gym.

- Automatic movements: options for the exergame personalization must include well-defined strategies to facilitate the interaction for people with several motor disabilities. Since the exergame includes 3 body movements (e.g. step, side step, and arm extension), health professionals should be able to activate/deactivate individual body gestures depending on users' abilities.
- Cognitive tasks: the inclusion of more cognitive-demanding activities in conjunction with the physical exertion in the Exergaming might enhance the health benefits and increase the likelihood of the long-term adoption of this technology.
- Control parameters: the inclusion of multiple game parameters might help to facilitate the personalization of activities' in terms of the fitness domains and training dimensions. By defining a set of game parameters, the difficulty of the exergame will be controllable allowing a more precise adaptation to specific motor and/or cognitive skills.

With these insights in mind, several features were added to the game. Cognitive challenges were added using game mechanics around wine recipes to stimulate visual processing and concentration. Three types of grapes are used: green, maroon and damaged (distractors). Users are encouraged to grab specific grape bunches following a recipe (e.g. 10 greens and 5 maroons) avoiding damaged bunches which appear randomly. Thus, the damaged bunches are used as distractors and their percentage can be defined in the initial menu. Optional tutorial and in-time instructions were also added. While the interactive video tutorial explains how to play the game at the start of the game, in-game videos are triggered if the game detects inactivity or unsuccessful movements being performed by the player. Thus, reinforcing the learning process of each gesture separately when the exergame is running. Moreover, a multiplayer option allows up to three users to be side by side in individual barrels to either collaborate or compete.

The final version of the game includes the following experience personalization parameters: duration (minutes), number of players and multiplayer mode (collaborative, cooperative), stepping (yes/no), pulling (yes/no), treadmill velocity (grape bunches/s), step height (cm), recipes (yes/no) and distractors (%).

7   Conclusions

Due to the growing number of elderly in developed countries and their specific needs we tried to get an insight of the desirability of different modes of controlling interaction in interactive floors. A medium which, by being scaled easily, can mitigate the visual perception deficits associated with old age, and can promote physical activity. Thus, in this work, two methods of interacting with virtual elements projected on the floor were developed and tested for differences in their usability, perceived workload and performance ratings by an elderly population. The interfaces consisted on either controlling the cursor with the direct mapping of feet position onto the projection surface or, alternatively, by mapping the cursor position to the participant's ray-casted forearm on the surface. These interfaces were tested on two different tasks, one mimicking a point-and-click interaction, the other a drag-and-drop. Although the NUI research field is extensive there is a lack of studies that approach the floor projected interfaces, and studies with the elderly are even rarer. This study gives an insight into the preferred modes of interaction for the elder population. Contrary to our initial guess, the results showed that from the two proposed methods the "*feet*" interface was superior in all the domains measured. It was shown that this method was perceived as more usable in both the tasks tested and at least less demanding in terms of workload for the drag-and-drop task. In terms of performance, a marginal advantaged was shown also for the "*feet*" method. This insight, triggered the development of a floor projection exergame focused on cardiorespiratory fitness training. The game was designed around the winemaking traditions of the Douro region in Portugal and the main interaction method used was virtual grape stomping. A game playtest session with the end-users provided feedback necessary to take the game further and allowed the addition of supplementary features, considered significant by both the target population and elderly sports professionals. The most important additions where difficulty/exertion parameterization, multiplayer support and guidance instructions.

Acknowledgment. The authors thank Funchal's Santo António municipal gymnasium for their cooperation, Teresa Paulino for the development of the experimental tasks, Fábio Pereira for his help during the data collection process, and Diogo Freitas and John Sousa for their contributions in the development of the first prototype of "Grape Stomping".

This work was supported by the Fundação para a Ciência e Tecnologia through the AHA project (CMUPERI/HCI/0046/2013) and LARSyS – UID/EEA/50009/2013.

Contributions. Afonso Gonçalves designed and carried out the floor projection interaction study, designed the "Grape Stomping" game and wrote the paper. Filipa Nóbrega developed the game and contributed to the writing of the paper. Mónica Cameirão supervised the study, contributed to the game design and writing of the paper. John Muñoz, Élvio Gouveia and Sergi Bermudez i Badia contributed to the game design and writing of the paper.

References

1. European Commission, Economic and Financial Affairs: The 2012 Ageing Report (2012)
2. Fozard, J.: Vision and hearing in aging. In: Birren, J.E., Schaie, K.W. (eds.) Handbook of the Psychology of Aging, pp. 143–156. Academic Press, San Diego (1990)
3. World Health Organization: Global recommendations on physical activity for health (2010). http://www.who.int/dietphysicalactivity/publications/9789241599979/en/
4. Microsoft News Center: Xbox Execs Talk Momentum and the Future of TV (2013). http://news.microsoft.com/2013/02/11/xbox-execs-talk-momentum-and-the-future-of-tv/
5. Microsoft's Q2: Record $24.52 billion revenue and 3.9 million Xbox One sales. http://www.theverge.com/2014/1/23/5338162/microsoft-q2-2014-financial-earnings
6. Wigdor, D., Wixon, D.: Brave NUI World: Designing Natural User Interfaces for Touch and Gesture. Elsevier, Amsterdam (2011)
7. Chen, C., Liu, K., Jafari, R., Kehtarnavaz, N.: Home-based Senior Fitness Test measurement system using collaborative inertial and depth sensors. In: 2014 36th Annual International Conference of the IEEE Engineering in Medicine and Biology Society (EMBC), pp. 4135–4138 (2014)
8. Gonçalves, A., Gouveia, É., Cameirão, M., Bermúdez i Badia, S.: Automating senior fitness testing through gesture detection with depth sensors. In: Proceedings of the IET International Conference on Technologies for Active and Assisted Living (TechAAL 2015). Institution of Engineering and Technology, London (2015)
9. Da Gama, A., Chaves, T., Figueiredo, L., Teichrieb, V.: Guidance and movement correction based on therapeutics movements for motor rehabilitation support systems. In: 2012 14th Symposium on Virtual and Augmented Reality (SVR), pp. 191–200 (2012)
10. Spasojević, S., Santos-Victor, J., Ilić, T., Milanović, S., Potkonjak, V., Rodić, A.: A vision-based system for movement analysis in medical applications: the example of Parkinson disease. In: Nalpantidis, L., Krüger, V., Eklundh, J.-O., Gasteratos, A. (eds.) ICVS 2015. LNCS, vol. 9163, pp. 424–434. Springer, Cham (2015). https://doi.org/10.1007/978-3-319-20904-3_38
11. Jones, B., et al.: RoomAlive: magical experiences enabled by scalable, adaptive projector-camera units. In: Proceedings of the 27th Annual ACM Symposium on User Interface Software and Technology, pp. 637–644. ACM, New York (2014)
12. Gonçalves, A., Cameirão, M.: Evaluating body tracking interaction in floor projection displays with an elderly population. In: Proceedings of the 3rd International Conference on Physiological Computing Systems - Volume 1: PhyCS, Lisbon, Portugal, pp. 24–32 (2016)
13. Nancel, M., Wagner, J., Pietriga, E., Chapuis, O., Mackay, W.: Mid-air pan-and-zoom on wall-sized displays. In: Proceedings of the SIGCHI Conference on Human Factors in Computing Systems, pp. 177–186. ACM, New York (2011)
14. Boulos, M.N.K., Blanchard, B.J., Walker, C., Montero, J., Tripathy, A., Gutierrez-Osuna, R.: Web GIS in practice X: a Microsoft Kinect natural user interface for Google Earth navigation. Int. J. Health Geogr. 10, 45 (2011)
15. Francese, R., Passero, I., Tortora, G.: Wiimote and Kinect: gestural user interfaces add a natural third dimension to HCI. In: Proceedings of the International Working Conference on Advanced Visual Interfaces, pp. 116–123. ACM, New York (2012)
16. Roupé, M., Bosch-Sijtsema, P., Johansson, M.: Interactive navigation interface for Virtual Reality using the human body. Comput. Environ. Urban Syst. 43, 42–50 (2014)
17. Tan, J.H., Chao, C., Zawaideh, M., Roberts, A.C., Kinney, T.B.: Informatics in radiology: developing a touchless user interface for intraoperative image control during interventional radiology procedures. RadioGraphics. 33, E61–E70 (2013)

18. Bigdelou, A., Schwarz, L., Navab, N.: An adaptive solution for intra-operative gesture-based human-machine interaction. In: Proceedings of the 2012 ACM International Conference on Intelligent User Interfaces, pp. 75–84. ACM, New York (2012)
19. Fikkert, W., van der Vet, P., van der Veer, G., Nijholt, A.: Gestures for large display control. In: Kopp, S., Wachsmuth, I. (eds.) GW 2009. LNCS (LNAI), vol. 5934, pp. 245–256. Springer, Heidelberg (2010). https://doi.org/10.1007/978-3-642-12553-9_22
20. Vatavu, R.-D.: User-defined gestures for free-hand TV control. In: Proceedings of the 10th European Conference on Interactive TV and Video, pp. 45–48. ACM, New York (2012)
21. Golod, I., Heidrich, F., Möllering, C., Ziefle, M.: Design principles of hand gesture interfaces for microinteractions. In: Proceedings of the 6th International Conference on Designing Pleasurable Products and Interfaces, pp. 11–20. ACM, New York (2013)
22. Lee, S.-S., Chae, J., Kim, H., Lim, Y., Lee, K.: Towards more natural digital content manipulation via user freehand gestural interaction in a living room. In: Proceedings of the 2013 ACM International Joint Conference on Pervasive and Ubiquitous Computing, pp. 617–626. ACM, New York (2013)
23. Bragdon, A., DeLine, R., Hinckley, K., Morris, M.R.: Code space: Touch + Air gesture hybrid interactions for supporting developer meetings. In: Proceedings of the ACM International Conference on Interactive Tabletops and Surfaces, pp. 212–221. ACM, New York (2011)
24. Hopmann, M., Salamin, P., Chauvin, N., Vexo, F., Thalmann, D.: Natural activation for gesture recognition systems. In: CHI 2011 Extended Abstracts on Human Factors in Computing Systems, pp. 173–183. ACM, New York (2011)
25. Krogh, P., Ludvigsen, M., Lykke-Olesen, A.: "Help Me Pull That Cursor" A collaborative interactive floor enhancing community interaction. Australas. J. Inf. Syst. **11**, 75–87 (2004)
26. Augsten, T., et al.: Multitoe: high-precision interaction with back-projected floors based on high-resolution multi-touch input. In: Proceedings of the 23nd Annual ACM Symposium on User Interface Software and Technology, pp. 209–218. ACM, New York (2010)
27. Larsen, L.H., Schou, L., Lund, H.H., Langberg, H.: The physical effect of exergames in healthy elderly—a systematic review. GAMES Health Res. Dev. Clin. Appl. **2**, 205–212 (2013)
28. Molina, K.I., Ricci, N.A., de Moraes, S.A., Perracini, M.R.: Virtual reality using games for improving physical functioning in older adults: a systematic review. J. Neuroeng. Rehabil. **11**, 156 (2014)
29. Vanden Abeele, V.A., Van Rompaey, V.: Introducing human-centered research to game design: designing game concepts for and with senior citizens. In: CHI 2006 Extended Abstracts on Human Factors in Computing Systems, pp. 1469–1474. ACM (2006)
30. Gerling, K., Masuch, M.: When gaming is not suitable for everyone: playtesting Wii games with frail elderly. In: 1st Workshop on Game Accessibility (2011)
31. Sayago, S., Rosales, A., Righi, V., Ferreira, S.M., Coleman, G.W., Blat, J.: On the conceptualization, design, and evaluation of appealing, meaningful, and playable digital games for older people. Games Cult. **11**, 53–80 (2016)
32. Folstein, M.F., Folstein, S.E., McHugh, P.R.: Mini-mental state. J. Psychiatr. Res. **12**, 189–198 (1975)
33. Roberta E. Rikli, C.J.J.: The Reliability and Validity of a 6-Minute Walk Test as a Measure of Physical Endurance in Older Adults (1998)
34. Brooke, J.: SUS-A quick and dirty usability scale. Usability Eval. Ind. **189**, 194 (1996)
35. Hart, S.G., Staveland, L.E.: Development of NASA-TLX (Task Load Index): results of empirical and theoretical research. In: Hancock, P.A., Meshkati, N. (eds.) Advances in Psychology, pp. 139–183. North-Holland, Amsterdam (1988)

36. Mousavi Hondori, H., Khademi, M., Dodakian, L., McKenzie, A., Lopes, C.V., Cramer, S. C.: Choice of human-computer interaction mode in stroke rehabilitation. Neurorehabil. Neural. Repair. **30**, 258–265 (2015)
37. Cunha, C.A., Cunha, R.: Culture and Customs of Portugal. ABC-CLIO (2010)
38. Oja, P., Tuxworth, B., et al.: Eurofit for adults: assessment of health-related fitness. Council of Europe (1995)
39. Rikli, R.E., Jones, C.J.: Development and validation of a functional fitness test for community-residing older adults. J. Aging Phys. Act. **7**, 129–161 (1999)
40. Bimber, O., Raskar, R.: Spatial Augmented Reality: Merging Real and Virtual Worlds. CRC Press, Boca Raton (2005)

Looking for Emotions on a Single EEG Signal

Roylán Quesada-Tabares[iD], Alberto J. Molina-Cantero[✉][iD],
José I. Escudero-Fombuena[iD], Manuel Merino-Monge[iD],
Isabel M. Gómez-González[iD], Clara Lebrato-Vázquez[iD],
and Juan A. Castro-García[iD]

Departamento de Tecnología Electrónica, Universidad de Sevilla, Seville, Spain
roylanqt@gmail.com, almolina@us.es

Abstract. This work aims at demonstrating that it is possible to detect emotions using a single EEG channel with an accuracy that is comparable to that obtained in studies carried out with devices that have a high number of channels. In this article the Neurosky Maindwave device, which only a single electrode at the FP1 position, the MatLab and the IBM SPSS Modeler were used to acquire, process and classify the signals respectively. It is remarkable the accuracy achieved in relation to the inexpensive hardware employed for the acquisition of the EEG signal. The result of this study allows us to determine when the brain response is more intense after undergoing the subject, in the experimentation, to the stimuli that generate those emotions. This let us decide which brain power bands are most significants and which moments are the most appropriate to carry out this detection of emotions.

Keywords: Emotions · Signal processing · Single EEG channel ·
Classification analysis · Dynamic properties

1 Introduction

Several theories have tried to explain the origin and nature of emotions. One of them posits the existence of a relative low number of basic emotions (families of emotions) which are universal for all human beings and independent of any cultural environment [8,12]. At least six emotional families have been proposed. They are: happiness, sadness, disgust, anger, fear and surprise. This theory includes, in turn, a locationist model that assumes that each emotional category starts from a specific place of the brain and body. Specifically, fear is located in the amygdala; disgust, in the insula; anger in the orbito-frontal cortex (OFC) and sadness in the anterior cortex of the cingulate (ACC) [28].

Another theory is based on the so-called constructionist model, in which it is asserted that emotions are psychological events that emerge from basic physiological operations and in which a large number of neural networks, spread in the

© Springer Nature Switzerland AG 2019
A. Holzinger et al. (Eds.): PhyCS 2016–2018, LNCS 10057, pp. 78–92, 2019.
https://doi.org/10.1007/978-3-030-27950-9_5

brain, work together to obtain a meaningful experience. In [13] the authors propose a model with four components: *core affect*, some body sensory input that is experienced as pleasant/unpleasant with some degree of excitation; *conceptualization*, which links the body sensations with previous experiences to endow them with meaning; *emotional words*, used as support of emotional categories that are not clearly differentiable from the sensitive point of view; and *executive attention*, which focuses on some of the incoming stimuli. Some neuroimaging results have corroborated that, unlike that the locationist model predicts, a region activated during a basic emotion, was also for at least one other emotion [13]. This suggests the existence of neural networks that interact with each other to generate the emotions, instead of precise places (locationist model). For example the amygdala is recruited for both fear and disgust, so it takes different functionalities depending on the neural network that uses it.

There is no a dominant theory about another, taking into account the results of some neuroimaging studies, which can be interpreted differently according to the procedure used for the treatment of the data. [11] summarizes the existing controversy pointing out that the future should include analysis with animal models and studies of patients with brain injuries, which have been reported a tendency towards a locationist theory.

The dimensional theory considers that emotions can be represented in an N-dimensional space, where two of the coordinate axis would explain most of the emotional variations. These axis are called Valence and Arousal [19]. Valence is related to pleasure and varies from low values (very unpleasant) to high values (very pleasant). Arousal is related to the intensity of emotion, ranging from very low to very high. The dimensional model is also called the circumplex model, which is a dimensional representation of the core affect in the constructionist model. Although it would seem more appropriate to use this representation for the constructionist model, in fact, the six basic emotions can also be characterized according to their valence and arousal.

Emotions can be detected in several ways: through the analysis of gestures (facial), speech [16] or the activity of various physiological signals, such as the electroencephalogram (EEG). In this work we analyze the EEG to obtain the activity of the brain during experiment in which specific emotions are elicited.

There are a large number of commercial devices for measuring and recording the EEG activity. They vary in price and the way in transmitting the information (wired or wireless). We opted for the use of a wireless device, for its advantages in mobility. Several devices with these characteristics can be found in the market: Emotiv [10], Neurosky Mindwave [10] and Enobio [9]. Emotiv offers better results than the Neurosky Mindwave when it is used for the evaluation of cognitive processes [7]. However, the Neurosky Mindwave usability and prices make it very competitive. This device has been widely used by the scientific community for the development of various applications such as the detection of sleepiness [27], level of attention [14], stress [6,17], and so on. It is a device that offers developers and researchers the possibility to make a treatment of the measured signal, but also comes integrated with a system that processes and delivers to the user characteristics of the post-processing, which will not be used in our case.

For the study and comprehension of the EEG signal, the analysis of the bands is widely used [20]. They are: δ (which ranges from 0 up to 4 Hz), θ (4–8 Hz), α (8–12 Hz), β (13–30 Hz) and γ (> 30 Hz). Another feature we have used to study the EEG signal is the fractal dimension [22,29]. The fractal dimension shows the complexity of the signal. There are several ways to calculate it, in this study we used the Higuchi's algorithm [26]. A fractal dimension close to 2 indicates that the signal is very complex, however a value close to 1 means that the signal is close to a line.

This study aims to keep on analyzing the features extracted from a single EEG signal, which started in our previous work [18], but adding the statistical significance when different temporal windows of data are used to make the classification of the emotional states elicited by sets of images.

2   Methodology

2.1   Materials

The EEG signal was captured using the Neurosky Mindwave, which has a fixed electrode located at Fp1, uses a sampling frequency at 512 Hz, a 12 bits analog-digital converter and a bluetooth interface to transmit the raw signal. To read, save, show the pictures and process data we used Matlab 8.4.0.150421 (R2014b). Finally, the IBM SPSS Modeler, a software with data mining tools, was employed to analyzed and classify the features extracted from raw EEG signals. IBM SPSS Modeler offers a wide variety of modeling methods from automated learning, artificial intelligence and statistics [5].

2.2   Experimentation

The experimentation consisted in showing 60 images (Table 1) selected from the IAPS (International Affective Picture System), grouped in three different sets of valence and arousal pairs (Fig. 1). An overall of three different arousal and valence values were chosen: 2.306 ± 0.43, 5.063 ± 0.24 and $6,921 \pm 0.032$ for valence and sets 1, 2 and 3 respectively, whereas for arousal, 6.1890 ± 0.04, $3,020 \pm 0.02$ and $4,551 \pm 0.02$ for respective sets.

Seven people took part in the experiment with a mean age of 29.85 and a standard deviation of 8.97. Before starting the experiment, the SAM test (*Self-assessment manikin*) was applied to each person to evaluate her/his initial valence and arousal at that moment.

Each picture was displayed on a computer screen for six seconds (Fig. 2) following the same experiment schedule performed in [1] with a resting period of time among images of 4 s, in which a cross was shown on the screen. A Matlab software application was responsible in displaying the images, registering the temporary marks to identify the time when the pictures appeared and were removed from the screen, and in receiving the raw EEG data sent by the Neurosky. All the information was stored for further processing.

Table 1. Selected pictures obtained from the IAPS database. The arousal and valance for each picture and its averages are also shown.

Set 1			Set 2			Set 3		
File	Valence	Arousal	File	Valence	Arousal	File	Valence	Arousal
2352.2	2.090	6.250	2038	5.090	2.940	1540	7.150	4.540
2683	2.620	6.210	2102	5.160	3.030	1731	7.070	4.560
3103	2.070	6.060	2381	5.250	3.040	2030	6.710	4.540
3150	2.260	6.550	2411	5.070	2.860	2152	6.930	4.500
3195	2.060	6.360	2850	5.220	3	2153	6.980	4.400
3550.1	2.350	6.290	2880	5.180	2.960	2306	7.080	4.460
6021	2.210	6.060	2890	4.950	2.950	2344	6.720	4.710
6022	2.140	6.090	6150	5.080	3.220	2362	6.740	4.600
6200	2.710	6.210	7003	4.970	3.160	2373	6.970	4.500
6213	2.190	6.010	7004	5	3.070	2391	7.110	4.630
6244	2.330	5.990	7010	4.930	3.010	2655	6.880	4.570
6350	2.310	6.380	7013	4.980	3	4616	6.860	4.430
6370	2.230	6.330	7018	5.180	3.120	5199	6.930	4.700
6570.1	2.190	6.240	7035	4.950	3.060	5300	6.910	4.360
6825	2.380	6.290	7054	5.220	2.950	5890	6.670	4.600
9301	2.260	6	7056	4.900	3.020	5994	6.800	4.610
9330	2.210	5.890	7057	5.070	3.070	7400	6.840	4.560
9610	2.480	6.460	7161	5.020	3.070	7430	6.910	4.550
9621	2.700	6.110	7165	4.980	2.980	7472	7.080	4.640
9903	2.330	6	7180	5.060	2.880	7481	7.080	4.550
mean:	2.306 ± 0.43	6.189 ± 0.040	**mean:**	5.063 ± 0.024	3.020 ± 0.020	**mean:**	6.921 ± 0.032	4.551 ± 0.020

A webcam recorded the experiment in order to contrast any possible anomaly in the signal. Finally, people were asked to fill in the SAM test for the 60 images. To do this, they were shown the same pictures again, in the same order.

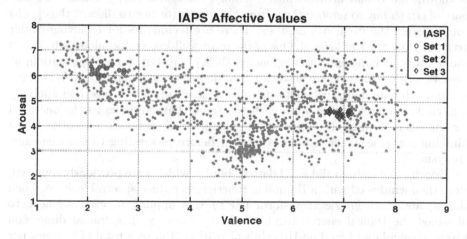

Fig. 1. Valence and arousal values of the selected pictures. Source [18].

2.3 Signal Processing

The EEG signal was split in epochs of 512 samples with an overlapping of 87.5% (or hop size of 64 samples). Then, each epoch was automatically analyzed to know if it was contaminated with artifacts: blinks, eye movements, muscle activity (EMG) or motion artifacts. In this specific case, the main source of artifacts are blinks and ocular movements, due to the electrode position, very close to the eye, although the electrical activity of the frontal an temporal muscles and motion artifacts are also important.

The automatic identification of contaminated epochs is based on obtaining two features: the difference between the maximum and minimum value (Min-Max) in the epoch and the total energy of the signal (ESF) after applying a Savitzky-Golay lowpass filter (order 2 and length 35) [21]. Figure 3 shows the feature space. Epochs contaminated by muscular activity have values of the Min-Max feature similar or a bit higher to those of the epochs with only EEG, but with more energy from the filtered signal (ESF). Blinking or EEG-only epochs have similar values in the ESF feature but differ from MinMax. Epochs with *motion artifact* contain values of these features that surround those obtained by other types of artifacts. An artificial neural network (ANN) was trained to detect epochs containing valid EEG data or blinks, but the results were similar to those obtained by setting thresholds in each dimension of the feature space (as shown in Fig. 3). Namely, the accuracy in detecting epochs contaminated with blinks was 98% whereas the accuracy in detecting valid EEG was of 96%. Setting thresholds in the feature space makes the identification method of valid epochs to be conservative, reducing the number of false positives at the cost of increasing the number of false negatives. This means that is better to reject some valid epochs than to accept contaminated epochs.

While motion and EMG artifact are infrequent, the ocular ones do not. It is known that ocular artifacts affect, mainly, the lowest energy bands (δ, θ and part of α), so not to remove them from the epoch (or not to discard the epoch) could distort the frequency analysis. There are techniques for removing ocular artifacts from the EEG signal. One of the most well-known technique is based on the analysis of independent components (ICA) [24], but, for its application, at least two EEG channels are needed, which do not exist in our case. [25] shows a technique to eliminate such artifacts in a single channel. It is based on applying a Savitzky-Golay low pass filter with the same characteristics as the one used for the calculation of the ESF feature. Therefore, if an epoch is identified as a blinking container, such a filter is applied before proceeding to the frequency analysis.

Epochs containing valid EEG data or blinks, which were previously removed, were then windowed with a Hamming function to reduce spectral leakage. Then the squared fast Fourier transform (FFT) was applied to each segment to obtained the typical energy bands: δ, θ, α, β and γ. The fractal dimension was also calculated based on Higuchi's algorithm [15], so a total of 6 values per epoch were obtained.

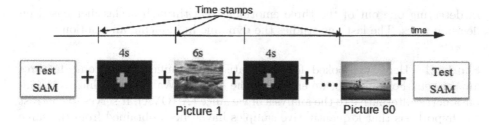

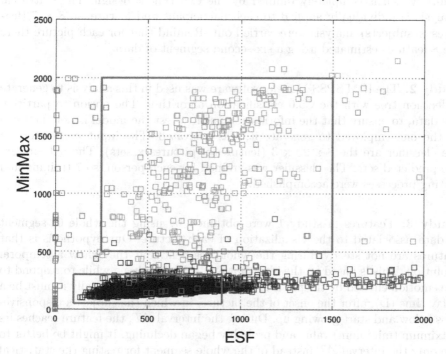

Fig. 2. Experimental sequence. Source [18].

Fig. 3. Feature spaces values for motion artifacts (pink), muscular activity (blue), blinks (green) and EEG (black). The selected areas to identify EEG and EEG+blinks epochs are also shown. Source [18] (Color figure online)

2.4 Analysis

For each subject, the average of five typical power bands, the fractal dimension and some ratios such as θ/β and θ/α for all valid epochs were obtained. This yields an overall of 60×8 numerical values for each subject, grouped into three sets, according to the valence/aerosal values shown in Table 1, or, in other words, $(3 \times 20 \times 8)$ features. Next, we applied three different types of analysis: statistical, classification and temporal. The first seeks to find significant differences among features and sets. The second analysis seeks to obtain the accuracy in detecting one out of the three emotional sets through a classifier based on decision trees. The last one studies the dynamic in inducing an emotion.

Study 1. Here, we looked for the statistical significance of some features among sets. For doing so, we employed the Kruskal-Wallis test, which is a non-parametric alternative to the analysis of variance (ANOVA). It serves to contrast the hypothesis that k quantitative samples haven been obtained from the same population. It requires samples (or features from pictures) to be obtained randomly, which is completely fulfilled by the experiment design. The statistical analysis is individually applied to each participant and feature, so 8 × 7 (features × subjects) analysis were carried out. Remind that for each picture there are 8 features estimated using a six-second segment of data.

Study 2. The IBM SPSS Modeler software was used in this analysis to generate a decision tree with the C5.0 classification algorithm. The option to partition the data, to ensure that the information used to test the model is not the same as the one employed to generate it, was activated. The input parameters to the classifier are the 8 x 20 x 3 (features x pictures x sets). The outputs are the predicted sets. The classifier was trained for each person, so 7 training and testing processes were accomplished.

Study 3. Features in study 1 were obtained by using the whole 6s segment of data associated to the visualization of each picture. Our hypothesis is that features are not steady during the whole segment, but they show a temporal evolution. This is based on the idea that any subject takes a while to respond to the emotion elicited by the picture. As can be seen in Fig. 4, initially it must be a delay time (D), after the onset of the picture, in which the subject's responsiveness is low and start growing up. During the interval ΔT, the feature reaches its maximum (minimum) value and probably began declining. It might be better to use only the interval ΔT instead of the whole segment for testing the statistical significance.

3   Results

3.1   Study 1

Table 2 shows the absolute values of the features obtained for Study 1, grouped according to the set of images and subject. Statistically significant values, with a $p < 0.05$ have been also highlighted. Subjects 3, 6 and 7 obtained values significant for the fractal dimension, subjects 5 and 7 in the α band and subject 5 in the γ power band too. There isn't a clear relationship between features' behavior and changes on valence and arousal. For example, for subject 3, the fractal dimension has a concave shape when moving from set 1 to set 3 whereas for the subject 6, the same feature, has a growing monotone behavior.

Table 2. Averaged values of each feature, subject and set of images. Values for power bands are scaled by 10^7. In bold the features that obtained significant results according to the Kruskal-Wallis test. Most of data contained in the table has been obtained from [18].

Subject	Set1								Set2								Set3							
	δ	θ	α	β	γ	$\frac{\varrho}{\beta}$	$\frac{\varrho}{\alpha}$	hfd	δ	θ	α	β	γ	$\frac{\varrho}{\beta}$	$\frac{\varrho}{\alpha}$	hfd	δ	θ	α	β	γ	$\frac{\varrho}{\beta}$	$\frac{\varrho}{\alpha}$	hfd
1	6,04	5,12	2,3	3,21	2,85	1,59	2,22	1,58	3,36	3,65	1,95	3,08	2,85	1,18	1,86	1,59	4,02	3,98	1,96	2,89	2,47	1,37	2,02	1,58
2	2,06	2,49	2,63	3,9	5,01	0,63	0,94	1,66	2,1	2,59	2,95	4,08	4,32	0,63	0,87	1,65	2,19	3,26	2,85	3,77	4,13	0,86	1,14	1,65
3	4,32	5,48	4,37	8,64	**3,73***	0,63	1,25	**1,57***	4,58	5,83	4,98	8,61	**3,34***	0,67	1,17	**1,55***	4,06	5,63	4,67	8,3	**3,81**	0,67	1,2	**1,58***
4	2,96	3,29	1,77	5,34	6,06	0,61	1,85	1,64	2,15	1,91	1,1	5,11	5,77	0,37	1,73	1,64	2,45	2,2	1,29	5,14	5,82	0,42	1,69	1,65
5	2,18	2,64	**1,56***	3,81	4,38	0,69	1,69	1,68	1,61	2,09	**1,1***	3,51	4,78	0,59	1,88	1,68	2,29	2,88	**1,47***	3,6	4,05	0,8	1,95	1,67
6	4,68	4,94	3,09	4,5	3,32	1,09	1,6	**1,58***	4,54	4,64	3,09	4,73	4,09	0,98	1,5	**1,6***	3,56	4,4	3,05	4,76	4,51	0,92	1,44	**1,63***
7	1,11	1,24	**0,69***	4,51	1,29	0,27	1,78	**1,71***	2,62	1,9	**1,32***	4,53	9,52	0,41	1,43	**1,68***	2,13	2,53	**1,64***	5,07	1,03	0,49	1,53	**1,69***

Subjects 5 and 7 show significant changes in the α band. However, like with the fractal dimension, there isn't a regular pattern in this feature. For example, while subject 7 shows an increase in α, subject 5, has a concave behavior.

Subject 3 also obtained significant values in γ band with a concave behavior among sets.

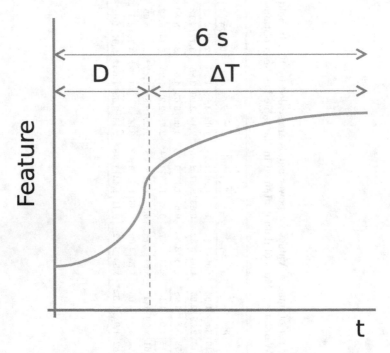

Fig. 4. Temporal evolution of a feature after the onset of the stimulus (t=0). There is an initial delay, D, followed by the interval of interest, ΔT, in which the feature reaches its maximum or minimum value.

3.2   Study 2

Table 3 shows the accuracy in classifying the 3 sets. For them all, the accuracy is over 70%, reaching up to near 92% for subject 5. In average, the accuracy was around 81%.

3.3   Study 3

We hypothesized that there must be a temporal evolution in any feature after the onset of the stimulus. To illustrate this Fig. 5 shows the average temporal evolution of α and γ power bands for subject 4 and set of pictures. It can be seen that power bands temporally changes as time goes by. For example, in set 3, it would be better to obtain this features in the middle of the interval for the α band.

Table 3. Accuracy in detecting emotional states.

Subject	Accuracy
1	78,33%
2	78,33%
3	76,67%
4	73,33%
5	91,67%
6	81.67%
7	85%
Mean	**80.71%**

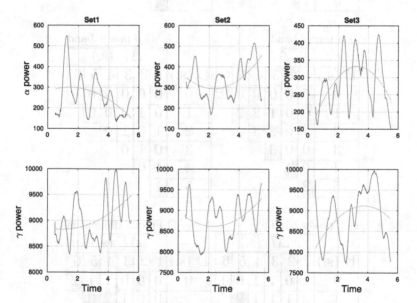

Fig. 5. Temporal evolution of α and γ power bands for participant 4 using 1s-length analysis windows. A parabolic interpolation curve is also shown.

Table 4 shows, for the different possible values of D and ΔT, how many statistically significant values ($p < 0.05$) are given in the different features under study (δ, θ, α, β, γ and hfd). The first thing to keep in mind is that in these tables the values below the diagonal do not make sense, since always $D + \Delta T$ must be less than or equal to 6 s. The most interesting results are obtained in the α and γ bands and hfd, and to a lesser extent in θ band. As seen, the β and δ bands are the least statistical relevance. It is also easily seen, that the best pair of values for (D, ΔT) are: (4,2); (3,3); (2,4) and to a lesser extent (1,5).

Table 4. Number of subjects with significant features according to the statistical analysis, the interval ΔT and the delay D.

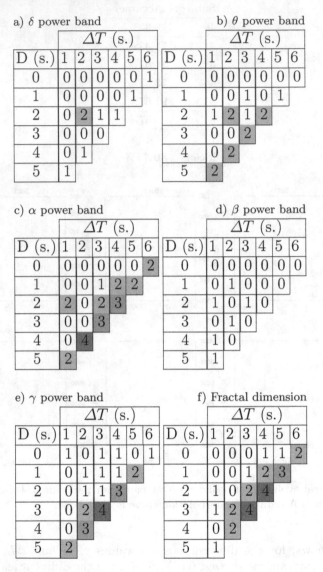

a) δ power band

D (s.)	ΔT (s.) 1	2	3	4	5	6
0	0	0	0	0	0	1
1	0	0	0	0	1	
2	0	2	1	1		
3	0	0	0			
4	0	1				
5	1					

b) θ power band

D (s.)	ΔT (s.) 1	2	3	4	5	6
0	0	0	0	0	0	0
1	0	0	1	0	1	
2	1	2	1	2		
3	0	0	2			
4	0	2				
5	2					

c) α power band

D (s.)	ΔT (s.) 1	2	3	4	5	6
0	0	0	0	0	0	2
1	0	0	1	2	2	
2	2	0	2	3		
3	0	0	3			
4	0	4				
5	2					

d) β power band

D (s.)	ΔT (s.) 1	2	3	4	5	6
0	0	0	0	0	0	0
1	0	1	0	0	0	
2	1	0	1	0		
3	0	1	0			
4	1	0				
5	1					

e) γ power band

D (s.)	ΔT (s.) 1	2	3	4	5	6
0	1	0	1	1	0	1
1	0	1	1	1	2	
2	0	1	1	3		
3	0	2	4			
4	0	3				
5	2					

f) Fractal dimension

D (s.)	ΔT (s.) 1	2	3	4	5	6
0	0	0	0	1	1	2
1	0	0	1	2	3	
2	1	0	2	4		
3	1	2	4			
4	0	2				
5	1					

4   Discussion

The fractal dimension is related to the complexity of the EEG signal, which is increased in neural activation processes. In our previous work [18], it was suspected the existence of a relationship between arousal and fractal dimension. In this new study we have included the γ power band which, in turn, can be also considered as an indicator of underlying neural activation. Only one subject obtained significant differences in this feature among sets, with a behavior that suggests a correlation with the arousal dimension. With respect to valence, [18] showed that it is very difficult to establish any kind of correlation with only one electrode since it does not capture lateralization effects. These effects between hemispheres have been found in some studies [1]. For negative valences it was observed a greater synchronization (activation) in the left hemisphere, whereas for positive valences, the same effect was observed in the opposite hemisphere.

The averaged accuracy in detecting these three emotional sets was approximately of 81% when using a decision tree as classifier. Table 5 summarizes a comparative between our results and other studies, highlighting the number of electrodes used and the emotions detected. As can be seen, our results outperforms previous work regarding the same number of electrodes [30] although the number of emotional states was slightly higher in such a study. Regarding to the same number of emotions to be detect, in this study we almost equal other works with higher number of electrodes [3]. For a more detailed discussion in this issue see [18].

Table 5. Accuracy in detecting emotional states.

Author	Number of electrodes	Number of emotions	Accuracy
H. Yoon [30]	1	4	66%
L. Brown [3]	9	3	82%
O. Sourina [23]	3	4	from 70% up to 100%
D. O. Bos [2]	3	5	92,3% (valence) 97,4% (arousal)
G. Chanel [4]	64	3	76% (valence) 67% (arousal)
R. Quesada [18]	1	3	80.71%

Data support the dynamic in the elicitation of an emotion. There exists an initial delay, which can vary between 1–2 s, wherein the physiological processes triggered by the picture visualization are emerging. When considering the whole interval of picture exposition, the estimated features may be pulled down by this initial phenomena. So, it is worthy to consider the assessment of the feature several seconds after the onset of the stimulus in order to give time to the internal process to get to a steady state.

An explanation of why there were only a few significant features can be seen in Fig. 6. It shows the averages of reported arousal and valence for each set of pictures per subject (circle) and the averages for all subjects (*).

Although it can be seen that averages per subject approximate to the values of the IAPS (except for set1, whose valence is greater and the arousal is lower), the dispersion of the values reported for each of the 20 pictures is quite higher than those indicated in the IAPS database. This could justify, in large part, why it has not been obtained significant variations among the measured features for the different sets of pictures.

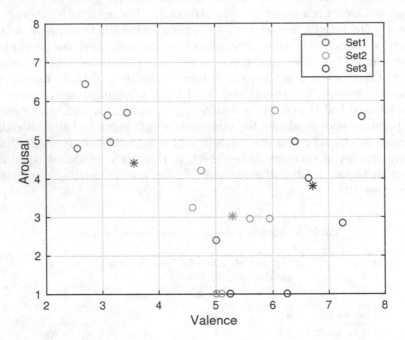

Fig. 6. Mean experimental valence and arousal values for each set of pictures and subject. Source [18].

5   Conclusions and Future Work

This study has shown the feasibility of using a device, with a single EEG at the frontopolar position, for registering the significant neural activity during experiments involving the elicitation of a small set of emotions. The detection accuracy was over 80%, which outperforms some results reported in the scientific literature. The most significant features were the α and γ power bands and the fractal dimension, hfd. It has also been proved that there is an improvement in the significance of results when the dynamic effect in inducing an emotion is considered. Namely, the number of subjects that obtained significant values in such bands increased when the delay D was higher than 2 s and the interval of analysis ΔT reduced to 2–4 s.

It is of interest for subsequent studies to make a similar investigation taking into account the following considerations: that the set of pictures vary in a single dimension of the circumplex model when passing from one set to another; increase considerably the number of people performing the experimental test;

use the incremental feature variation between the the analysis window and the preceding resting period; and finally take into account the values of D and ΔT to improve the classification results.

Acknowledgments. We sincerely and deeply thank the people involved in the realization of this study and the anonymous reviewers who helped us improve this document with their comments.

References

1. Aftanas, L., Varlamov, A., Pavlov, S., Makhnev, V., Reva, N.: Affective picture processing: event-related synchronization within individually defined human theta band is modulated by valence dimension. Neurosci. Lett. **303**(2), 115–118 (2001)
2. Bos, D.O., et al.: EEG-based emotion recognition. The Influence of Visual and Auditory Stimuli, pp. 1–17 (2006)
3. Brown, L., Grundlehner, B., Penders, J.: Towards wireless emotional valence detection from EEG. In: 2011 Annual International Conference of the IEEE Engineering in Medicine and Biology Society. pp. 2188–2191. IEEE (2011)
4. Chanel, G., Ansari-Asl, K., Pun, T.: Valence-arousal evaluation using physiological signals in an emotion recall paradigm. In: 2007 IEEE International Conference on Systems, Man and Cybernetics, pp. 2662–2667. IEEE (2007)
5. Corporation, I.: Manual de usuario de IBM SPSS Modeler 15, p. 280 (2012). ftp://public.dhe.ibm.com/software/analytics/spss/documentation/modeler/15.0/ es/UsersGuide.pdf
6. Crowley, K., Sliney, A., Pitt, I., Murphy, D.: Evaluating a brain-computer interface to categorise human emotional response. In: 2010 10th IEEE International Conference on Advanced Learning Technologies. pp. 276–278. IEEE (2010)
7. Das, R., Chatterjee, D., Das, D., Sinharay, A., Sinha, A.: Cognitive load measurement-a methodology to compare low cost commercial EEG devices. In: 2014 International Conference on Advances in Computing, Communications and Informatics (ICACCI), pp. 1188–1194. IEEE (2014)
8. Ekman, P., et al.: Universals and cultural differences in the judgments of facial expressions of emotion. J. Pers. Soc. psychol. **53**(4), 712 (1987)
9. Enobio: http://www.neuroelectrics.com/products/enobio/
10. Epoc, E.: www.emotiv.com
11. Hamann, S.: Mapping discrete and dimensional emotions onto the brain: controversies and consensus. Trends Cogn. Sci. **16**(9), 458–466 (2012)
12. Levenson, R.W.: Basic emotion questions. Emot. Rev. **3**(4), 379–386 (2011)
13. Lindquist, K.A., Wager, T.D., Kober, H., Bliss-Moreau, E., Barrett, L.F.: The brain basis of emotion: a meta-analytic review. Behav. Brain Sci. **35**(03), 121–143 (2012)
14. Liu, N.H., Chiang, C.Y., Chu, H.C.: Recognizing the degree of human attention using eeg signals from mobile sensors. Sensors **13**(8), 10273–10286 (2013)
15. Liu, Y., Sourina, O.: EEG-based subject-dependent emotion recognition algorithm using fractal dimension. In: 2014 IEEE International Conference on Systems, Man, and Cybernetics (SMC). pp. 3166–3171. October 2014. https://doi.org/10.1109/ SMC.2014.6974415

16. Liu, Y., Sourina, O., Nguyen, M.K.: Real-time EEG-based emotion recognition and its applications. In: Gavrilova, M.L., Tan, C.J.K., Sourin, A., Sourina, O. (eds.) Transactions on Computational Science XII. LNCS, vol. 6670, pp. 256–277. Springer, Heidelberg (2011). https://doi.org/10.1007/978-3-642-22336-5_13
17. Maki, Y., Sano, G., Kobashi, Y., Nakamura, T., Kanoh, M., Yamada, K.: Estimating subjective assessments using a simple biosignal sensor. In: 2012 13th ACIS International Conference on Software Engineering, Artificial Intelligence, Networking and Parallel & Distributed Computing (SNPD), pp. 325–330. IEEE (2012)
18. Quesada-Tabares, R., Molina-Cantero, A.J., Gómez-González, I., Merino-Monge, M., Castro-García, J.A., Cabrera-Cabrera, R.: Emotions detection based on a single-electrode EEG device. In: Proceedings of the 4th International Conference on Physiological Computing Systems, vol. 1: PhyCS, pp. 89–95. INSTICC, SciTePress (2017). https://doi.org/10.5220/0006476300890095
19. Russell, J.A., Barrett, L.F.: Core affect, prototypical emotional episodes, and other things called emotion: dissecting the elephant. J. Pers. Soc. Psychol. **76**(5), 805 (1999)
20. Sanei, S., Chambers, J.: EEG Signal Processing. Wiley, New Jersey (2007)
21. Schafer, R.: What is a savitzky-golay filter? [lecture notes]. Signal Process. Mag., IEEE **28**(4), 111–117 (2011). https://doi.org/10.1109/MSP.2011.941097
22. Siamaknejad, H., Loo, C.K., Liew, W.S.: Fractal dimension methods to determine optimum EEG electrode placement for concentration estimation. In: 2014 Joint 7th International Conference on Soft Computing and Intelligent Systems (SCIS), and 15th International Symposium on Advanced Intelligent Systems (ISIS), pp. 952–955. December 2014. https://doi.org/10.1109/SCIS-ISIS.2014.7044757
23. Sourina, O., Liu, Y.: A fractal-based algorithm of emotion recognition from EEG using arousal-valence model. In: BIOSIGNALS, pp. 209–214 (2011)
24. Stone, J.V.: Independent Component Analysis: A Tutorial Introduction. MIT Press, Cambridge (2004)
25. Szibbo, D., Luo, A., Sullivan, T.J.: Removal of blink artifacts in single channel EEG. In: 2012 Annual International Conference of the IEEE Engineering in Medicine and Biology Society. pp. 3511–3514 August 2012. https://doi.org/10.1109/EMBC.2012.6346723
26. Cervantes-De la Torre, F., González-Trejo, J., Real-Ramírez, C., Hoyos-Reyes, L.: Fractal dimension algorithms and their application to time series associated with natural phenomena. In: Journal of Physics: Conference Series. vol. 475, p. 012002. IOP Publishing (2013)
27. Van Hal, B., Rhodes, S., Dunne, B., Bossemeyer, R.: Low-cost EEG-based sleep detection. In: 2014 36th Annual International Conference of the IEEE Engineering in Medicine and Biology Society (EMBC), pp. 4571–4574. IEEE (2014)
28. Vytal, K., Hamann, S.: Neuroimaging support for discrete neural correlates of basic emotions: a voxel-based meta-analysis. J. Cogn. Neurosci. **22**(12), 2864–2885 (2010)
29. Wang, Q., Sourina, O.: Real-time mental arithmetic task recognition from EEG signals. IEEE Trans. Neural Syst. Rehabil. Eng. **21**(2), 225–232 (2013). https://doi.org/10.1109/TNSRE.2012.2236576
30. Yoon, H., Park, S.W., Lee, Y.K., Jang, J.H.: Emotion recognition of serious game players using a simple brain computer interface. In: 2013 International Conference on ICT Convergence (ICTC), pp. 783–786. IEEE (2013)

Detection of Artifacts Using a Non-invasive BCI on the Basis of Electroencephalography While Utilizing Low-Cost Off-the-Shelf Equipment

Patrick Schembri[✉], Richard Anthony, and Mariusz Pelc

Department of Computer and Information Systems, University of Greenwich, Greenwich, London, UK
{P. Schembri, R. J. Anthony, M. Pelc}@greenwich.ac.uk

Abstract. Brain Computer Interface (BCI) on the basis of Electroencephalography (EEG) has gained prominence over the past decade, especially with the proliferation of cheap EEG devices including user-made equipment. The main shortcoming of EEG, particularly with this type of equipment, is that it is frequently contaminated by various artifacts. Moreover a number of researchers and end users are currently using off-the-shelf equipment as a "black box" approach without any qualitative testing. This exposed an evident necessity to validate the equipment's suitability. In this paper we provide vital groundwork by identifying and categorizing artifacts using our specific low fidelity equipment. This work forms part of a wider project where we assess the viability of this equipment, primarily in the artifacts domain, as a precursor for further studies. Our promising results show that we were able to effectively identify and categorize the most commonly encountered artifacts with the aforementioned equipment.

Keywords: Brain Computer Interface · Electroencephalography · EEG · Artifacts

1 Introduction

This paper investigates the ability of our specific low fidelity equipment to successfully detect the most common artifacts, observed in a non-clinical environment. Our research makes use of a non-invasive Brain Computer Interface (BCI) on the basis of Electroencephalography (EEG). The aim of this paper is to assess the functionality and reliability of our low cost equipment in its ability to detect rudimentary signals such as artifacts. The work presented here is part of a wider EEG project where the ensuing phase is to utilize this equipment to perform several different EEG tasks; with varying degrees of success; comparable to medical grade equipment. These include different domains such as P300 and Motor activity.

An artifact is a signal that is detected by EEG equipment, which is not of cerebral origin but from various different sources. In the context of EEG, artifacts are unwanted since they mask the brain wave signals and have always been given a great deal of attention due to the undesirable affect that these have on the signal of cerebral origin.

A. Holzinger et al. (Eds.): PhyCS 2016–2018, LNCS 10057, pp. 93–109, 2019.
https://doi.org/10.1007/978-3-030-27950-9_6

In this paper we prepare the groundwork for filtering and using these artifacts, through categorization of artifacts, and their manifest characteristics, using specific low fidelity equipment. The work presented here is part of a larger EEG based project and in continuation and as a precursor of our papers [1–3].

2 Experimental Methodology

Our work is concerned with exploring the capabilities and limitations of low cost off the shelf equipment which in return will facilitate and increase accessibility for EEG applications. We aim to compensate for the low fidelity aspect of this equipment with enhanced software filtering and analysis. This particular part of the work sets the foundations for further work by investigating the way in which various artifacts are detected, identified and categorized with low fidelity equipment.

A way in which an electrode (input1) is connected relative to another electrode (input2) is called a derivation. A collection of derivations are called a montage and there are several different ones in popular use. The intention of using a specific montage is to keep the experiments tractable and to avoid unnecessary complexity. Moreover other types of montage; even the more complex such as Laplacian and Common Average Reference; can be derived from the collected data, since montage reformatting is achieved by performing a simple mathematical operation. In fact [4] states that *"for this reason, digital EEG systems store the original EEG signal in a referential montage containing all electrodes"*. This is of course possible as long as all the electrodes that need to be combined have in some way been referred to each other in the original recording.

For instance when labeling a channel montage as $Fp1 - A1$, a mathematical expression is being created which implies that the signal displayed will be Fp1 minus A1. If a recording has been obtained from $Fp1 - A1$ and $Fp2 - A1$ then $Fp1 - Fp2$ can be derived from:

$$(Fp1 - A1) - (Fp2 - A1) = Fp1 - Fp2 + A1 - A1 = Fp1 - Fp2 \tag{1}$$

This formula (1) is extracted from [1]. Although montage reformatting is possible to be performed instantaneously, this is ideally used for recorded sessions and is not suggested for real-time streaming.

2.1 Equipment Used

The work reported herein is based on an OpenBCI[1] 32-bit board called *Cyton Biosensing Board* (referred to as *Cyton* in this paper), connected with an Electro-Cap[2] using the international 10/20 system for scalp electrode placement in the context of EEG experiments. A basic overview of the equipment being used is shown in Fig. 1.

---

[1] http://openbci.com/.

[2] http://electro-cap.com/.

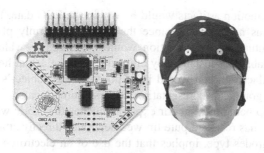

Fig. 1. Cyton board and Electro-CAP.

The *Cyton*'s board microcontroller is the PIC32MX250F128B[3] which includes a 32-bit processor with a maximum speed of 50 MHz; storage of 32 KB of memory and is *Arduino* compatible. The board uses the ADS1299[4] IC developed by Texas Instruments, which is an 8-Channel, 24-Bit, simultaneous sampling delta-sigma, Analogue-to-Digital Converter used for bio potential measurements such as in EEG and Electrocardiography (ECG). The 24-bit resolution gives a huge range of microvolts (μV) that covers ±187 mV (187000 μV) - *refer to* Sect. 2.3. When considering that EEG data ranges are typically between ±100 μV, it clearly illustrates that it is able to provide a broad spectrum of flexibility and scalability. Moreover this chip is capable of supporting up to 16,000 Hz although the transfer of that much data through an Arduino would be impracticable. There is the ability to use the SD card for faster sample rates, which is discussed below.

The board comes with eight bio potential input channels which can be increased to sixteen channels with the addition of a *Daisy Module*; which plugs itself onto the existing *Cyton* board. Our current experiments do not make use of the daisy module, although future experiments may need these extra channels.

The system comes with a pre-programmed USB dongle for wireless communication which communicates with the low cost RFDuino[5] RFD22301 microcontroller built on the *Cyton* board. This microcontroller can communicate wirelessly with any device compatible with Bluetooth Low Energy (BLE). In addition a local Secure Digital (SD) slot is built-in the board, which gives it the ability to store recorded data on SD memory card. This is particularly useful when requiring improved portability and highest data rates.

An additional feature which is included in the *Cyton* board is a 3-axes accelerometer from *ST* with model LIS3DH[6]. This accelerometer is capable of 16 bit data output and of measuring accelerations with output data rates from 1 Hz to 5.3 kHz. This can prove to be quite useful; such as, for sensing change in orientation of the head or sensing rough motion. In these cases the value from the accelerometer

[3] http://www.microchip.com/wwwproducts/en/en557425.

[4] http://www.ti.com/product/ADS1299.

[5] http://www.rfduino.com/.

[6] http://www.st.com/en/mems-and-sensors/lis3dh.html.

would suggest that motion artifacts would be within the EEG data. In our experiments this information was not required, since the board was firmly placed on the desk. However, in the future, this information would be extremely valuable if the *Cyton* board is made portable; for instance, by attaching it to the actual headset. This would lead to motion artifacts since it would be exposed to the subject's head movements. Figure 2 depicts a graphical representation of these components.

The Electro-Cap being used in our experiments has the fabric which is made from elastic spandex and has recessed pure tin wet electrodes directly attached to the fabric. The term wet electrodes type, implies that the use of an electrolyte gel is required to make effective contact with the scalp; otherwise it may result in impedance instability.

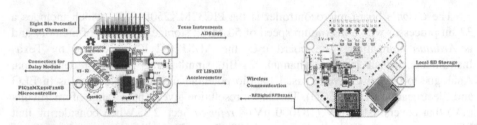

Fig. 2. Cyton board (front and back) components.

2.2 Experimental Setup

The EEG signals where sampled at 250 Hz (this being OpenBCIs default value) while the sampling precision was 24-bit. The recordings where stored anonymously as raw data in text, comma separated value (csv) files. Eight EEG electrodes where used in different regions of the scalp according to the International 10–20 System as shown in Fig. 3(a). This system is the de facto standard for the placement of electrodes along the head. Each electrode is assigned a letter to identify the lobe and a number to identify the hemispheric location. The letters F, P, T and O stand for Frontal, Parietal, Temporal and Occipital lobes. In addition, letter C refers to the central area of the brain. The even numbers represent the electrodes positioning on the right hemisphere, while the odd numbers represent the electrodes positioning on the left hemisphere. The Xz stands for a zero and represents an electrode placed on the midline such as Fz, Cz and Pz. In addition the letter A can represent the reference electrode which will measure the potential difference between itself and the other electrodes and/or the ground electrode for common mode rejection.

The equipment we are using supports the use of eight electrodes. The electrode positions Fp1, Fp2, C3, C4, T5, T6, O1 and O2 are selected because they provide good coverage for detecting these artifacts. These are referenced to the electrode A1 as follows: Channel 1: Fp1; Channel 2: Fp2; Channel 3: C3; Channel 4: C4; Channel 5: T5; Channel 6: T6; Channel 7: O1; Channel 8: O2 as shown in Fig. 3. A referential montage was selected to analyze how artifacts are exposed with this setup, even though no single reference electrode is ideal for all situations. Nonetheless and if required, other types of montage can be reconstructed from the chosen montage by executing a simple mathematical operation; as previously explained. The reference electrode was placed on the left earlobe A1 as shown in Fig. 3(b).

EEG signals where obtained from a healthy human subject; male in the age group between 30 and 40 years old and on three different sessions with a few days apart. Before the start of the experiments, the subject was asked to calm down in a seated position and relax for a few minutes. The subject was seated one meter away from the equipment. The researcher and his equipment where situated on the left side of the subject. Then, the subject was instructed on a series of tests such as muscle movement that are designed to detect the artifacts which are discussed in Sect. 3.

Three trials where conducted for these experiments. The first session results and recordings where archived. The second session was done on a separate day with the same conditions of the first session and the results where archived for comparisons. These two sessions were carried out to familiarize the user with the equipment and the methodology of the experiments. The third session was done a day later with the same conditions of the first and second session and the results are shown in this paper. During the recording the subject received a 2 s beep sound to perform the requested trial and a 1 s beep sound to stop.

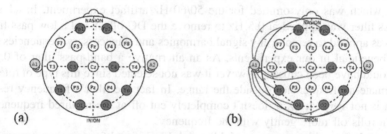

Fig. 3. (a) Electrode placement following the International 10–20 system (b) Referential montage used.

2.3 Processing

The data that was transmitted from the RFDuino module found on the *Cyton* board is considered as 'raw' EEG data in ADC counts. These where transferred as 24-bit integer, since it's the native format used by the ADS1299 chip. Since this is an unusual format, it was immediately converted via the OpenBCI open-source JAVA function '*interpret24bitAsInt32*' into a 32-bit signed integer [5].

Subsequently the *scale factor* was required, which is the multiplier used to convert the EEG values from counts to scientific units like volts. This is found by following the formula extracted from [1] and found in the ADS1299 datasheet table number 7:

$$Scale\ Factor = V_{REF}/(2^{23} - 1)/Gain * 1000000 \qquad (2)$$

The datasheet also states that the voltage reference input is hardware bound to 4.5 V, while we used the maximum and default gain factor of 24-bit. Thus the formula (2) can be reformed into formula (3) which is extracted from [1].

$$Scale\ Factor = 4.5\ V/\left(2^{23} - 1\right)/24 * 1000000 \tag{3}$$

Hence the scale factor value is 0.02235 per count. Therefore the 32-bit signed integer is multiplied by the scale factor and we get the EEG data values in microvolts (μV). This is the actual stored data in the *csv* file. The full scale of $\pm$187 mV (187000 μV) discussed in Sect. 2.1 is achieved by $2^{23} * 0.02235 = \pm187485.388$ μV.

As previously mentioned the ADS1299 chip is capable of a sample rate of up to 16,000 Hz; however in our experiments we used OpenBCIs default rate of 250 Hz especially when considering that the data was being transmitted wirelessly through the RFDuino module.

The captured raw data was imported in MATLAB R2014a[7] via the *csvread* command into a MATLAB matrix and any unnecessary rows and columns were removed. These consisted of the first five rows which are superfluous comments; the first column which stored the sample index/packet counter and the last three columns which stored the auxiliary data of the accelerometer.

The MATLAB array was later imported into EEGLAB[8] for processing and for offline qualitative and quantitative analysis. The first process was to apply a 50 Hz (60 Hz in some countries) notch filter to eliminate the environmental electrical interference, which was only omitted for the 50/60 Hz artifact experiment. In addition a high pass filter was applied at 0.5 Hz to remove the DC offset and a low pass filter of 49 Hz was applied to remove any signal harmonics and unnecessary frequencies which are not beneficial in our experiments. As an alternative a band-pass filter of 0.5 Hz– 49 Hz could have been chosen, however it was not selected since this type of filter does not attenuate all frequencies outside the range. In fact the filter's frequency response function is not very steep; it doesn't completely cut-off at the required frequency, but instead it rolls off more gently with the frequency.

The result from this processing yields a rich EEG signal for our experiments which can be analyzed with different tools. The screenshots presenting the EEG signal (see Figs. 4, 5, 6, 7, 8, 9, 10, 11, 12 and 13) where plotted by using the EEGLAB *Plot: Channel Data (Scroll)* menu option. The frequency-time domain screenshots where produced by the *Time-Frequency transforms: Channel-time frequency* menu option. The plot Event Related Spectral Power (ERSP) was employed since it is a statistical measure; the mean of a distribution of single-trial time/frequency transform [6]. In our processing we used the Fast Fourier Transform (FFT) option; 400 time points for the time-frequency decomposition and the frequency was set between one and forty which provides us with enough information for artifacts detection. The baseline was set to the default of 0 for pre-stimulus and the single trial DIV baseline option was used. Subsequently the choice of channel number and time range in relation to the experiment being analyzed where entered (such as Channel 1 for FP1; time range 5000 ms–9000 ms).

The spectrogram frequency-domain screenshots were produced in Matlab; outside of EEGLAB using a customized code. This is shown in the code snippet below.

---

[7] https://www.mathworks.com/products/matlab.html.
[8] https://sccn.ucsd.edu/eeglab/.

The data was filtered using Butterworth filter design of the second order. First a notch filter was used followed by a low pass and a high pass filter; with the same values used for EEGLAB.

```
fs = 250;
nfl = 49;
nfh = 51;
fl = 49;
fh = 0.5;
order = 2;

%Butterworth notch filter
[bn,an]=butter(order,[nfl nfh]/(fs/2),'stop');

%Butterworth low pass filter
[b,a]=butter(order,lp/(fs/2),'low');

%Butterworth high pass filter
[b,a]=butter(order,fh/(fs/2),'high');

%Spectrogram
spectrogram
(eegdata_f,hanning(256),255,[1:40],250,'yaxis');
```

3 Results

Although a number of research papers have been published showing different types of artifacts such as [7] and [8]; these were presented with a "black box" approach or using medical equipment, or otherwise, mentioned in a different context. What we present in this paper are results that are relevant to our own specific low fidelity hardware.

An EEG device is very sensitive and it is easily susceptible to disruption from other electrical activities. Moreover some artifacts are easily distinguishable while others closely resemble cerebral activity and are very challenging to be recognized. Artifacts are usually categorized as physiological (biological) and non-physiological (extra physiological) [9]. The classification mentioned below is not rigorous; for instance, if the subject makes a movement, this may lead to artifacts originating as electrode artifact.

Table 1 represents the classification of the most common artifacts which are observed in a non-clinical environment and which will be discussed in this paper. This does not imply that our list is a rigorous classification, but we are merely classifying the artifacts that are most commonly encountered in a non-clinical environment. This list is also extensible for future work and/or fellow researchers. We have not included artifacts of clinical nature, since our main aim is to steer away from medical environments.

Table 1. Artifacts classification.

Physiological	Non-physiological
Ocular artifacts	Environmental electrical interference
• Blink	• 50/60 Hz artifact
• Eye flutter	• Radio frequency
• Lateral eye movement	• Mains-Borne
• Slow roving eye movement	
Muscle (EMG) artifacts	Equipment artifacts
• Surface EMG	• Electrode pop
– Clench teeth	• Electrode contact and lead movement
• Glossokinetic	• Salt bridge
• Intermittent Photic Stimulation (IPS)	• Perspiration
Movement artifacts	
Cardiac artifacts	
Pulse wave artifacts	
Skin potential artifacts	

3.1 Physiological Artifacts

Physiological artifacts are bioelectrical signals that are generated from the user's body excluding the brain. These are usually embedded along the electrical cerebral bio-signals in an EEG session. The physiological artifacts include, but are not limited to:

Ocular Artifacts. Ocular artifacts are essentially a result from the eyeball acting as a dipole which becomes pertinent when it develops into a moving electrical field such as when the subject opens and closes his eyes and/or the EMG potentials from muscles in and around the orbit. These generate signals that are detected predominantly by electrodes Fp1/Fp2 and F7/F8.

Blink. Blink/blinking which is the most common ocular artifact, occurs spontaneously and is very challenging for the subject to control even for short periods of time. When the subject blinks, the eyeball triggers an instinctive upward movement (Bells phenomenon) and hence produces a positive potential in the frontal lobe which is displayed in EEG as a transient, diphasic, synchronous slow wave [10–12] as shown in Fig. 4. This image also shows that, the faster the blink the shorter the wavelength, as depicted by the first blink occurrence which was faster than the second blink. When the subject performs a number of repetitive blinks, the displayed EEG could mimic a triphasic wave or resemble rhythmic delta activity as shown in Fig. 5. Additional and more frequent blinking can simulate theta activity as shown in Fig. 6.

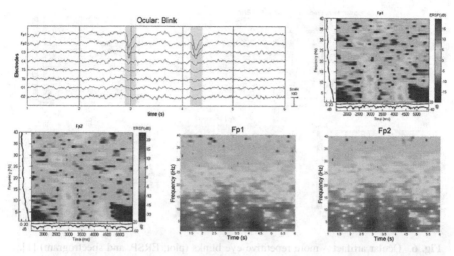

Fig. 4. Ocular artifact – eye blink predominantly on electrodes Fp1 and Fp2 (plot, ERSP, and spectrogram) [1].

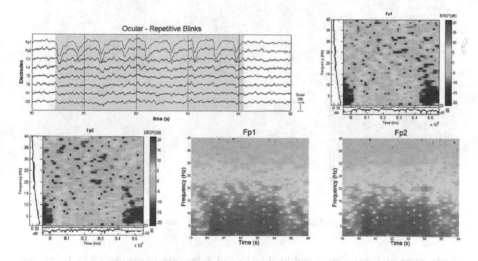

Fig. 5. Ocular artifact – repetitive eye blinks (plot, ERSP, and spectrogram) [1].

Eye Flutter. Eye Flutter produces an ocular artifact that is more rhythmic, with higher frequency and lower amplitude as shown in Fig. 7.

Lateral Eye Movement. Lateral Eye movement artifact is mostly detected in a bipolar longitudinal montage using Fp1 − F7 and Fp2 − F8 and may start off with a single sharp muscle potential called lateral rectus spike. In this type of montage a left lateral eye movement will have a positive potential in electrode F7 and an opposite negative potential in electrode F8. In our referential montage, the frontal origin of eye movement

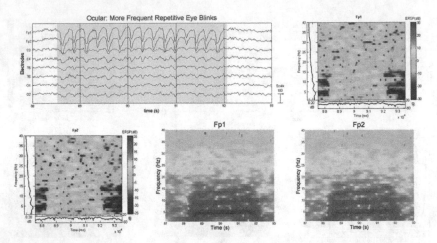

Fig. 6. Ocular artifact – more repetitive eye blinks (plot, ERSP, and spectrogram) [1].

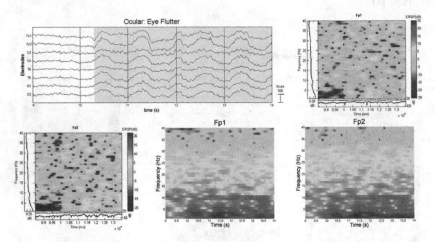

Fig. 7. Ocular artifact – eyeflutter (plot, ERSP, and spectrogram) [1].

artifacts remained indistinguishable due to the reference electrode (A1) being contaminated by eye movements [9].

Slow Roving Eye Movement. Slow Roving eye movement differs from lateral eye movement since no saccades occur; consequently resulting in no abrupt changes. On a bipolar montage these are reflected as smooth lateral movements with phase reversing. On a referential montage using low fidelity equipment, this artifact was not detected.

Muscle Artifacts - EMG (Electromyography) Activity. EMG activity produces artifacts that are due to muscle contraction and are the most common and significant noise source in the context of EEG. Although EMG in itself is useful for electromyography; they are considered noise in EEG, since they overlap and obscure the

EEG signal due to their higher amplitude and frequency. If, however, this signal is passed through a low-pass filter set at 35 Hz or less, this will change their form and caution is required since these may transpire as beta activity or like abnormal epileptiform spikes. The extent of a muscle artifact depends on the duration of the muscle activity, which might be less than a second and/or throughout the entire session [9–11].

Surface EMG. Surface EMG activities generally occur in regions with underlying muscle such as the masseter and temporalis muscle, which affect the frontal and temporal electrodes. These may also disseminate and diffuse to other channels. Electrodes Fz, Cz and Pz can provide a reasonably pure EEG signal. Figure 8 shows an EMG effect when the subject clenches his teeth. ERSP screenshot doesn't show any recognizable activity.

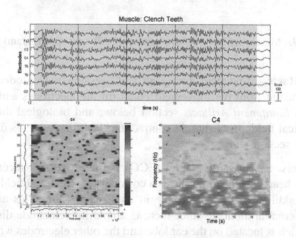

Fig. 8. Muscle artifact – clench teeth (plot, ERSP, and spectrogram) [1].

Glossokinetic. Glossokinetic is an artifact arising from the movement of the tongue. It is similar to the eyeball movement in ocular artifacts, though less sharp. The tongue functions as a dipole where the tip acts as a negative with respect to the positive base. This results in the surging of diffuse delta like activity, which is frequently supplemented by muscle artifact. The tongue has a DC potential and equipment running on DC amplifiers will not record its potential as is the case in the equipment being used for this experiment. Figure 9 shows the effect of swallowing in our subject which affects the oropharyngeal muscle. This experiment could have been included in the Surface EMG section, since no tongue potential is being recorded, but is being listed here for classification reasons.

Intermittent Photic Stimulation (IPS). Intermittent Photic Stimulation (IPS)/is a photomyogenic/photomyoclonic response to a visual stimulation where the subject eyes are presented with intermittent flashes of light. This results in an involuntary time linked facial muscle response to the flash of light which affects the frontal and periorbital regions, specifically the frontalis and orbicularis muscles [13]. At this stage in our work we don't include this.

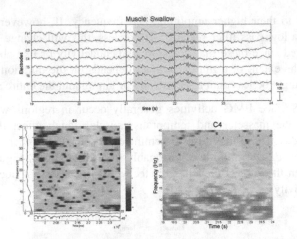

Fig. 9. Muscle artifact – swallow (plot, ERSP, and spectrogram) [1].

Movement Artifacts. Movement during an EEG session may produce two distinct artifacts; instrumental from the movement effect on the electrodes and their leads as discussed in the *Equipment Artifacts* section below; and biological through the generation of electrical fields from muscle contraction; EMG activity; as discussed in the *Muscle Artifacts* section above.

Cardiac Artifacts. Electrocardiography (ECG) is the process of recording electrical activity from the heart. The heart produces a considerable electrical field that spreads to the base of the skull, which is detectable in an EEG session. This artifact is easily detected in a referential montage since there is ample interelectrode distance between the reference which is located on the ear lobe and the other electrodes which are located on the scalp. In addition this artifact is most prominent in subjects with a short neck. This artifact appears as a QRS complex which represents three graphical deflections in an ECG diagram. The QRS complex is preceded by a P wave and followed by a T wave as shown in Fig. 10. With clinical EEG equipment using a referential montage setup; a poor QRS complex was formed. This was due to the distance from the heart where the P wave and T wave are not visible [9, 11]. ECG artifact may be reduced or removed by adding a second reference; however it will only work if both reference electrodes are able to detect a pulse [14]. Unfortunately we were unable to reproduce this artifact using low fidelity equipment. It is true that the artifact is a poorly formed QRS complex which is most prominent in short necks and could have been easily concealed within the noise; but that does not negate the fact that we should have at least encountered it even as a low amplitude signal. We have tried several types of filters but without any apparent result. We were however able to produce an ECG signal on purpose; not as an artifact; with a different set-up, which however is beyond the scope of this paper.

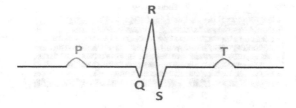

Fig. 10. QRS complex [1].

Pulse Wave Artifact. Pulse artifact mainly occurs when electrodes are placed over a pulsating artery manifesting a regular pulse beat. These pulsations instigate periodic slow waves that can be misidentified as EEG activity. There is a direct link between ECG and pulse waves; where the QRS complex happens right before (about 200 ms) the pulse waves. In our experiments the electrodes where not placed over a pulsating artery and thus it did not show in our experiments.

Skin Potential. Skin potentials where discussed in *Non-Physiological Artifacts*, explicitly under *Equipment Artifacts* which included *Perspiration* and *Salt bridges*.

3.2 Non-physiological Artifacts

Non-Physiological artifacts are externally generated outside the user's body such as artifacts arising from environmental electrical interference and artifacts relating to the equipment being used.

Environmental Electrical Interference

Environmental Electrical Interference 50/60 Hz Artifact. The most common electrical interference artifacts usually emanate from electrical devices and in close proximity to power lines. The greatest contributor is the alternating current (AC) with a monomorphic frequency of either 60 Hz (ex. United States) or 50 Hz (ex. Europe). These artifacts can be introduced either electromagnetically, where the strength of the field is determined by the current flowing through cables or by the equipment such as transformers and TV power supplies; and electrostatically due to the capacitance property of objects where the subject or electrodes pick up capacitance potentials from other sources which are in their proximity such as the movement of any charged bodies or objects (ex. plastic, rubber, synthetic fibres) near the subject [9, 15]. Figure 12 shows the effect of a 50 Hz noise on our EEG signal. This artifact can be reduced by grounding the equipment, moving the subject away from power lines and sources that can generate electrostatic interference and keeping electrodes impedance to less than 5 KΩ which is the leading cause of the 50/60 Hz artifact [14]. Should these methods not suffice; the artifact can be eliminated by a notch-filter (or similar) which will only remove the 50 Hz or 60 Hz activity from the signal. The filter should only be used if necessary.

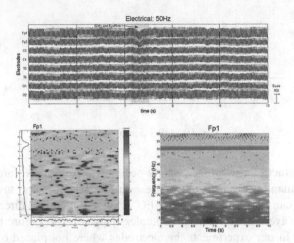

Fig. 11. Electrical artifact: 50 Hz (plot, ERSP, and spectrogram) [1].

Radio Frequency/Mains-Borne. Other electrical interferences which are less prominent include Radio Frequency when they are modulated in a lower frequency and Mains-Borne interference arising from fluctuating power supplies.

Equipment Artifacts. A number of different artifacts can be caused from the recording electrodes and the equipment being used. Electrode artifacts can manifest as two dissimilar waveforms; low frequency rhythms amidst a scalp area and brief transient morphology which would be limited to one electrode [11].

Electrode Pop. Electrode Pop can occur occasionally when there is an instantaneous change in the electrical potential between the electrode and the scalp, where it is typically followed by a sudden, high amplitude spike in the EEG recording [16] as shown in Fig. 11. This may occur when electrodes are not firmly attached and/or when direct pressure is applied on the electrodes.

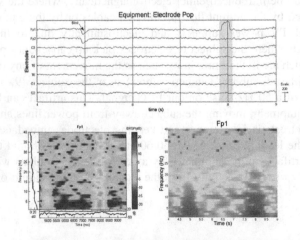

Fig. 12. Equipment artifact: electrode pop (plot, ERSP, and spectrogram) [1].

Electrode Contact and Lead Movements. A weak Electrode Contact and Lead Movements generate a different artifact that has a less sustained morphology compared to electrode pop as shown in Fig. 13. The weak electrode contact results in impedance instability, which will produce waves with fluctuating amplitude and morphology; although if there is a context of rhythmic movement such as from tremors, the resulting waves may be rhythmic as well. Lead movements do not resemble any true EEG activity where the morphology of the wave is incoherent [11].

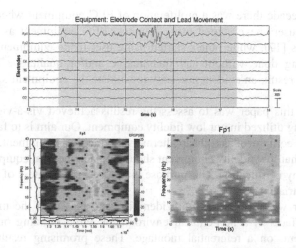

Fig. 13. Equipment artifact: electrode contact and lead movement (plot, ERSP, and spectrogram) [1].

Salt Bridge. A Salt Bridge artifact can occur when smearing the electrolyte gel between two electrodes or by applying an excessive amount of electrolyte gel, which may result in an inadvertently overlap, thus creating a short circuit between the electrodes. This artifact is usually channel specific and manifested as a low amplitude wave compared to the background. Salt bridge artifact will eventually be prevented by use of dry electrodes; which we plan to do in our future experiments.

Perspiration. Perspiration artifact although not as stable, is similar to a salt bridge artifact where the salinity between electrode locations will merge the affected electrodes as a single entity. It is usually manifested as a slow wave that is typically greater than 2 s in duration which is out of the frequency scope of EEG [9, 11].

Salt Bridge and Perspiration artifacts can be easily recognized in an EEG session and should be resolved prior to commencement. The salt bridge artifact is eliminated by cleaning the excess electrolyte between the affected electrodes and wiping the subjects forehead with a spirit solution, while the perspiration artifact can be eliminated by providing a cooler environment and reducing the emotional stress of the subject. The experiments reported here where based on a referential montage, where these artifacts where not present. The lack of these findings suggests that an electrolyte bridge is only present amongst electrodes such as in a bipolar montage.

4 Conclusion

The detection and categorization of artifacts is predominately performed using medical grade EEG equipment and are usually categorized with different type of montages such as referential or bipolar. This makes comparison of artifacts between devices, a challenging task. Moreover only a few artifacts have been documented properly using low cost equipment and this has usually been done ad hoc and without any proper categorization.

In the past decade there was a proliferation of EEG equipment where a number of researchers and users have started using low cost EEG equipment as a "black box" approach such as [17], while others started using user-made equipment such as [18]. This was/is being done without any quantitative and/or qualitative testing on the equipment. As a result, an evident necessity to validate the equipment's suitability was present.

The goal of this paper was to assess the results achieved vis-à-vis the hardware components being utilized in our low fidelity equipment. Our aim is to facilitate the use of low cost EEG equipment as a cheap alternative to medical equipment. However, this does not imply that low fidelity equipment should replace medical equipment; in fact it does not have any certification. Our purpose is to assess the aptness of our equipment for non-clinical trials.

In this paper we have successfully identified and classified the most commonly encountered artifacts in a non-clinical environment while utilizing our specific low fidelity equipment, on a referential montage. These promising results allow us to proceed with our project, where we plan to assess the viability and performance of the aforementioned equipment in different domains such as P300 and motor activity. Successively, we plan to introduce a number of distractions and assessing the ways and extents to which different degrees of distractions affect the detection success of the particular domain while using our low cost equipment.

References

1. Schembri, P., Anthony, R., Pelc, M.: Detection of electroencephalography artefacts using low fidelity equipment. In: Proceedings of the 4th International Conference on Physiological Computing Systems, pp. 65–75 (2017)
2. Schembri, P., Anthony, R., Pelc, M.: The viability and performance of P300 responses using low fidelity equipment. In: 5th International Conference on Biomedical Engineering and Systems (2018)
3. Schembri, P., Anthony, R., Pelc, M.: The feasibility and effectiveness of P300 responses using low fidelity equipment in three distinctive environments. In: 5th International Conference on Physiological Computing Systems (2018)
4. Fisch, B.: Basic Principles of Digital and Analog EEG. Elsevier, Amsterdam (1999)
5. Chip Audette. Data Format for OpenBCI V3 (2014). https://github.com/OpenBCI/OpenBCI-V2hardware-DEPRECATED/wiki/Data-Format-for-OpenBCI-V3
6. Neuper, C., Klimesch, W.: Event-Related Dynamics of Brain Oscillations. Elsevier, Amsterdam (2006)

7. Aydemir, O., Pourzare, S., Kayikcioglu, T.: Classifying various EMG and EOG artifacts in EEG signals, pp. 218–222 (2012)

8. Begum, B.S.: A review on machine learning algorithms in handling EEG artifacts. In: The Swedish AI Society (SAIS) Workshop SAIS, p. 14 (2014)

9. Fisch, B.: EEG Artifacts. LSU Medical Center (2000)

10. Misra, U.K., Kalita, J.: Clinical Electroencephalography. Elsevier, Amsterdam (2005)

11. Stern, J.M.: Atlas of EEG Patterns. Lippincott Williams & Wilkins, Philadelphia (2005)

12. Sovierzoski, M.A., Argoud, F.I.M., de Azevedo, F.M.: Identifying eye blinks in EEG signal analysis, pp. 406–409. IEEE (2008)

13. Shamsaei, G.R.: Review of clinical electroencephalography. Jundishapour University of Medical Sciences (2014)

14. Spriggs, W.H.: Essentials of Polysomnography. Jones and Bartlett Publishers, LLC, London (2010)

15. Binnie, C.D., Rowan, A.J., Gutter, T.H.: A Manual of Electroencephalographic Technology. Cambridge University Press, Cambridge (1982)

16. Barlow, J.S.: Automatic elimination of electrode-pop artifacts in EEG's. IEEE Trans. Biomed. Eng. **BME-33**(5), 517–521 (1986)

17. Lecoutre, L., Lini, S., Bey, C., Lebour, Q., Favier, P.A.: Evaluating EEG measures as a workload assessment in an operational video game setup. In: PhyCS, pp. 112–117 (2015)

18. Wang, P., Li, S., Shao, M., Liang, C.: A low-cost portable real-time EEG signal acquisition system based on DSP. Int. J. Signal. Process. Image Process. Pattern Recogn. **9**, 239–246 (2016)

A Data-Driven Model Based on Support Vector Machine to Identify Chronic Hypertensive and Diabetic Patients

Cristina Soguero-Ruiz[1]([✉]) [ID], Pablo de Miguel-Bohoyo[2] [ID],
and Inmaculada Mora-Jiménez[1] [ID]

[1] Department of Signal Theory and Communications, Telematics and Computing,
Universidad Rey Juan Carlos, Madrid, Spain
{cristina.soguero,inmaculada}@urjc.es
[2] University Hospital of Fuenlabrada, Fuenlabrada, Madrid, Spain
pablo.miguel@salud.madrid.org

Abstract. Hypertension and diabetes are chronic conditions that have a considerable prevalence in the elderly. It is estimated that both hypertensive patients and people with diagnosed diabetes double cost of normotensive individuals and those in the absence of diabetes, respectively. It is therefore important to pay attention to these chronic conditions, both from a health and economical point of view, especially in scenarios with budget limitations.

Clinical identification of chronic patients can be performed by feeding data of the patient encounters with the healthcare system to population classification systems such as Clinical Risk Groups (CRGs). CRGs classify individuals in unique and excluding health status categories taking both demographic and clinical information during certain period of time.

In this work, we characterize healthy and chronic hypertensive and diabetic population at different chronic statuses (CRG) according to gender, age, diagnoses and drugs. After this characterization, we propose to use a supervised machine learning approach, in particular Support Vector Machines, to construct a data-driven model identifying the patient health status. We conclude that drugs and diagnoses are quite informative to discriminate patients with hypertension and diabetes, achieving promising results with the use of data-driven models.

Keywords: Hypertension · Diabetes · Chronic condition ·
Clinical Risk Groups · ICD9-CM diagnosis codes · ATC drug codes ·
Prediction · Machine learning · Support Vector Machines

This work has been partly supported by Research Project TEC2016-75361-R and by Network of Excellence TIN2017-90567-REDT, from the Spanish Government, and by Research Project DTS17/00158 from Institute of Health Carlos III.

A. Holzinger et al. (Eds.): PhyCS 2016–2018, LNCS 10057, pp. 110–129, 2019.
https://doi.org/10.1007/978-3-030-27950-9_7

1   Introduction

Financial crisis and budgetary adjustments have caused a deep concern among the population, in terms of access to basic social services. In this sense, health services have been profoundly affected by budget cuts [15], and the question about the sustainability of the health system has reappeared. Several initiatives have emerged in order to improve the efficiency and the use of resources management. In this sense, the health status evolution of chronic patients is vital for the adequate allocation of available resources, and hence, for the sustainability of the health system.

Given that aging and chronicity go hand in hand [1], the joint impact on health spending is an important task to deal with. In fact, more than 80% of the expenditure of the healthcare system is related to chronic diseases, and it is estimated that 75% of the population will suffer from a chronic condition anytime in their lives.

Two of the chronic conditions with more prevalence are arterial hypertension (AHT) and diabetes mellitus (DM). AHT is characterized by high blood pressure on the walls of the arteries (in particular, systolic/diastolic pressure greater than 140/90 mm Hg). It is generally named a "silent disease" because it rarely shows symptoms alerting the patient, and therefore it is usually non-detected. Regarding DM, it is characterized by high concentrations of glucose in the blood, persistently or chronically, due either to a defect in the production of insulin, to a resistance to the action of it to use glucose, to an increase in the production of glucose or to a combination of them. Clinically speaking, the relevance of controlling arterial hypertension is high, since AHT is one of the risks for a cardiovascular accident and can be associated to the onset of other chronic conditions such as chronic kidney or heart diseases. On the other hand, diabetes can be associated to visual problems, chronic kidney disease, heart diseases or depression, among others. It is also known that AHT is also related to diabetes, and their joint presence is known to have dreadful outcomes [16]. From an economical point of view, in 2016 the average annual expense per hypertensive patient is about $776, and $2.565 for DM, with high costs in dispensation of medical drugs [29].

Nowadays, a large number of developed countries use Patient Classification Systems (PCSs) as a basic tool for cost management and resource allocation [10,17]. Within the different PCSs, we focus on those which take into account all the patient encounters with the health system during a period of time. These are called Population Classification Systems or Population Groupers, and are very useful to provide information on the general morbidity of the population as well as to identify specific groups of patients with important care needs and high consumption of resources. From the viewpoint of financing, they can be used as a means to allocate the necessary resources in different areas or health centers [32]. There are several Population Groupers, among them: Adjusted Clinical Groups (AGS), mainly used for reimbursement in primary care, Diagnosis Cost Groups (DCGs), and Clinical Risk Groups (CRGs), oriented to the chronic population.

In this work, we consider the CRGs as the most suitable system for patient classification [4,14]. Since CRGs are also the most extensively used grouper, we will consider it for research purposes. The CRGs take into account all the information available in the different areas of care (inpatients, outpatients, pharmacy dispensation or functional health status) during a certain period of time (normally one year) and classify each patient into a single mutually exclusive category (risk groups) with clinical logic. In terms of economical cost, patients in the same category have a similar resource consumption.

Since different codification systems of diagnosis can be available according to the area of attention, a previous stage of code standardization has to be performed by a clinical coding expert. The International Classification of Diseases - 9th revision-Clinical Modification - (ICD9-CM) [7] has been considered in this work for diagnosis coding in primary and specialized care. For pharmacy dispensation, the Anatomical, Therapeutic, Chemical (ATC) [22] classification system has been taken into account.

The powerful of machine learning techniques to predict the patient health status has been validated in several works [12,28]. For example, in [12], age, gender and diagnosis codes were used in order to classify patients into three health statuses (healthy, hypertensive, and hypertensive with comorbidities) by using Support Vector Machines (SVMs). SVM provides good theoretical properties for discovering hidden knowledge in data.

The aim of this work is twofold. On the one hand, to provide an explanatory analysis of demographic data, ATC drug codes and ICD9-CM diagnosis codes related to healthy, chronic hypertensive and diabetic patients. On the other hand, to apply machine learning techniques, specifically, Support Vector Machines (SVM) to predict the health status of a patient. In the long term, the goal is to analyze clinical data for a long enough period to find patterns identifying potential patients related to chronic conditions highly prevalent in the population. The creation of predictive models could allow us to identify population groups on which act in the early stages of the disease. This could help to avoid the worsening of their health status and quality of life, as well as to reduce the impact that chronic diseases has on the health expenditure. In this sense, the work presented here can be considered as one of the first stages, since only coded contacts for one year have been considered.

The rest of the paper is organized as follows. Section 2 describes the chronic conditions and its importance from a clinical point of view. The PCSs are presented in Sect. 3, and the database in Sect. 4. Section 5 presents a descriptive population analysis of ICD9-CM diagnosis and ATC codes and their evolution for different health status. A predictive analysis based on Support Vector Machines (SVM) considering demographic data, ICD9-CM and ATC drug codes is provided in Sect. 6. Finally, conclusions are presented in Sect. 7.

2   Chronic Conditions: Hypertension and Diabetes

Chronic conditions are diseases lasting three months or more according to the definition of U.S. National Center for Health Statistics. Life expectancy, together with tobacco and alcohol use, lack of physical activity as well as unhealthy eating habits are major contributors to leading chronic conditions [5]. Previous studies have shown that 88% of the population aged 65 years and older have at least one chronic condition [13]. Furthermore, the prevalence of chronic diseases is increasing, expecting alarmed figures like by 2020 nearly 50% of the population will have at least one chronic condition [34]. Therefore, it is not surprising that considerable efforts have been oriented towards preventing the progression of specific chronic diseases such as AHT and DM [12, 28].

A patient is considered hypertensive when the force that the blood exerts against the vessel walls (blood pressure) is higher than a certain value, and it happens repeatedly when measuring the arterial tension. This can increase the risk of suffering from heart attacks, strokes and others [16]. Some factors, such as age or gender can increase the risk of suffering from AHT [21]. Specifically, blood pressure increases with age [24]. Regarding gender [3], women who are older than 55 are more likely to develop AHT than men, though men younger than 55 have more risk to develop ATH.

Regarding diabetes, the number of people suffering from diabetes has increased from 108 million in 1980 to 422 million in 2014 [18], with a higher increase in low-middle income countries. Millions of deaths have been attributable to high blood glucose in the last decade, occurring almost half of them before patients aged 70 years old. Indeed, the World Health Organization estimates that diabetes will be the seventh leading cause of death by 2030 [18]. In general, diabetes can be the trigger for several comorbidities related to the heart, the blood vessels, the nerves and the eyes. For example, patients suffering from diabetes are more likely to have heart attacks and strokes [9]. Kidney failure or breathing problems are also diabetes-related complications [31]. Furthermore, diabetes with reduced blood flow increased the risk of infections and amputations. On the other hand, more than 2% of blindness is associated to diabetes [6].

Apart from that, it is known that DM is a complication of AHT and that DM is complication of AHT [23]. It is important to note that the number of patients suffering more than one disease (i.e., comorbidity) is increasing due to population aging [33]. Therefore, efforts to treat and research the relationship of DM, AHT and other diseases are needed to achieve a good quality of life [8]. For these reasons, in this work we focused on AHT and DM.

3   Patient Classification Systems

Developed countries use PCSs for clinical purposes and also as a basic tool for cost management. PCSs are based on the idea that diagnoses, procedures and drugs are good at predicting health spending, so it is possible to obtain clinical information and expenditure with the same data set. PCSs are built from a set of clinical rules that assign each patient to one of a limited collection of homogeneous groups in terms of resources use and/or health status. There are different families of PCS, those based on diagnosis/procedure and severity called

Diagnosis Related Groups (DRGs), those based on clinical risk called Adjusted Clinical Groups (ACGs) and, in a residual way, those based on disability (DPs).

The family based on DRGs is the most used all over the world [25] to analyze the hospital case mix, as well as for reimbursement and financing healthcare processes. DRGs were created in Yale University at the end of 60's as a system to classify each healthcare episode at a hospital, creating groups with clinical coherence and similar use of hospital resources [2]. The final goal was to obtain a capitation payment system for MEDICAID, a state program in the U.S. that help covering medical costs to people with limited income or resources. In PCSs, every episode of the same patient can create a different DRG, being the same or different depending on the diagnoses assigned. So we will find a DRG for each inpatient. Associated to each DRG there is a weight reflecting the consumption of resources respect to an average DRG, which is considered as a comparison unit. Some countries use this weight, along with other metrics (hospital stay, and others), to compare hospital activity and funding them.

The main limitation of DRGs is that they only consider inpatients, but in the healthcare system there is much more activity (primary care, outpatients, pharmacy). Additionally, DRGs just analyze information for healthcare episodes, without considering data during a period of time. The identification of chronic conditions based on DRGs can be a difficult task since these diseases tend to be reflected in certain diagnosis and pharmacy dispensation. Therefore, for chronic patients identification, it would be more appropriate to use a system considering all encounters of the patient with the health system. PCSs that are prepared to take into account all encounters of the patient with the health system are named Population Classification Systems or Population Groupers. As previously indicated in Sect. 1, Population Groupers usually consider age, gender, diagnoses and procedures and other factors that affect the health status during a certain period of time [10]. Over the last years, pharmacy dispensation has also been incorporated to the clinical rules of some Population Groupers, transforming the drug into a diagnosis code when there is a direct relationship between them, in order to obtain a more complete knowledge about the health status.

Population Groupers named CRGs (developed by 3M^{TM}) are a population classification system using inpatient and ambulatory diagnosis and procedure codes, pharmaceutical data and functional health status for a period of time (usually one year [20]) to assign each patient to a single, severity-adjusted group. Each 3M CRG represents a clinically meaningful group of individuals who require similar amount and types of resources. 3M CRGs describe the health status and burden of illness of individuals in a population, and can help identify medically complex individuals with different chronic conditions and severity levels within a population. This will allow an individual to be related to the amount and type of healthcare resources that the patient will need in the future [2].

There are 1080 different groups (health statuses) in the CRG classification system. Each health status, called CRG from now on, is identified by 5 digits. There are 9 core health status groups (first digit), which are subdivided into 272 chronic condition categories (CCC, next three digits). Categories, in turn, are subdivided into severity levels (SL, last digit), yielding a total of 1080 groups. The core groups are hierarchically organized as follows: CRG-1 (healthy/non-user) composed by 2 CCC, without SL; CRG-2 (significant acute) with 6 CCC and without SL; CRG-3 (single minor chronic), 41 CCC and 2 SL; CRG-4 (multiple minor chronic pair), 1 CCC and 4 SL; CRG-5 (single dominant/moderate chronic) 107 CCC and 2 or 4 SL; CRG-6 (multiple significant chronic pair), 61 CCC and 2 or 4 SL; CRG-7 (chronic triplet), 21 CCC and 6 SL; CRG-8 (metastatic malignancy), 22 CCC and 4 SL; and CRG-9 (catastrophic), 11 CCC and 4 SL. As an example, CRG-51913 corresponds to the group of single dominant/moderate chronic diseases (first digit), and specifically refers to coronary atherosclerosis (next three digits), with the third level of severity (last digit).

Owing to the limitation in the number of patients with multiple chronic conditions, we discarded the SL and created new groups named base-CRGs. This way, base-CRGs will have a reasonable size (higher than original CRG groups) to apply data-driven techniques. In particular, we considered just the first four digits of the original CRG name to create the base-CRGs. Thus, for example, base-CRG 5192 encompasses patients with AHT and four severity levels (CRG-51921, CRG-51922, CRG-51923, and CRG-51924).

4 Database Description

Our database comes from the Electronic Health Record (EHR) of the University Hospital of Fuenlabrada (UHF) in Madrid, Spain, during the year 2012. Specifically, demographic data (age and gender) and clinical encounters (diagnoses, procedures and pharmacy dispensation) were considered from individuals categorized by the CRG system as healthy, hypertensive, diabetic, and with multiple chronic conditions related to AHT and DM.

Four different base-CRG associated to diabetic and hypertensive patients, coded by four numbers, were analyzed: base-CRG 5192 (hypertension), base-CRG 5424 (diabetes), base-CRG 6144 (hypertension and diabetes), and base-CRG 7071 (hypertension, diabetes and other dominant chronic disease). Patients classified in CRG-1 (healthy, base-CRG 1000) have been also considered in our study, providing a total of 65174 individuals, as detailed in Table 1.

Table 1. Number of patients per base-CRG during the year 2012 in UHF.

Base-CRG	Individuals in 2012
1000	46835
5192	12447
5424	2166
6144	3179
7071	547
Total	65174

Table 2 shows the gender and age distribution per base-CRG. In general, there is a balance between both genders except for base-CRG 5424, with the highest proportion for men. For base-CRG 7071 the proportion of women is slightly higher than men. In this CRG, the mean age is higher than in the others, with a higher life expectancy for women. This can be the reason to explain this fact.

Regarding the age distribution, Table 2 shows that healthy patients are younger than chronic ones, what is quite reasonable. In general, patients with AHT and DM (no comorbidity, just one chronic condition) tend to be younger than individuals with comorbidities (base-CRG 6144 and base-CRG 7071).

Table 2. Gender distribution (in %) and age (mean and std) per base-CRG.

Base-CRG	Gender		Age Mean (std)		
	Men	Women	Men	Women	Total
Base-CRG 1000	47.3	52.7	26.09 (15.9)	26.56 (15.4)	26.34 (15.7)
Base-CRG 5192	48.0	52.0	54.3 (12.3)	53.3 (16.1)	53.8 (14.4)
Base-CRG 5424	65.2	34.8	49.7 (14.2)	48.9 (17.5)	49.4 (15.5)
Base-CRG 6144	55.2	44.8	59.9 (9.9)	64.35 (11.8)	61.9 (11.1)
Base-CRG 7071	44.2	55.8	64.0 (11.3)	68.0 (12.1)	66.2 (11.9)

On the other hand, Fig. 1(a) and (b) show the distribution of patients per health status with an specific number of different ICD9-CM and ATC codes, respectively. Horizontal axis indicates the number of different codes per patient during 2012. Note that healthy individuals have a lower number of ICD9-CM and ATC codes than chronic patients, what seems quite reasonable. Additionally, the mode in the number of different codes per patient increases with the number of chronic conditions, being higher for ATC than for diagnosis codes. Specifically, the modes for diagnosis codes and base-CRG are: 1, 3, 3, 4, and 6, respectively; whereas for ATC codes are: 0, 3, 4, 6, and 9. Note also that the distribution tends to be heavy-tailed in the right hand side as the number of chronic conditions increases. These results are consistent with the comorbidity associated to each base-CRG.

5   Health Status Analysis in Terms of Diagnostics and Drugs

A population analysis to get the clinical profile per CRG-base, as well as the most frequent codes, is first presented in Sect. 5.1. Then, the evolution of codes associated to health statuses is analyzed in detail in Sect. 5.2.

5.1   Medical Profiles

Diagnostics and medications are described according to international medical coding systems: ICD9-CM and ATC, respectively. The syntax of ICD9-CM is based on categories (the three first digits), subcategories (the next digit after a dot) and sub-classifications (the second digit after the dot). For example,

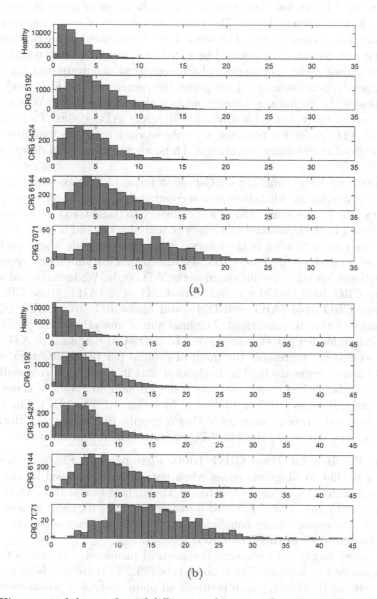

(a)

(b)

Fig. 1. Histogram of the number of different codes per patient assigned to each health status: (a) diagnosis codes; and (b) ATC codes.

diagnoses codes (000-999) can be written as "XXX.XX", V codes (V01-V89) as "VXX.XX", E codes (E800-E999) as "EXXX.X", and M codes (M8000-M9970) as "MXXXX.XX", where X is a digit number between 0 and 9. As for the case of CRG-base, to have a higher number of patients with a specific diagnosis code, in this work we will consider just the categories. Thus, considering just the codes before the dot, there are 1517 different ICD9-CM diagnosis codes.

Regarding ATC codes, their syntax is a combination of seven letters/digits, organized in five different levels. The first level consists of one letter and refers to the anatomical main group. The second level indicates the therapeutic subgroup and consists of two digits. The third and fourth levels consist of one letter and indicate the therapeutic/pharmacological subgroup and the chemical/therapeutic/pharmacological subgroup, respectively. The fifth level of the code indicates the chemical substance and consists of two digits. When considering all levels, there are a total of 3430 different ATC codes. To reduce the number of ATC codes for analysis, we only worked with the four first levels, i.e., we omitted the chemical substance. Thus, we work with 746 different ATC codes.

To have a medical profile per CRG-base in terms of diagnoses and drugs, we compute the average profile taking into account the presence of codes per patient in a group. The profile associated to a specific group (base-CRG in this case) is a graph showing in the horizontal axis every potential code, and in the vertical axis the presence rate (a number in the interval $[0, 1]$) of every code when considering patients associated to that base-CRG, see also [12]. This number represents the rate of patients having a specific diagnosis or ATC code. We focus on individuals from base-CRG 1000 (healthy users), base-CRG 5192 (AHT), base-CRG 5424 (DM), base-CRG 6144 (AHT and DM), and base-CRG 7071 (AHT, DM and other dominant chronic condition). The final aim of analyzing these profiles consists of finding hidden patterns associated to ICD9-CM diagnosis or ATC codes. Figure 2(a) and (b) represents the medical profiles per base-CRG for diagnosis and ATC codes, respectively. The horizontal axis in Fig. 2(a) correspond to an index for the ICD9-CM codes: diseases codes (from 1 to 1000), V codes (from 1001 to 1091), E codes (1092 to 1319) and M codes (1320 to 1517). The vertical axis represents the rate of patients having a specific diagnosis code. Horizontal axis in Fig. 2(b) represents the 746 ATC codes considered in this work.

Medical Profiles for Base-CRG 1000. First panel in Fig. 2(a) shows the profile for ICD9-CM diagnosis codes when patients are classified by the CRGs system as healthy. According to this figure, the highest rate is 15%, which corresponds to *jaws issues* (526), followed by *common cold* (460) and *general symptoms* (780). As expected, we conclude that there is no diagnosis code with an outstanding presence in this base-CRG.

First panel in Fig. 2(b) presents the medical profile of ATC codes for individuals classified as healthy. The highest rate (29.2%) corresponds to *propionic acid derivatives* (M01AE), which includes all plain ibuprofen preparations even if they are only intended for use as pain relief. The second ATC code most frequent is *anilides* (N02BE), including common drugs such as paracetamol. The rate for the other ATC codes is lower than 15% for healthy patients.

In general, these results seem reasonable, since the most common diagnoses are acute diseases and they can be considered as normal issues in healthy individuals. Clinicians and experts validated that these codes are related to common diseases.

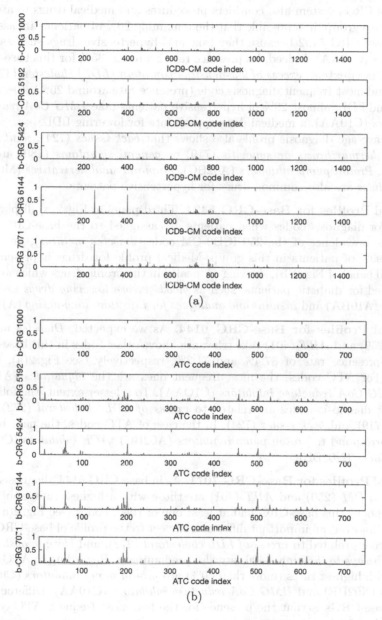

Fig. 2. Medical profile per base-CRG considering: (a) ICD9-CM diagnosis codes; and (b) ATC codes.

Medical profiles for Base-CRG 5192. Second panel in Fig. 2(a) and (b) shows the presence rate of diagnosis and drug codes, respectively, for patients assigned to the base-CRG 5192. Different from base-CRG 1000, now there is a dominant diagnosis code, *essential hypertension* (401), with a presence rate about 80%. This was expected since base-CRG 5192 refers to hypertensive patients. However, since the CRGs system also considers procedures and medical drugs to assign a patient to a group, it is possible that the remaining 20% of patients are assigned to the base-CRG 5192 because they take anti-hypertensive drugs such as *ACE inhibitors* (C09AA). Indeed, its presence rate is around 35% for this base-CRG.

To a lesser extent, *excess of low-density lipoprotein (LDL) cholesterol* (272) is the second most frequent diagnosis code (presence rate around 20%). Regarding ATCs and LDL, almost 29% of hypertensive patients take *HMG CoA reductase inhibitors* (C10AA), a medical drug appropriate for lowering LDL.

The average diagnosis profile also shows that *back issues* (724), *joint issues such as hermarthrosis or synovitis* (719) or *general symptoms* (780) are also relevant. *Proton pump inhibitors* (A02BC), *propionic acid derivatives* (M01AE) and *anilides* are also common drugs for hypertensive patients.

Medical Profiles for Base-CRG 5424. Third panel in Fig. 2(a) displays the profile for diagnosis codes when patients are assigned to the base-CRG 5424. Note the prevalence of the 250 ICD9-CM code (*diabetes mellitus*), present in almost 90% of patients in this group. Medical profile for drugs is presented in the third panel of Fig. 2(b), showing as 'peaks' in the profile drugs which are only prescribed for diabetic patients, such as *blood glucose lowering drugs excluding insulins* (A10BA) and *insulins and analogues for injection, long-acting* (A10AE).

Medical Profiles for Base-CRG 6144. As we expected, *Diabetes mellitus (DM)* (250) and *AHT* (401) take relevance above other codes in this base-CRG, with a presence rate of 87.4% and 71.3%, respectively (see Fig. 2(a), fourth panel). For ATC codes, the most frequent ones are the *biguanides* (A10BA) and *HMG CoA reductase inhibitors* (C1OAA). To a lesser extent, the following rates for diagnosis codes are related to *excess of LDL cholesterol* (272), *joint issues* (719) and *back issues* (724). In the case of ATC codes, the next highest rates correspond to *proton pump inhibitors* (A02BC), *ACE inhibitors* (C09AA) and *anilides* (N02BE).

Medical Profiles for Base-CRG 7071. As in base-CRG 6144, diagnosis codes related to *DM* (250) and *AHT* (401) are those with a highest rate: about 80% of patients in this base-CRG had at least one of these codes (see Fig. 2(a), fifth panel). However, an important difference respect to the profile of base-CRG 6144 is that codes related to *excess of LDL cholesterol* (272), and *chronic obstruction of the airways to the lungs* (496) are also predominant. Regarding to ATC codes, those with highest rates (more than 60%) are *proton pump inhibitors* (C09AA), *anilides* (N02BE) and *HMG CoA reductase inhibitors* (C10AA). Different from other base-CRGs is that the presence for the five most frequent ATC codes is higher than 50%.

As a summary, Table 3 lists the five most probable diagnosis and drug codes per base-CRG. Several conclusions can be obtained: (1) base-CRG 1000 do not get a high percentage of common diseases or drugs; meaning that patients in this group have high variability and there is no characteristic pattern; (2) the variability in the ATC codes for all base-CRGs, and specifically for those associated to a better health status, is higher than that of ICD9-CM codes. For example, in base-CRG 1000, the most common diagnosis code has a prevalence lower than 15%, corresponding to *jaws issues* (14.8%). However, for the other base-CRGs, the prevalence rate is higher. For example, AHT is coded as a diagnostic for (74.9% of the patients in base-CRG 5192, for 71.7% in base-CRG 6144, and for 69.2% in base-CRG 7071); whereas DM appears in the (89.8% of patients in base-CRG 5424, 87.4% in base-CRG 6144 and 86.8% in base-CRG 7071).

Table 3. More frequent ICD9-CM and ATC codes, expressed as % of patients in base-CRG 1000, base-CRG 5192, base-CRG 5424, base-CRG 6144, and base-CRG 7071.

	ICD9-CM Code	Description	%	ATC Code	Description	%
base-CRG 1000	526	Jaws issues	14.8	M01AE	Propionic acid derivatives	29.2
	460	Common cold	12.3	N02BE	Anilides	19.2
	780	General symptoms	6.1	J01CA	Penicillins with extended spectrum	11.4
	463	Acute tonsillitis	8.8	J01CR	Combinations of penicillins	11.1
	558	Other issues related with gastroenteritis	8.6	R06AX	Other antihistamines	10.7
base-CRG 5192	401	Essential hypertension	74.9	N02BE	Anilides	28.2
	272	Excess of LDL (cholesterol)	20.3	C09AA	ACE inhibitors	35.3
	724	Back issues	14.0	A02BC	Proton pump inhibitors	30.7
	719	Joint issues	12.9	C10AA	HMG CoA reductase inhibitors	28.7
	780	General symptoms	10.5	M01AE	Propionic acid derivatives	27.4
base-CRG 5424	250	DM	89.8	A10BA	Biguanides	54.3
	272	Excess of LDL (cholesterol)	20.0	C10AA	HMG CoA reductase inhibitors	43.0
	719	Joint issues	12.8	M01AE	Propionic acid derivatives	28.5
	724	Back issues	10.4	N02BE	Anilides	27.8
	526	Jaws issues	9.4	A10AE	Insulins and analogues for injection, long-acting	27.4
base-CRG 6144	250	DM	87.4	A10BA	Biguanides	70.6
	401	Essential hypertension	71.3	C10AA	HMG CoA reductase inhibitors	66.4
	272	Excess of LDL (cholesterol)	27.3	A02BC	Proton pump inhibitors	48.4
	724	Back issues	13.8	C09AA	ACE inhibitors	43.9
	719	Joint issues	17.1	N02BE	Anilides	42.0
base-CRG 7071	250	DM	80.8	A02BC	Proton pump inhibitors	72.9
	401	Essential hypertension	69.2	N02BE	Anilides	64.2
	780	General symptoms	31.1	C10AA	HMG CoA reductase inhibitors	62.5
	272	Excess of LDL (cholesterol)	28.7	A10BA	Biguanides	59.4
	496	Chronic obstruction of the airways to the lungs	20.1	N02BB	Pyrazolones	59.4

Continuing with the analysis of Table 3, it may be observed that the ATC code *anilides* (N02BE) appears in all the considered CRGs: 19.2% in base-CRG 1000, 28.2% in base-CRG 5192, 27.8% in base-CRG 5424, 42.0% in base-CRG 6144, and 64.2% in base-CRG 7071. This is an expected result, since most individuals take *anilides* such as paracetamol, independently of the health status of the patient. However, the ATC code *HMG CoA reductase inhibitors* (C10AA) appears in all base-CRGs, but not in the one related to healthy patients.

5.2   Evolution of ICD9-CM and ATC Codes

Figure 3(a) and (b) show the evolution of the diagnosis and ATC codes, respectively, with higher presence rate according to the health status (base-CRG) in 2012.

For the evolution of diagnosis codes, note that nearly 75% of the hypertensive patients (base-CRG 5192) have the diagnosis code '401' (AHT), while DM ('250') is present in more than 85% of patients assigned to base-CRG 5424, base-CRG 6144 and base-CRG 7071. It is clear from Fig. 3(a) how *excess of LDL* (cholesterol, diagnosis code '272') increases its prevalence with the number of the health core status (from groups CRG-base 5192 to CRG-base 7071). It is in base-CRG 7071, associated to the worst chronic condition among those considered here, where *excess of LDL* takes the highest presence rate (about 30%). Regarding the diagnosis code '526' (*jaws issues*) with the highest rate in the group of healthy patients, it appears at a similar rate in all base-CRGs (presence rate lower than 15%). Code of *general symptoms* ('780') is also present in every group, with the highest rate in base-CRG 7071 (about 30%), nearly tripling its presence regarding healthy patients. This fact can be justified by the fact that patients in the seventh core group have a high number of comorbidities, and so the *general symptoms* code is quite frequent when attending to the doctor. We conclude stating that the evolution of the diagnosis codes with the health status was as expected: AHT has a high presence over acute diseases in base-CRGs 5192, 6144 and 7071, getting a similar behavior for DM in the last two base-CRGs. Besides, we verify the relationship between healthy patients and acute diseases, these being present in a low rate.

Respect to the evolution of ATC codes, note that the presence rate for *propionic acid derivatives* (M01AE), which includes drugs such as ibuprofen, is similar for all base-CRGs, around 30%. However, the rate for *anilides* (N02BE), which includes paracetamol, is higher for patients assigned to base-CRG 6144 and base-CRG 7071. This behavior is similar for *proton pump inhibitors* (A02BC), which is used to treat gastro-oesophageal reflux diseases. With lower presence rate, the dispensation of other analgesis and antipyretics such as *pyrazolones* (N02BB) is common for all base-CRGs, though there is an increase for base-CRG 7071. On the other hand, there are certain drugs not prescribed to healthy patients. For example, the *HMG CoA reductase inhibitors* (C10AA), used to treat the hypercholesterolemia, or the *ACE inhibitors* (C09AA), considered as an antihypertensive drug but can be indicated for other pathologies (this is the reason why it appears in the profile of patients associated to base-CRG 5424). There are

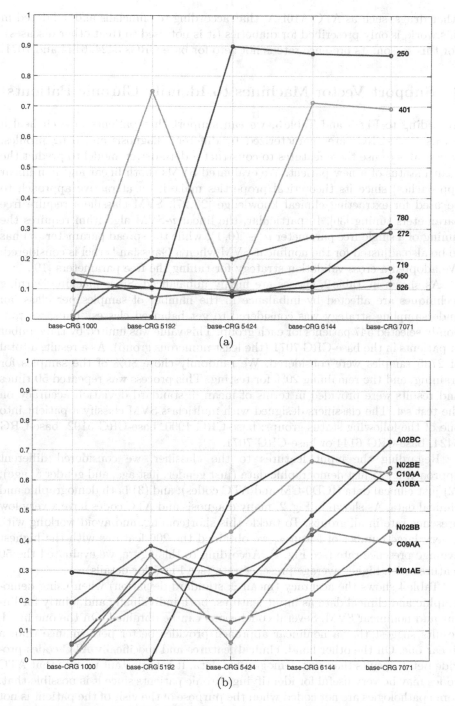

Fig. 3. Evolution of the ICD9-CM diagnosis codes (a) and ATC codes (b) with the highest presence rate in terms of health status (base-CRG).

other drugs, such as ATC A10BA, that according to clinicians and validated in this work, is only prescribed for diabetics (it is not used to treat other diseases). For this reason, its presence rate is not zero for base-CRGs 5424, 6144 and 7071.

6   Support Vector Machines to Identify Chronic Patients

According to Fig. 3 and Table 3, we can support that patients in each health status (base-CRG) are characterized by different diagnosis and drug profiles. Our goal is to use these features to construct a data-driven model to predict the health status of a new patient. We evaluated SVMs (both linear and non-linear approaches) since its theoretical properties make it an attractive approach to be used for extracting clinical knowledge [26,27]. SVM classifiers require free parameters tuning [30]. In particular, the linear ν-SVM algorithm requires the tuning of a single free parameter $\nu \in (0,1)$, while the spread parameter (σ) has to be also adjusted for the nonlinear SVM when a Gaussian kernel is considered. We adopted a cross-validation strategy for tuning the free parameters [19].

As shown in Table 2, classes are highly unbalanced. Since machine learning techniques are affected by imbalance in the number of samples per class, an undersampling strategy was considered to get balanced classes. Thus, we randomly selected 547 patients for each group. This value was limited by the number of patients in the base-CRG 7071 (the least numerous group). As a result, a total of 2735 samples were considered. We randomly chose 80% of the samples for training, and the remaining 20% for testing. This process was repeated 50 times and results were provided in terms of mean ± standard deviation accuracy on the test set. The classifiers designed with multiclass SVM classify a patient into one of the following status groups: base-CRG 1000, base-CRG 5192, base-CRG 5424, base-CRG 6144 or base-CRG 7071.

Regarding the input features to the classifier, we considered different approaches: (1) just demographic data (just gender, just age, and gender & age); (2) just clinical data (ICD9-CM and ATC codes); and (3) both demographic and clinical data. As shown in Fig. 2, many diagnosis and ATC codes have a very low presence rate in all groups. To tackle this shortcoming, and avoid working with a very large number of features, we obtained the 200 features with the highest average presence rate (see Fig. 4). According to this figure, we evaluated the 50 features with higher average presence rate (see Fig. 5 for details).

Table 4 shows the accuracy (mean ± standard deviation) when using demographic and clinical data as input features, both individually and jointly for linear and nonlinear SVM. Several conclusions can be obtained. On the one hand, results suggest that a nonlinear approach provides better performance than a linear one. On the other hand, clinical features and specifically ATC codes provide better results than just demographic data. It is important to note that ATC codes may be very useful for identifying chronic patients since it is possible that, some pathologies are not coded when the purpose of the visit of the patient is not the chronic disease. This result also validates the claim that drug information is better coded than that related to diagnostics. This can be based on the fact

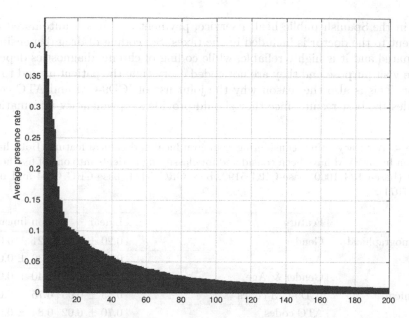

Fig. 4. Sorted average presence rate for the 200 most frequent features taking into account both diagnosis and ATC codes.

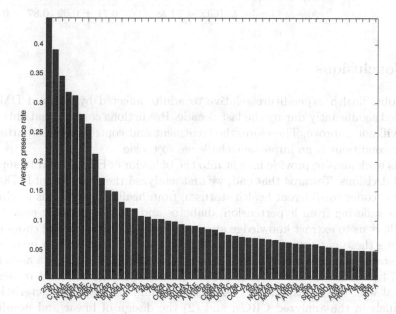

Fig. 5. Average presence rate and ICD9-CM and ATC description for the 50 codes with higher rate.

that, in the Spanish public health service, payment of drugs is automated and payment to the doctor is included in the taxes. So, coding of drug dispensing is automated and it is highly reliable, while coding of chronic diagnostics depends on the visit purpose and they are not coded every time the patient attend to the doctor. This is also the reason why the joint use of ICD9-CM and ATC codes provides the best result, since they should provide supplementary information.

Table 4. Accuracy values considering demographical and clinical feature. Both linear and non linear SVM have been considered for classifying patients into one of five health status (base-CRG 1000, base-CRG 5192, base-CRG 5424, base-CRG 6144 and base-CRG 7071).

	Feature	Linear	Non linear
Demographical	Gender	0.20 ± 0.02	0.21 ± 0.02
	Age	0.25 ± 0.09	0.39 ± 0.01
	Gender & Age	0.25 ± 0.06	0.40 ± 0.02
Clinical	ICD9-CM codes	0.55 ± 0.05	0.75 ± 0.01
	ATC codes	0.70 ± 0.02	0.84 ± 0.03
Demographical and Clinical	Age & Gender & ICD9-CM	0.60 ± 0.05	0.68 ± 0.03
	Age & Gender & ATC	0.70 ± 0.02	0.76 ± 0.03
	Age & Gender & ICD9-CM & ATC	0.71 ± 0.02	0.87 ± 0.01

7   Conclusions

The global health expenditure relative to adults affected by EH and DM has increased significantly during the last decade. Predictions confirm that this situation will not improve. Therefore, the treatment and control of these particular chronic conditions is an important challenge to tackle.

This work aims to provide insight into the behavior of EH and DM to support clinical decisions. Towards that end, we first analyzed the evolution of ICD9-CM and ATC codes by different health statuses: from healthy individuals to chronic patients suffering from hypertension, diabetes and multiple chronic conditions. This allows us to extract knowledge about the most common clinical codes characterizing these patients. Then, a data-driven model is designed to predict the health status of a new patient. To this end, we considered EHRs data associated to 65174 patients of UHF during 2012. The methodology followed to achieve this goal was: (1) an exploratory analysis to summarize the characteristics of individuals in the analyzed CRGs; and (2) the design of linear and non-linear models based on SVM.

For the exploratory analysis, we first focus on gender and age. Regarding the gender, the percentage of diabetic men is slightly higher than that of diabetic women in our population. The national diabetes statistic report (2017) about the estimates of diabetes and its burden in the United Stated provides similar percentages [11]. Regarding the age, our analysis confirmed that the older the patients are, the more comorbidities they have. We also analyzed the number of diagnosis and drug codes per patient and health status by means of a population analysis. We can claim that patients in CRG-1000 are characterized by less diagnosis and ATC codes compared to other CRGs.

For the predictive analysis of the health status, linear and nonlinear SVM classifiers were designed. Demographic and clinical features were considered, both individually and jointly. The highest accuracy is obtained when a nonlinear SVM is trained with ATC codes, considering also age and gender. Compared to previous results obtained without considering medical drugs [12], we can conclude that when including information about ATC codes, we enhance the classifier performance and we are able to extract more knowledge about chronic conditions.

In conclusion, our analysis has allowed us to describe and verify the relationship that demographic and standardized clinical data, collected from patient encounters with primary and specialized care, have with the patient health status.

References

1. Anderson, G., Horvath, J.: The growing burden of chronic disease in America. Public Health Rep. **119**(3), 263–270 (2004)
2. Averill, R.F., et al.: Development and evaluation of clinical risk groups (CRGs). 3M Health Information Systems, Wallingford, CT (1999)
3. Banegas, J.B.: Epidemiology of arterial hypertension in Spain. Present situation and perspectives. Hipertensión **22**(9), 353–362 (2005)
4. Berlinguet, M., Preyra, C., Dean, S.: Comparing the value of three main diagnostic-based risk-adjustment systems (DBRAS). Technical report, Canadian Health Services Research (2005)
5. Booth, F.W., Roberts, C.K., Laye, M.J.: Lack of exercise is a major cause of chronic diseases. Compr. Physiol. **2**(2), 1143 (2012)
6. Bourne, R.R., et al.: Causes of vision loss worldwide, 1990–2010: a systematic analysis. Lancet Glob. Health **1**(6), e339–e349 (2013)
7. Centers for Disease Control and Prevention: International Classification of Diseases, Ninth Revision, Clinical Modification (ICD-9-CM) (2011). http://www.cdc.gov/nchs/icd/icd9cm.htm. Accessed Mar 2018
8. Chin, Y.R., Lee, I.S., Lee, H.Y.: Effects of hypertension, diabetes, and/or cardiovascular disease on health-related quality of life in elderly Korean individuals: a population-based cross-sectional survey. Asian Nurs. Res. **8**(4), 267–273 (2014)
9. Emerging Risk Factors Collaboration and others: Diabetes mellitus, fasting blood glucose concentration, and risk of vascular disease: a collaborative meta-analysis of 102 prospective studies. Lancet **375**(9733), 2215–2222 (2010)
10. Davis, N.A., LaCour, M.: Foundations of Health Information Management. Elsevier Health Sciences, Amsterdam (2016)
11. Centers for Disease Control and Prevention and others: National diabetes statistics report. Centers for Disease Control and Prevention, Atlanta, GA (2017)

12. Fernández-Sánchez, J., et al.: Clinical risk groups analysis for chronic hypertensive patients in terms of ICD9-CM diagnosis codes. In: Proceedings of the 4th International Conference on Physiological Computing Systems, vol. 1, pp. 13–22 (2017)
13. Hoffman, C., Rice, D., Sung, H.Y.: Persons with chronic conditions: their prevalence and costs. JAMA **276**(18), 1473–1479 (1996)
14. Hughes, J.S., et al.: Clinical risk groups (CRGs): a classification system for risk-adjusted capitation-based payment and health care management. Med. Care **42**(1), 81–90 (2004)
15. Karanikolos, M., Heino, P., McKee, M., Stuckler, D., Legido-Quigley, H.: Effects of the global financial crisis on health in high-income OECD countries: a narrative review. Int. J. Health Serv. **46**(2), 208–240 (2016)
16. Mancia, G., et al.: 2007 guidelines for the management of arterial hypertension. Eur. Heart J. **28**(12), 1462–1536 (2007)
17. Marazzi, A., Gardiol, L., Duong, H.D.: New approaches to reimbursement schemes based on patient classification systems and their comparison. Health Serv. Manage. Res. **20**(3), 203–210 (2007)
18. Mathers, C.D., Loncar, D.: Projections of global mortality and burden of disease from 2002 to 2030. PLoS Med. **3**(11), e442 (2006)
19. Nasrabadi, N.M.: Pattern recognition and machine learning. J. Electron. Imag. **16**(4), 049901 (2007)
20. Newhouse, J.P., Buntin, M.B., Chapman, J.D.: Risk adjustment and medicare: taking a closer look. Health Affairs **16**(5), 26–43 (1997)
21. NHLBI: Risk Factors for High Blood Pressure (2016). http://www.nhlbi.nih.gov/health/health-topics/topics/hbp/atrisk. Accessed 29 May 2016
22. Norwegian Institute of Public Health: WHO Collaborating Centre for Drug Statistics Methodology, Guidelines for ATC classification and DDD assignment, Oslo (2016)
23. Ohishi, M.: Hypertension with diabetes mellitus: physiology and pathology. Hypertens. Res. **41**, 389 (2018)
24. Pinto, E.: Blood pressure and ageing. Postgrad. Med. J. **83**(976), 109–114 (2007)
25. Rice, N., Smith, P.C.: Capitation and risk adjustment in health care financing: an international progress report. Milbank Q. **79**(1), 81–113 (2001)
26. Soguero-Ruiz, C., et al.: Support vector feature selection for early detection of anastomosis leakage from bag-of-words in electronic health records. IEEE J. Biomed. Health Inform. **20**(5), 1404–1415 (2016)
27. Soguero-Ruiz, C., et al.: Predicting colorectal surgical complications using heterogeneous clinical data and kernel methods. J. Biomed. Inform. **61**, 87–96 (2016)
28. Soguero-Ruiz, C., et al.: On the use of decision trees based on diagnosis and drug codes for analyzing chronic patients. In: Rojas, I., Ortuño, F. (eds.) IWBBIO 2018. LNCS, vol. 10814, pp. 135–148. Springer, Cham (2018). https://doi.org/10.1007/978-3-319-78759-6_14
29. Soni, A., Mitchell, E.: Expenditures for commonly treated conditions among adults age 18 and older in the U.S. civilian noninstitutionalized population (2016), statistical Brief, 487, May 2016. Agency for Healthcare Research and Quality, Rockville, MD. Accessed 22 Feb 2017
30. Steinwart, I., Christmann, A.: Support Vector Machines. Springer, New York (2008). https://doi.org/10.1007/978-0-387-77242-4
31. United States Renal Data System: 2015 USRDS annual data report: epidemiology of kidney disease in the United States (2015)

32. Vivas-Consuelo, D., Usó-Talamantes, R., Guadalajara-Olmeda, N., Trillo-Mata, J.L., Sancho-Mestre, C., Buigues-Pastor, L.: Pharmaceutical cost management in an ambulatory setting using a risk adjustment tool. BMC Health Serv. Res. **14**(1), 462 (2014)

33. Weale, R.A.: A note on age-related comorbidity. Arch. Gerontol. Geriatr. **49**(1), 93–97 (2009)

34. Wu, S.Y., Green, A.: Projection of chronic illness prevalence and cost inflation. RAND Health, Santa Monica, CA, 18 2000

Inner Flower: Design and Evaluation
of a Tangible Biofeedback for Relaxation

Morgane Hamon[1], Léo Cousin[2], Rémy Ramadour[1], and Jérémy Frey[1]([⊠])

[1] Ullo, 40 rue Chef de Baie, La Rochelle, France
{morgane.hamon,remy.ramadour,jeremy.frey}@ullo.fr
[2] Inria Bordeaux, 200 avenue de la Vieille Tour, Talence, France
leo.cousin@inria.fr

Abstract. Anxiety is a common health issue that can occur throughout one's existence. In this paper we describe the process design and the evaluation of Inner Flower, a tangible biofeedback device aimed at reducing anxiety. Inner Flower is meant to be used during daily life to help users regulate their anxiety and improve their overall mental health. It serves as a breathing guide that is being adapted to users through heart rate measurements. The Inner Flower does not intrude into users' routine, instead it acts as an ambient display that operates in the peripheral vision. The Inner Flower was evaluated through two studies. The first one took place in a replica apartment in order to assess its usability and how people would appropriate the device. The second study assessed the effect of the device when stressors were presented to participants. We show how the final design of the Inner Flower was praised by users and how it can reduce symptoms of stress when users focus their attention on it. We then draw future research directions to further assess the effect of an ambient display and determine the importance of the biofeedback component of the device.

Keywords: Biofeedback · Tangible interface ·
Relaxation ambient display · Interoception · Design

1 Introduction

At times, to endure fear might be beneficial, when one is facing dangerous situations or unknown events. "Fight or flight" responses were proven important for survival. However if stress becomes chronic and is not treated, it can be a factor of sleep disorders or cardiovascular disease [13]. It can also lead to a pathological state of anxiety when the anticipation of stressing stimuli is sufficient to trigger the same symptoms as with the actual appearance of stimuli. Finding effective and lasting solutions to reduce stress is necessary to alleviate this public health problem, which impedes the lives of many. Treatments exist against stress and anxiety, but they might require a strong and timely involvement (i.e. therapies) or provoke side effects (i.e. drugs). Studying anxiety and offering alternative

© Springer Nature Switzerland AG 2019
A. Holzinger et al. (Eds.): PhyCS 2016–2018, LNCS 10057, pp. 130–157, 2019.
https://doi.org/10.1007/978-3-030-27950-9_8

solutions to drugs (sport, yoga, mindfulness) is a growing body of research, and nowadays tools exist to let people autonomously reflect on their states and better act upon themselves. This paper describes the design process and the assessment of the Inner Flower, a tangible and ambient biofeedback aimed at relaxation that was first described in [8].

1.1 Biofeedback

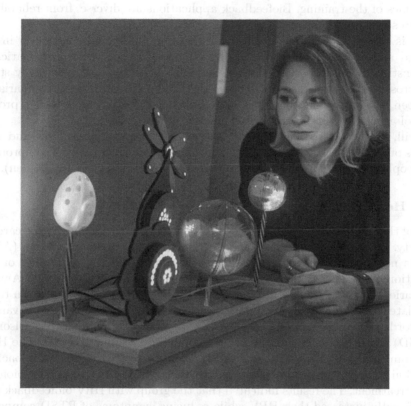

Fig. 1. In this example heart-rate is measured through a smartwatch; tangible interfaces serve both as breathing guides for the user and as biofeedback devices (image © Inria, photograph C. Morel, extracted from [8]).

Biofeedback is a method that enables users to learn to control autonomous bodily processes. Biofeedback is part of a larger notion known as "interoception" which is defined by [5] as *"the sense of signals originating within the body"* or *"the process of receiving, accessing and appraising internal bodily signals"*. Biofeedback relies on physiological measurements and is getting more and more popular thanks to the increasing availability of non-invasive sensors (Fig. 1). Most of the time, signals originate from respiration, electrodermal activity (EDA) or heart rate (HR) [19].

While these processes are mostly involuntary and with weak level of consciousness, through physiological sensors it becomes possible to visualize them in real-time. Users are then able to view effects of a particular behavior on their physiology. For example if a person wearing a HR sensor begins to run, HR is going to increase suddenly. Connected to a biofeedback display, the increase of HR could be symbolized by a color change, a blinking light, or simply seen as a graph. This information can then be used to help users regulate their state, for example staying within a specific HR range to prevent injuries or maximize the outcomes of the training. Biofeedback applications are diverse, from rehabilitation to stress management [19].

It is worth noting that despite the fact that biofeedback has been investigated and applied for decades, its effectiveness has not been systematically demonstrated. Notably, even though a review such as [32] presents many studies across a variety of medical applications, there are hardly any comparisons between biofeedback and sham feedback, which is the only way to form a proper control group and pin-point the real efficacy of the technique.

Still, as a drug-free and a non-invasive approach, potential risks and side effects of Biofeedback are small. With a medical opinion it could be a compromise for people who can not or do not want to take drugs (e.g pregnant women).

1.2   Heart Rate Variability: A Marker of Anxiety

One of the most studied case of biofeedback for stress management is the cardiac activity. Heart Rate is under control of the autonomous nervous system (ANS) and is not constant at rest. Heart Rate Variability (HRV) – a marker of the evolution of HR over time – is a representative index of ANS activity. Among the variety of factors that could influence HR, a low HRV has been shown to be correlated with impaired parasympathic activity, higher anxiety, and a variety of disorders [30]. [29] showed that veterans with Post Traumatic Stress Disorder (PTSD) had a HRV significantly lower than subjects without PTSD. The HRV was compared between veterans with PTSD who received HRV biofeedback in addition to their regular treatment and veterans without the additional biofeedback treatment. The results indicated that the group with HRV biofeedback had significantly increased their HRV while reducing symptoms of PTSD compared to the other group. Finding ways to assist people to learn to increase their own HRV and improve their health is one of the motivations of our study.

1.3   Increasing Heart Rate Variability

Deep breathing is a well documented manner to increase the HRV. "Cardiac Coherence" is a notion according to which respiration and cardiovascular functions are synchronized. That means the HR increases during the inhalation and decreases during exhalation, and so periodically [18]. Authors proposed that 6 breaths per minute is the respiratory frequency that allows one to reach cardiac coherence and the highest amplitude in heart rate oscillations (hence the highest HRV) [3]. Cardiac Coherence is then *a priori* obtained when breathing at a 0.1 Hz frequency which corresponds to six 10-s breathes per minute.

Several studies have investigated a static breathing guidance at 6 breaths per minute to reduce stress. For example in [31], where authors showed that HRV was higher after the breathing exercise, while subjective impressions – as measured by the State Trait Anxiety Index questionnaire, or STAI [28] – were not different. In [4] authors designed an immersive system which is composed of a blanket containing small vibrating motors (haptic stimulus) and headphones (audio stimulus). Haptic and audio stimuli are synchronized and generated at such a frequency that the user can follow them as a breathing guidance. One of the studied frequency modality was 6 breaths per minute. Some participants reported the frequency as too fast or too slow. The Authors highlighted that a poorly adapted frequency can potentially create hypo/hyperventilation.

Even if a static guidance might on average be optimal for the population, it is not the best way to maximize HRV for each individual. As a matter of fact, [30] found that resonant frequency (equivalent to the cardiac coherence) differs according to each person. By exposing a breathing guidance from 4.5 to 6.5 breaths per minute to their participants, they managed to define the best frequency for each subject.

As such, we opted for an adapted breathing guidance to create our biofeedback; in our current study we compare it with a fixed breathing feedback (i.e. "Dynamic" vs "Static" feedback) in order to have a better grasp on the effect of an adapted biofeedback.

1.4   Shaping the Best Biofeedback

[23] proposed a certain type of biofeedback to achieve higher HRV and reach a resonant frequency. In this study, a graph based on HR fluctuations was created, having users inhaling until the HR reaches a "peak" and exhaling until it reaches a "pit". Because of the improved HRV as compared to breathing exercises agnostic to HR, we also designed a biofeedback device that would use HR measurements to propose an adapted breathing guide.

However, the feedback modality used to convey the information back to the user is important, and graphs are not the only way to present a breathing guidance. Actually, such kind of feedback might even impede acceptability because it could appear as being too judgmental due to its close relationship to a metric. In order to craft a more "organic" and yet informative biofeedback, we decided instead to rely on a physical object to present the feedback.

Indeed, thanks to recent advances in human-computer interaction, it is now possible to directly integrate digital information within users' surroundings, for example through the use of tangible interfaces. These interfaces have been proven effective to help people learn about bodily processes – see e.g. [6]. Through tangible interfaces, biofeedback can then be more easily integrated in the natural settings of users, and become part of a specific scenario.

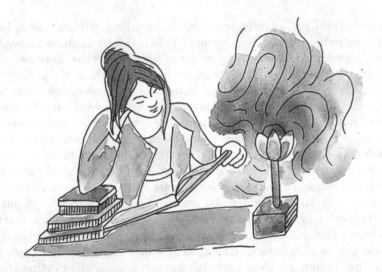

Fig. 2. Illustration of an ambient device; the person is focused on another task but is still able to receive peripheral information.

1.5   Ambient Feedback

Ambient computing contrasts with disrupting notifications. In this context "ambient" refers to information that is being presented in the peripheral attention of users [16]. Ambient devices do not mobilize attention. They require minimal efforts from the user and yet they provide informative feedback; rather than "pushing" a notification it is up to users to "pull" information when they require it. Figure 2 illustrates this notion.

Along those lines, [22] highlights two ways to train respiration: consciously thinking about it or learning to follow an external stimulus such as a pacing light or an auditory guide. While the former method implies focus of attention, the latter, if proven effective, could alleviate the required amount of cognitive resources [10].

In [22], authors investigated whether a breathing guidance at the periphery of the screen during work had an influence on respiratory rate. As this type of guide does not require full attention they called it *Peripheral Paced Respiration (PPR)*. This ambient guide can be very useful by allowing the user to fully commit to another task. The guide rate setting was 20% below the user baseline. They showed significant difference on breath rate depending on the activation of the PPR. The same thinking led [1] to develop a wearable device that delivers tiny vibrations on the wrist with a frequency 20% slower than the participant resting HR. Users didn't know the function of the device and were preparing an oral presentation (to induce stress). Results showed that the control group had significantly higher anxiety according to questionnaires (STAI) and physiological data (EDA).

[27] investigated in a longitudinal study if a device called BIM (for Breathe with Interactive Music) had a positive influence on Blood Pressure (BP). The BIM device creates a musical pattern which is related to the user breathing rate. A 10 min long quiet synthesized music recording was used as an active control. Results showed BP reduction was greater in the experimental group compared to the control, and seem to have a long-term effect (significantly different 6 months after).

Based on these various findings, we decided to investigate not only a "Focus" but an "Ambient" utilization of a tangible biofeedback device as well. In order to better frame our experimental design, we turned to previous work from psychology and physiological computing that aimed at investigating various dimensions of stress.

1.6   Evaluating and Inducing Stress

Inducing stress to evaluate short-term effects of biofeedback devices is common in the literature. To artificially put participants in a more stressed state increases the range of measurements and help to reduce variability between subjects. Different type of stress can be induced, physical (e.g. extreme heat or cold), psychological (e.g. increase in mental workload) or psychosocial (e.g. public speaking) [24]. Psychosocial stress can be induced by faking an interview – Trier Social Stress Test [12] – or simply asking participants to prepare a speech, as in [1].

In [31] authors induced psychological stress with a mathematical task for a ten-minutes period. Several manners exist to check if the stress inducing task had an effect. First, it can be detected by recording physiological data, for example with HRV as a marker of anxiety. EDA is also a common recorded measure – e.g. [26] – to detect arousal. Because physiological signals might have poor specificity, those indicators do not represent how participants are feeling, what is their state of mind. Questionnaires can compensate for this situation. To measure anxiety the most frequently used questionnaire is the STAI as in [1,31], or [24]. In the latter work authors compared the robustness of various physiological signals to detect stress. They crossed psychosocial stress (TSS) with psychological stress, by manipulating the amount of cognitive workload endured by participants. To do so, they employed the N-back task, which leverage on memory load [25]. We chose to use the N-back task as well to induce stress in our study since it is effective in doing so and since we can easily compute a performance metric to sense how participants might be affected by the exposition to a tangible biofeedback.

1.7   Objectives

In the present paper, our first objective is to describe the design process of a tangible device meant to regulate anxiety. Users were presented to the device in an ecological environment, that let them better express how they would use it during their daily life. Using questionnaires and a semi-structured interview, we assessed the usability and the perception of the device.

Our second objective is to investigate if an ambient modality could have positive effects on stress. To explore this issue we compared two modalities: Ambient *vs* Focus. "Ambient" stands for the presence of the device during the whole experiment (30 min) in the peripheral visual field of the participant. "Focus" refers to a short (6 min) utilization in the middle of the experiment requiring full-attention.

Our third objective is to check the relevance of breathing guidance based on HR. Indeed, as we propose a new device it is important to consider that any observable effect might be due to a "novelty effect". Moreover, we wanted to assess the usefulness of actually measuring physiological activity. Hence we compare a true biofeedback ("Dynamic" condition, where the breathing guide is adapted using HR) with a sham biofeedback, or "pseudofeedback" ("Static" condition, where the breathing guide is set to a fixed rate). As explained by [11], a *"pseudofeedback is defined as a non contingent stimulus presented in exactly the same manner as the true biofeedback and with the intention of having subjects believe that it is true biofeedback"*.

2   Designing the Inner Flower

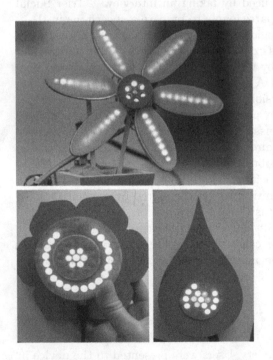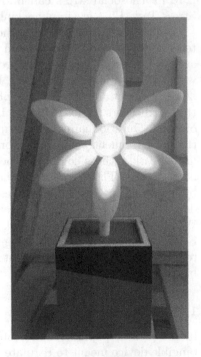

Fig. 3. *Left*: Examples of prototypes toward a tangible biofeedback. *Right*: Design of the Inner Flower used in the study. From [8].

To design the Inner Flower we investigated features as the shape, the color, or the way it conveys information. As our long-term objective is to deploy the device outside the laboratory, we assessed its relevance, its usability and asked people how they would used it. Among the key questions we tried to answer: "Is this device useful? For who? Where the user is going to use it? What time of the day? For which reason?". In this section we try to answer them, focusing on the user experience, while in Sect. 3 we describe a second study where we assess the effect of the device in various conditions when users are presented with a stressor.

2.1   Prototyping

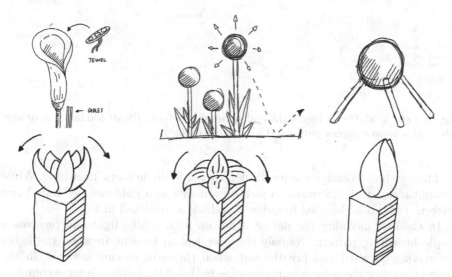

Fig. 4. *Top*: Examples of prototypes toward an abstract shape. *Bottom*: Sketches of a mechanic flower acting as a breathing guide.

We iterated over various form factors to craft a tangible biofeedback that could both act as an ambient feedback and as a breathing guide. Among the biofeedback modalities that are traditionally employed – visual, audio or haptic – [7] suggests that there is little difference regarding the effectiveness of conveying a breathing feedback. We chose to rely on visuals with color LEDs since they offered many degrees of freedom to work with (e.g. location of the lights, intensity, color, speed of the animation) and since it was easy to implement. We employed laser cutting, Arduino-based micro-controllers (Arduino mini), and Adafruit[1] Neopixel LEDs to prototype several artifacts (Fig. 3).

---

[1] https://www.adafruit.com/.

It quickly became apparent that frosted plastic was the best material to work with in order to improve the LEDs' diffusion, smooth the light and prevent an impression of a pixelated display, which would be too much reminiscence of a desktop display. Regarding the actual appearance of the object, after having explored more abstract shapes (as shown in Fig. 4), we decided to create a somewhat stereotypical flower in order to convey a sense of well-being. Additionally, as one might want to smell the scent of a flower, it is in a way a valid proxy for breathing.

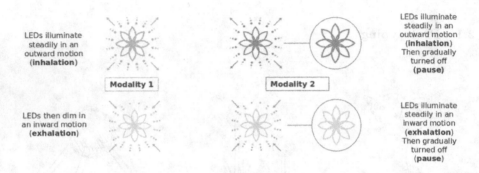

Fig. 5. *Left:* Modality 1: blue light and a simple pattern, *Right:* Modality 2: orange light and a more complex pattern. (Color figure online)

Then we had to design the feedback that would guide users' breathing. While it might seem straightforward to pick movements as a guidance, we tested two patterns that could be used to guide breathing as depicted in Fig. 5.

In the first modality the device lights up with a blue light and presents a simple breathing pattern. Namely the user has to breathe in when the lights are moving outward and breathe out when they are moving inwards. In the second modality, the color is warm (orange-red) and the pattern is more complex. The inhalation and exhalation have to be performed in a two steps: breathe in, hold breath, breathe out, pause before a new inhalation. The light pattern for this modality had accordingly two phases per inhalation and exhalation: lights gradually turn on outwards (breathe in) then gradually turn off (pause), then they turn on gradually inwards (breathe out), and finally they turn off (pause before a new cycle).

Even when the use of the Inner Flower is coupled with a smartwatch measuring heart rate, there was no direct representation of this metric (e.g. no light blinking upon detection of heartbeats) so as not to overwhelm users with information not related to current usage scenarios.

2.2   Measures

SUS. To assess usability we chose to use different standardized scales. The System Usability Scale (SUS) [2] is a 10-item short form to evaluate the general opinion of the user about the device. Statements like "I think this device is easy to use" have to be rated by users according to a 5-point Likert Scale. A resulting score over 100 is computed by averaging all items of the questionnaire.

Context of Use. To evaluate the interest of such a device we designed our own questionnaire to ask participants the context of use of this type of device. As shown in Fig. 6, each statement is combined with a sketch. Questions about where to use the device, what time of the day, how many times a day are part of this form. An additional question asked which modality and which color the user preferred.

If I had to use the device, I would put it...

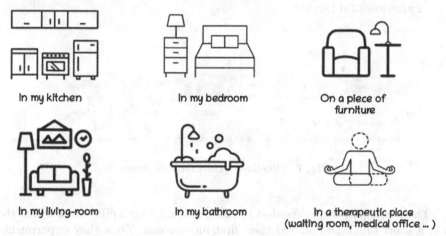

In my kitchen	In my bedroom	On a piece of furniture
In my living-room	In my bathroom	In a therapeutic place (waiting room, medical office ...)

Fig. 6. To evaluate the context of use we asked participants to imagine where they would put the device.

AttrakDiff. We chose the AttrakDiff questionnaire [9] to measure the pertinence, the hedonic qualities and the attractiveness of the device. AttrakDiff enables the designer to gain a deeper insight about how users perceive a device, how likeable it is and if it answers their needs. The questionnaire is a 7-point Likert scale with 28 items presenting two words semantically antagonist. It is scored from −3 to 3.

As the study took part in France we used a validated French version [14]. The form assesses usability according to 4 categories (7-item each): Pragmatic Quality, Hedonic Quality-Identity, Hedonic Quality-Stimulation and Attractiveness.

2.3   Procedure

A total of 13 participant took part in the study. They all went through the same procedure, and experienced the two modalities we described earlier.

This design study took place in the replica of an apartment, that was recreated within the host research facility in order to create more ecological scenarios. The apartment was equipped with a kitchen, a bedroom, and a living-room with a table, one couch and a TV.

The procedure, depicted in Fig. 7, comprised the following main steps:

First, the user was welcomed and led to the apartment (see Fig. 8). A short explanation about the experiment was given to the user, after which they fulfilled the information consent form. We then explained how the Inner Flower worked. As the device acts as a breathing guidance, we ensured that the participant understood both display modalities before proceeding.

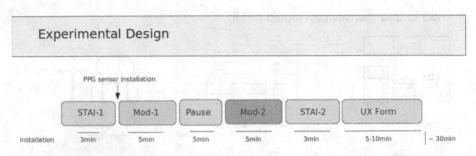

Fig. 7. Timeline of the first experiment.

The participant experimented the first modality for 5 min, after which they had a short break and shared their first impressions. Then they experimented

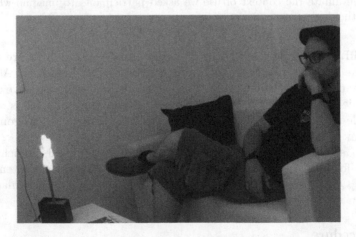

Fig. 8. A participant evaluating the Inner Flower during the design study that took place in the replica of an apartment.

the second modality for 5 min. Lastly they fulfilled the various questionnaires described previously (AttrakDiff, SUS, context). The whole experiment duration was about 30 min.

Note that during this study participants also fulfilled a STAI questionnaire at the beginning and at the end of the session. Moreover, they were equipped with smartwatch measuring heart rate. This was aimed at controlling their stress level. Since a dedicated study investigating reaction to stress is related in the next section, we deliberately chose to focus here on the design considerations associated with the Inner Flower.

2.4   Results and Discussion

Context of Use and Personal Preferences. When we asked participants about where they would use the device, 75% would use it in the bedroom and 57% in the living room. The bathroom was among the least cited (15%) location, and only 4% of participants would place the Inner Flower on a desk – maybe due to the configuration of the replica apartment. About the usage scenarios, 66% would use it during a stress episode and 42% would use it in order to better sleep. That is being reflected by the reported preferred time to use the device, 70% would use it before going to bed while 30% would use it after upon getting up in the morning. Interestingly, 50% of users envisioned a therapeutic use of the Inner Flower. Despite the fact that after the sessions with the Inner Flower 87% of participants reported being more relaxed, only a minority (23%) would use it several times a day, while 67% would use it once over the course of the day and 14% would have a more moderate utilization of the device. These numbers have to be put in perspective with the fact that the Inner Flower is meant to be used as an ambient display, i.e. functioning while users perform other activities. Most likely participants could not fully grasp such scenario over such a short exposition.

Participants preferred the blue color over the orange color (8/13, including 2 non-respondent), blue possibly being more easily associated to a breathing exercise or to a relaxing environment. Participants were ambivalent about the modalities. Despite the fact that the second modality was more complex and might appear less intuitive, half participants (7/13) preferred it over the first modality. We hypothesized that the increased complexity of the pattern was more involving for participants. An alternative and complementary hypothesis is that this particular breathing pattern, with a pause between each inhalation and exhalation, felt more natural. Overall, the diversity of users' preferences highlights how customization would play an important role to ensure the acceptability of the device. In the future we will create tools so that users can easily switch colors and patterns in order to adapt the Inner Flower to their taste and preferred breathing.

SUS and AttrakDiff. The average SUS score was 62.15 (SD: 15.11), as depicted by Fig. 9. That denotes a rather good usability of the system.

Results of the AttrakDiff questionnaire are presented Fig. 10. The average Pragmatic Quality was 1.32 (SD: 0.72). While the Inner Flower was perceived as "simple" or "straightforward", a majority of users reported its unpredictability. This might be related to the comprehension of the various modalities, as discussed in the previous section.

The average Hedonic Quality-Identity was 0.37 (SD: 0.73). This is the lowest score of the 4 dimensions that were measured by the AttrakDiff. It is caused by the fact that users perceived the Inner Flower as being both isolating and separating. The very nature of the activity, that is meant to focus users on their own breathing through a biofeedback, could explain this result. There are however ways to use biofeedback to improve in social settings. In [26] for example an ambient device embedded in the workplace informed those around about one's state, which resulted in colleagues being more sensitive to the emotional states

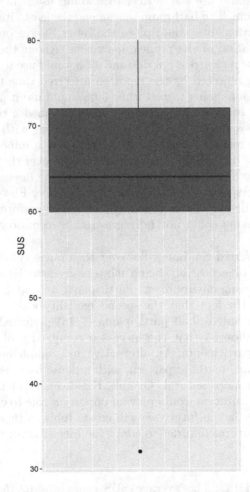

Fig. 9. Usability as measured by SUS during the first study.

of others. We discuss in Sect. 4 how we envision a social utilization of the Inner Flower.

The average Hedonic Quality-Stimulation was 1.75 (SD: 0.51), with the Inner Flower described as something new or creative, while users are mixed regarding its challenging aspect, maybe due to the unchanging nature of the device that they tested.

When the pragmatic and hedonic qualities of the Inner Flower are weighted one against the other (Fig. 11), the Inner Flower lean toward being a desired object.

The average Attractivity was 2.19 (SD: 0.56). This was the dimension most praised by users, who were unanimous concerning qualities such as its likeability or its appeal. This result is a milestone toward the validation of the current form factor of the Inner Flower, that will be evaluated as a relaxation device in the next section.

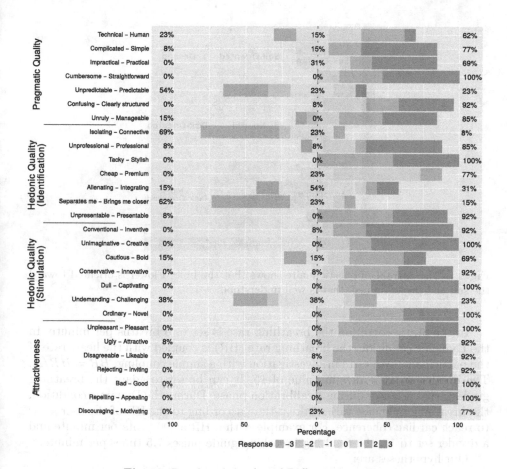

Fig. 10. Results of the AttrakDiff questionnaire.

3   Investigating the Inner Flower as a Relaxation Device

In this section, we investigate the effect of the Inner Flower when users are exposed to a stressor. The form factor was identical to the device used in the previous section. For this study we chose to use a blue light and the breathing guidance pattern from the second modality, both of which were preferred in the design study.

This study possesses a 2 (Attention: Ambient *vs* Focus) × 2 (Biofeedback: Dynamic *vs* Static) between-subject experimental plan. As a result we split our participants into four distinct groups: Ambient-Dynamic, Ambient-Static, Focus-Dynamic and Focus-Static.

Because in the Focus group the device is used only mid-experiment, the first part of the experiment in Focus serves as a control group (no device) for the investigation of attention.

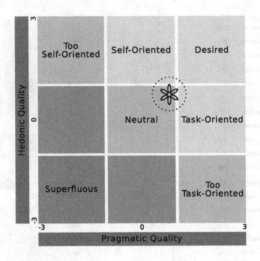

Fig. 11. The AttrakDiff questionnaire shows that the Inner Flower is oriented toward the self and present a task that is well understood.

In the Static condition the breathing rate is set to 6 breaths per minute. In the Dynamic condition, the breathing rate (BR) is coupled with the heart rate of the participant. We start our investigation with a simple coupling: $BR = HR/\Delta$. The divider Δ has a default value of 15. It can be set to adapt the breathing guidance to each user during a calibration phase. During the Dynamic condition, the breathing guidance varies in real-time according to the HR of the user so as to reach cardiac coherence. For example with a HR at 90 beats per minute and a divider set to 12, the resulting breathing guide pulses 7.5 times per minute.

Our hypotheses are:

H1. Exposition to an Ambient feedback (H1a) or to a Focus feedback (H1b) reduces psychological stress.

H2. An adapted breathing guidance with a biofeedback device (Dynamic) will reduce stress as compared to a pseudofeedback (Static).

H3. The usability resulting from the use of a biofeedback device is improved as compared to a pseudofeedback (Focus-Dynamic *vs* Focus-Static).

3.1 Measures

During the study we were interested in collecting two types of data: the (psychological) stress level of participants, and a usability index related to the tangible biofeedback. Stress was assessed along three dimensions: physiological activity (HR), behavioral measures (performance in a N-back task) and questionnaires (STAI). Usability was assessed through a questionnaire (USE) administered at the end of the experiment for those groups that explicitly used the device (i.e. Focus groups).

Heart Rate. Each participant was equipped with a smartwatch measuring heart rate ("Link" from Mio[2]), placed on their non-dominant hand. Mio smartwatches employ photoplethysmography (PPG) to compute heart-rate, a technique which basically detects variations in skin's color to assess heartbeats. This solution was preferred over electrocardiography (ECG) to improve comfort and acceptance of the system, which is meant to be used in ecological settings, outside the laboratory. Even though PPG is less robust than ECG, being that the participants are steady and seated, i.e. without the risk of creating motion artifacts throughout this study, PPG is a sufficiently good sensor. During pilot studies, we validated that the instantaneous HR measured by this particular smartwatch was accurate enough to detect changes in HRV associated with deep relaxation.

Data was collected over Bluetooth, processed in real-time in the Dynamic condition and stored for further analysis. From HR measurements we focused our investigation on one index of HRV: RMSSD – root mean sum of the squared differences. RMSSD takes as input the inter-beat interval (the inverse of the instantaneous HR measured by the smartwatch). It is one of the best indicator of cognitive workload [20], a specific type of psychological stress induced during the experiment.

N-Back. The N-back task served both to induce psychological (cognitive) stress, and to evaluate the cognitive load of participants. The latter is revealed by calculating participants' performances. During this task, as in [24], each letter appears on the screen for 0.5 s every 2 s. Participants have to determine whether the current letter is the same as the one they saw N steps before (left click on a mouse) or not (right click). We employed a 2-back task (Fig. 12), which showed to induce a high workload level [24]. Typically, when workload increases the performance during the task decreases.

---

[2] https://www.mioglobal.com/.

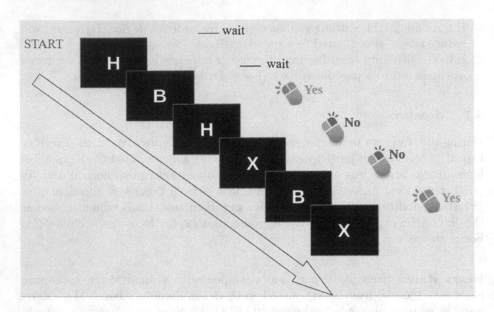

Fig. 12. 2-back task. Participants have to click left when the displayed letter is the same as two steps before (from [8]).

An immediate feedback is provided to inform participants whether their answers are correct or not. Two N-back tasks were presented to each participant, denoted as "N-back1" and "N-back2". Each task is comprised out of three sequences of one minute (30 letters). The first task (N-back1) includes an additional sequence at the beginning that acts as a training session. Over each N-back task we measured participants' performance (percentage of correct answers).

STAI. The State Trait Anxiety Index (STAI) enables the measurement of self-reported anxiety levels [28]. The STAI Y-A version of the questionnaire measures anxiety as a state (about one's current endeavor). The classical version is composed of 20 items (e.g. "I am tense"; "I feel content") that participants rate on a 4-point Likert scale. A higher score reflects a higher anxiety state. Because we administrated multiple times the STAI during the experiment, we favored a six-item short-form [17]. It was faster to fill by participants and still produced similar scores to those obtained with the full-form.

Usability. In order to assess the usability of the device, we adapted the USE questionnaire [15]. We removed the "Usefulness" subscale because it was not relevant to our study – participants did not use the device long enough. Questions were translated to French. The resulting questionnaire comprises three subscales: "Ease of use", "Ease of learning" and "Satisfaction". Each is composed of three items (e.g. "I easily remember how to use it", "It is simple to use"). Participants had to state their agreement to each sentence on a 4-point Likert scale

("Not at all" ... "Very much"). Since such usability questionnaire is poorly suited to assess an ambient device, with which users merely interact directly and/or consciously, the USE was only administrated to participants of the Focus groups.

3.2   Participants

A total of 36 volunteers (18 females) took part in the study. Overall the mean age was 23.80 years old (SD = 4.82). The demographics per group is depicted in Fig. 13.

3.3   Procedure

The timeline of the experiment is presented Fig. 14. The experiment took place in a quiet room, deprived of distractions, and we detail it step by step as follows.

Upon entering the room and sitting at a table, participants signed a consent form. Afterwards we proceeded to explain briefly how the experiment would take place and equipped participants with the smartwatch. The Inner Flower was then switched on and its core functionalities were explained to participants. In the Focus-Dynamic group, a calibration phase occurred in order to determine a pace that would suit users (i.e. obtaining a breathing guide that would not appear too fast nor too slow). After the calibration, the device was switched off. On the other hand, the Focus-Static group had no calibration, hence the device was simply switched off. Lastly in the Ambient groups the device was left active on the side of the table, in the peripheral vision of participants.

Device modality	Feedback modality	
	Dynamic	Static
Ambient	10 people (5 ♀ - 5 ♂) mean age = 21.1 sd = 4.54	9 people (5 ♀ - 4 ♂) mean age = 24.5 sd = 4.99
Focus	8 people (4 ♀ - 4 ♂) mean age = 24.8 sd = 6.28	9 people (4 ♀ - 5 ♂) mean age = 21.5 sd = 2.78

Fig. 13. Demographics of our groups in the second study (from [8]).

Afterwards, to induce psychological stress and control for the effect of the N-back task participants fulfilled a first STAI (STAI-1), performed a first N-back task (N-back1) and finally fulfilled a second STAI (STAI-2). At this point of the experiment, by comparing Ambient groups (active device on the side) with Focus groups (devices turned off) we are able to investigate the effect of an ambient breathing guide.

In order to assess how much the Inner Flower would affect HRV while employed as an explicit breathing guide, further in the experiment we switched-on the device in the Focus groups and participants carried out the breathing exercise. In the Ambient groups participants performed a substitute task instead; they read the short story "The Oval Portrait" by Edgar Allan Poe. Both tasks lasted 6 min and were designed to equally involve users' attention. At the end of the task, the device was switched-off in the Focus groups.

Then, all participants performed a second N-back task (N-back2). Their performance, during this test would enable us to assess the efficacy of the Inner Flower as a tool to reduce psychological stress and improve cognitive availability.

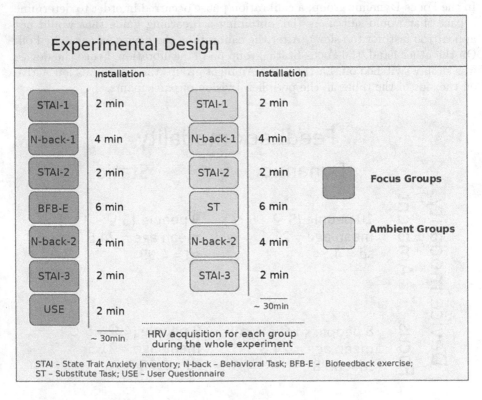

Fig. 14. Timeline of the second study (from [8]).

Finally, participants filled out a third STAI (STAI-3). Additionally, in the Focus groups, participants answered the USE questionnaire.

3.4   Results

Due to the nature of the data and the modest number of participants per group, we used non-parametric statistical tests to analyze the data. For studying HRV, N-back and STAI, we performed resampling (permutation) statistics using the Minque[3] package from R. Answers to the USE questionnaire were analyzed with a Wilcoxon rank sum test. When applicable, we tested for the effect of each main factor (Attention, Biofeedback and moment of measurement) as well as for the interaction of thereof.

HRV. HRV was computed during both N-back tasks (*time1* and *time3*) and during the breathing exercise (*time2*). There was a significant interaction between the Attention factor and time, with a difference between Focus during the breathing task ($M = 1.47 \times 10^{-2}$, $SD = 0.67 \times 10^{-2}$) and the rest of the conditions ($M = 1.07 \times 10^{-2}$, $SD = 0.48 \times 10^{-2}$, $p < 0.05$, Fig. 15). Across other factors and interactions there were no significant differences in HRV.

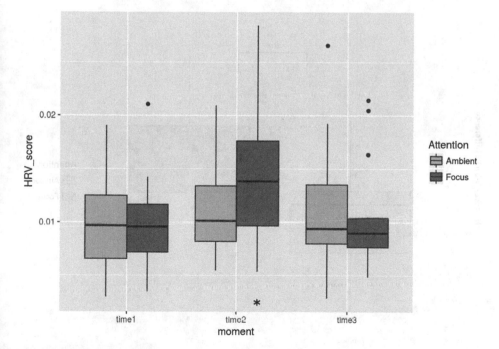

Fig. 15. HRV across Attention factor and time (i.e. during N-back1, exercise, N-back2). "*": p-value < 0.05. From [8].

---

[3] https://cran.r-project.org/web/packages/minque/minque.pdf.

Note that due to technical issues the HR data is incomplete for 5 participants (out of 36).

N-Back. We investigated the evolution of the percentage of accuracy during the N-back between the first and the second test (i.e. N-back2 - N-back1). Overall performance increased between those two tests; with a significant effect of the Attention factor. Performance increased more sharply in Focus groups (M = +11.23pp, SD = 8.36) as compared to Ambient groups (M = +4.21pp, SD = 7.03, p < 0.01, Fig. 16). Across other factors and interactions there was no significant differences in the evolution of N-back performance.

STAI. There was a significant effect of time. STAI-2 scores (after the first N-back task) were higher (M = 42.4, SD = 9.08, p < 0.01) when compared to the other scores (M = 34.8, SD = 8.57, Fig. 17, top). There was a significant interaction between Attention and time, with lower scores in the Focus groups in STAI-3 at the end of the experiment (M = 30.8, SD = 5.92), when compared to the rest of the conditions. (M, 38.5, SD = 9.48, p < 0.01, Fig. 17, bottom). Across other factors and interactions there was no significant differences.

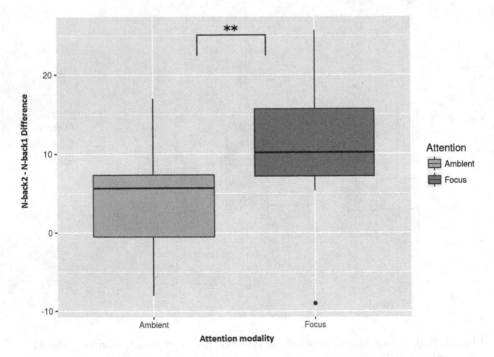

Fig. 16. Evolution of the performance between the first and the second N-back task. Performance increased further in the Focus groups. "**": p-value < 0.01. From [8].

USE Questionnaire. As mentioned earlier the USE questionnaires were fulfilled only in Focus groups. There was no significant difference between Static (M = 32.8, SD = 2.92) and Dynamic (M = 28.9, SD = 6.79, p = 0.26) groups.

3.5 Discussion

The N-back task had a significant effect on the perceived anxiety, as the STAI-2 was higher than the STAI-1. This replicates the validity of such task to induce stress.

As opposed to previous work – e.g. [31], which employed arithmetic tasks between breathing exercises – we did not measure a noticeable effect of the Ambient condition and could not validate H1a. There was no significant difference within any marker of stress (HRV, N-back performance, STAI) between participants with an active ambient device and participants with no device (beginning of the study). We would need longer experiments, or even longitudinal studies, to better grasp the influence and the dynamic of an ambient (and subtle) biofeedback. Interestingly, when asked after the experiment during informal interviews, participants in the Ambient groups reported that they did not pay attention to the device – an indicator that at the very least it was not disruptive. Still, it is possible that such an ambient biofeedback might reduce stress even more than a short explicit breathing exercise when users are exposed for a couple hours, or over the course of several days.

In contrast, over the 6-min breathing exercise participants of the Focus group demonstrated a lower level of stress on all three markers – H1b is validated. Not only did the breathing exercise increased HRV and helped participants to feel less anxious, but it also induced a higher performance during the N-back task. This scenario mirrors the (negative) effects that might arise when a psychological test is administered to a sensitive population in a stressful environment (e.g. elderly in a hospital). In similar situations, the use of a device alike the Inner Flower might increase patients' cognitive availability before a test and prevent biases during a psychological evaluation.

Since there was no effect of the Feedback modality over the course of the experiment, we cannot validate H2. An actual biofeedback did not perform better (or worse) than a simple breathing exercise based on a fixed breathing rate. There are however multiple factors that could explain this outcome and that would need further investigations.

First, by trying to give more freedom to users and finely adapt the breathing guide (i.e. calibration phase in Focus-Dynamic group) we might have introduced a higher between-subject variability, as we observed more variability in the Focus-Dynamic group.

Second, the N-back task might have resulted in a ceiling effect with some participants. While overall participants tended to improve their scores between N-back1 and N-back2, those who already had a good score (i.e. > 80%, n = 17) had difficulties to improve afterward. This plateau is among the confounding factors that we would need to control more finely during recruitment for future work, alongside personality traits.

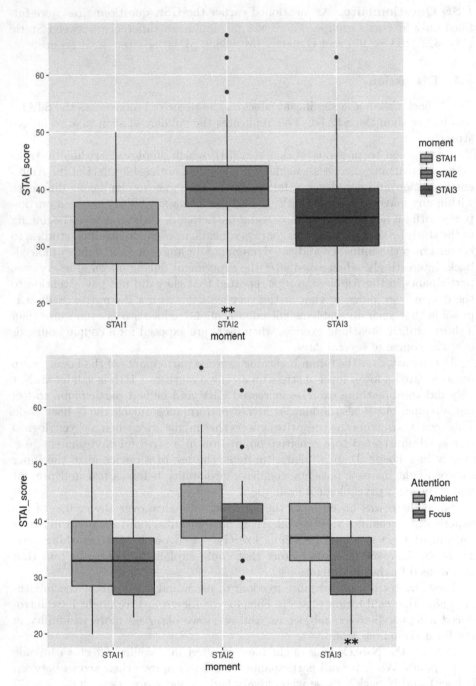

Fig. 17. *Top*: STAI scores across time (lower score: less anxiety). *Bottom*: STAI scores across Attention factor and time. "**": p-value < 0.01. From [8].

Third, and maybe most importantly, our choice of biofeedback might not have been perceived as an actual manifestation of user's physiology. While we did not want to overwhelm users with too many stimuli, the absence of a dedicated HR biofeedback might have impeded their sense of agency, i.e. users did not realize that they were actually "connected" with the device.

This latter interpretation would be on par with the fact that there was no significant difference in the usability questionnaire. With current results we cannot validate H3, since Focus-Dynamic and Focus-Static groups rated equally high the device, between 80% and 90%. We would expect a higher sense of agency (i.e. in Focus-Dynamic) to be reflected on "Ease of use" and "Ease of learning" subscales of USE.

Despite the encouraging effect on relaxation and cognitive availability of the Focus groups, when users are presented with an explicit breathing guide, the absence of results between a coupled (Dynamic) and a fixed (Static) breathing guidance highlights once again how much rigor is needed when assessing the effect of physiological measures and the resulting benefit of biofeedback.

4   Conclusions

In this paper, we shared the design process of the Inner Flower and how users perceived it when it was being used in an home studio replica, a more ecological environment than a traditional laboratory settings. While most participants envisioned using the device daily, either to help them cope with anxiety or to sooth them before going to sleep, this part of the study was limiting due to the short exposition with the device. Participants could not really grasp the fact that the device can be used as an ambient display.

In the lab study assessing its effect on stress, it is likely than an analogous limitation prevented to draw conclusions when being left activated in the peripheral vision. Still, we demonstrated how a tangible device could help to reduce

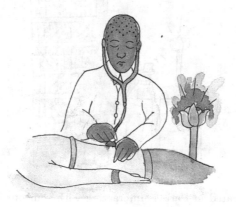

Fig. 18. The Inner Flower being used as a proxy between a caregiver and a patient.

perceived anxiety (measured with STAI) and alleviate a physiological symptom of stress (increase in HRV). Moreover, it enabled participants to improve performance in a cognitive task. Increasing cognitive availability before a psychological test is one of the most promising applications of this technology.

As shown by [10] it is difficult to evaluate ambient technology on a one-time basis because it has to be by definition blended into the environment. In the second study, conditions were maybe not ecological enough in the sense that experiments took place in a small and impersonal room. Encouraged by the important attractiveness measured during the design study, in the future we expect to deploy the device in participants home in order to both ensure an ecological scenario and a prolonged exposition. While it is harder to bring the technology outside the laboratory, longitudinal studies, over several days

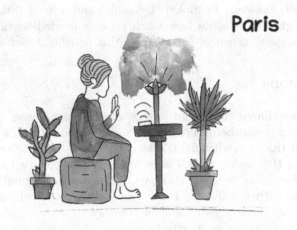

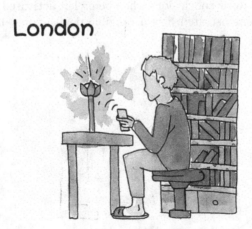

Fig. 19. A person located in Paris is interacting with someone in London using the device as a mean of communication.

or weeks, would inform us about the required amount of time for an ambient biofeedback to become effective.

While the Inner Flower was well received by participants, its main limitation pertains to how it is being employed. Indeed, despite the high usability scores and the many positive associations, it was perceived as isolating people. With the proper set of features, we do believe, though, that such technology can be employed to bring people together and increase connectedness. We recently proposed several projects in this direction: a pendant letting close ones share breathing in real time at a distance [7] or a breathing pacer triggered through heart-rate measurements that could also foster remote and yet shared relaxation sessions [21].

We furthermore hypothesize that a social usage of the Inner Flower is a way to reinforce the association with an actual biofeedback, which in turn will have positive impact on the users. Hence, we created a collaborative scenario where users would try to synchronize their heart rate through the device, with a color-based HR feedback. We envision such exercise as a way to establish trust between people. The Inner Flower could then become both a tool to manage stress and a proxy for communication, for example in situations involving patients and care givers (Fig. 18) or when people are living apart (Fig. 19).

References

1. Azevedo, R.T., Bennett, N., Bilicki, A., Hooper, J., Markopoulou, F., Tsakiris, M.: The calming effect of a new wearable device during the anticipation of public speech. Sci. Rep. **7**(1), 1–7 (2017). https://doi.org/10.1038/s41598-017-02274-2
2. Brooke, J.: SUS - a quick and dirty usability scale. In: Usability Evaluation in Industry, pp. 189–194. CRC Press (1996). https://doi.org/10.1002/hbm.20701
3. DeBoer, R.W., Karemaker, J.M., Strackee, J.: Hemodynamic fluctuations and baroreflex sensitivity in humans: a beat-to-beat model. Am. J. Physiol. Heart Circ. Physiol. **253**(3), H680–H689 (1987). https://doi.org/10.1152/ajpheart.1987.253.3. H680. http://www.physiology.org/doi/10.1152/ajpheart.1987.253.3.H680
4. Dijk, E.O., Weffers, A.: Breathe with the ocean: a system for relaxation using audio, haptic and visual stimuli. In: Special Symposium at EuroHaptics 2010: Haptic and Audio-Visual Stimuli: Enhancing Experiences and Interaction, Amsterdam, The Netherlands. Univ. Twente (2011)
5. Farb, N., et al.: Interoception, contemplative practice, and health. Front. Psychol. **6**(June), 763 (2015). https://doi.org/10.3389/fpsyg.2015.00763. http://www.pubmedcentral.nih.gov/articlerender.fcgi?artid=4460802&tool= pmcentrez&rendertype=abstract
6. Fleck, S., Baraudon, C., Frey, J., Lainé, T., Hachet, M.: "Teegi's so Cute!": assessing the pedagogical potential of an interactive tangible interface for schoolchildren. In: IDC 2018–17th Interaction Design and Children Conference. Trondheim, Norway, June 2018. https://doi.org/10.1145/3202185.3202731, https://hal.inria. fr/hal-01804324
7. Frey, J., Grabli, M., Slyper, R., Cauchard, J.R.: Breeze: sharing biofeedback through wearable technologies. In: CHI 2018 (2018). https://doi.org/10.1145/ 3173574.3174219

8. Hamon, M., Ramadour, R., Frey, J.: Exploring biofeedback with a tangible interface designed for relaxation. In: PhyCS-International Conference on Physiological Computing Systems. SCITEPRESS (2018)
9. Hassenzahl, M., Burmester, M., Koller, F.: AttrakDiff: Ein Fragebogen zur Messung wahrgenommener hedonischer und pragmatischer Qualität, pp. 187–196. Vieweg+Teubner Verlag, Wiesbaden (2003). https://doi.org/10.1007/978-3-322-80058-9_19
10. Hazlewood, W.R., Stolterman, E., Connelly, K.: Issues in evaluating ambient displays in the wild: two case studies. In: Proceedings of the SIGCHI Conference on Human Factors in Computing Systems, pp. 877–886. ACM (2011)
11. Health, T., The, S.A., Hatch, J.P.: Controlled group designs in biofeedback research: ask, "what does the control group control for?". Biofeedback Self-Regul. **7**(3), 377–401 (1982)
12. Kirschbaum, C., Pirke, K.M., Hellhammer, D.H.: The "trier social stress test" - a tool for investigating psychobiological stress responses in a laboratory setting. Neuropsychobiology **28**(1–2), 76–81 (1993). https://doi.org/10.1159/000119004
13. Kivimäki, M., Leino-Arjas, P., Luukkonen, R., Riihimäi, H., Vahtera, J., Kirjonen, J.: Work stress and risk of cardiovascular mortality: prospective cohort study of industrial employees. BMJ **325**(7369), 857 (2002). https://doi.org/10.1136/bmj.325.7369.857. https://www.bmj.com/content/325/7369/857
14. Lallemand, C., Koenig, V., Gronier, G., Martin, R.: Création et validation d'une version française du questionnaire AttrakDiff pour l'évaluation de l'expérience utilisateur des systèmes interactifs. Revue Europeenne de Psychologie Appliquee **65**(5), 239–252 (2015). https://doi.org/10.1016/j.erap.2015.08.002. http://dx.doi.org/10.1016/j.erap.2015.08.002
15. Lund, A.M.: Measuring usability with the use questionnaire12. Usability Interface **8**(2), 3–6 (2001)
16. MacLean, K.E.: Putting haptics into the ambience. IEEE Trans. Haptics **2**(3), 123–135 (2009). https://doi.org/10.1109/TOH.2009.33
17. Marteau, T.M., Bekker, H.: The development of a six-item short-form of the state scale of the Spielberger State-Trait Anxiety Inventory (STAI). Br. J. Clin. Psychol. **31**(3), 301–306 (1992). https://doi.org/10.1111/j.2044-8260.1992.tb00997.x. http://doi.wiley.com/10.1111/j.2044-8260.1992.tb00997.x
18. McCraty, R., Atkinson, M., Tomasino, D., Bradley, R.T.: The coherent heart: heart-brain interactions, psychophysiological coherence, and the emergence of system-wide order. Integr. Rev. **5**(2), 10–115 (2009). Publication No. 06–022
19. McKee, M.G.: Biofeedback: an overview in the context of heart-brain medicine. Clevel. Clin. J. Med. **75**(SUPPL.2), 31–34 (2008)
20. Mehler, B., Reimer, B., Wang, Y.: A comparison of heart rate and heart rate variability indices in distinguishing single task driving and driving under secondary cognitive workload. In: Proceedings of the Sixth International Driving Symposium on Human Factors in Driver Assessment, Training and Vehicle Design, pp. 590–597 (2011). http://drivingassessment.uiowa.edu/sites/default/files/DA2011/Papers/085_MehlerReimer.pdf
21. Mladenović, J., Frey, J., Cauchard, J.R.: Dišimo: Anchoring our breath. In: Extended Abstracts of the 2018 CHI Conference on Human Factors in Computing Systems, p. D208. ACM (2018)
22. Moraveji, N., et al.: Peripheral paced respiration: influencing user physiology during information work. In: The 24th Annual ACM Symposium on User Interface Software and Technology, pp. 423–428 (2011). https://doi.org/10.1145/2047196.2047250

23. Muench, F.: HRV: the manufacturers and vendors speak. Assoc. Appl. Psychophysiol. Biofeedback **36**(1), 35–39 (2008). www.aapb.org
24. Mühl, C., Jeunet, C., Lotte, F.: Eeg-based workload estimation across affective contexts. Front. Neurosci. **8**, 114 (2014). https://doi.org/10.3389/fnins.2014.00114. https://www.frontiersin.org/article/10.3389/fnins.2014.00114
25. Owen, A.M., McMillan, K.M., Laird, A.R., Bullmore, E.: N-back working memory paradigm: a meta-analysis of normative functional neuroimaging studies. Hum. Brain Mapp. **25**(1), 46–59 (2005)
26. Roseway, A., Lutchyn, Y., Johns, P., Mynatt, E., Czerwinski, M.: BioCrystal: an ambient tool for emotion and communication. Int. J. Mob. Hum. Comput. Interact. **7**(3), 20–41 (2015). https://doi.org/10.4018/ijmhci.2015070102
27. Schein, M., et al.: Treating hypertension with a device that slows and regularises breathing: a randomised, double-blind controlled study. J. Hum. Hypertens. **15**(4), 271–278 (2001). https://doi.org/10.1038/sj.jhh.1001148. http://www.nature.com/articles/1001148
28. Spielberger, C.D., Gorsuch, R.L., Lushene, R.E.: Manual for the State-Trait Anxiety Inventory. Consulting Psychologists Press, Palo Alto (1970)
29. Tan, G., Dao, T.K., Farmer, L., Sutherland, R.J., Gevirtz, R.: Heart rate variability (hrv) and posttraumatic stress disorder (ptsd): a pilot study. Appl. Psychophysiol. Biofeedback **36**(1), 27–35 (2011). https://doi.org/10.1007/s10484-010-9141-y
30. Vaschillo, E.G., Vaschillo, B., Lehrer, P.M.: Characteristics of resonance in heart rate variability stimulated by biofeedback. Appl. Psychophysiol. Biofeedback **31**(2) (2006).https://doi.org/10.1007/s10484-006-9009-3, https://pdfs.semanticscholar. org/f3e4/76002c25b6b331bf3700d94c4603f3cbd0fc.pdf
31. Yu, B., Feijs, L., Funk, M., Hu, J.: Breathe with touch: a tactile interface for breathing assistance system. In: Abascal, J., Barbosa, S., Fetter, M., Gross, T., Palanque, P., Winckler, M. (eds.) INTERACT 2015. LNCS, vol. 9298, pp. 45–52. Springer, Cham (2015). https://doi.org/10.1007/978-3-319-22698-9_4
32. Yucha, C.B., Montgomery, D.: Evidence-Based Practice in Biofeedback and Neurofeedback. AAPB, Wheat Ridge (2008)

Towards Industrial Assistance Systems: Experiences of Applying Multi-sensor Fusion in Harsh Environments

Michael Haslgrübler[1,2,3]([⊠]), Bendikt Gollan[2], and Alois Ferscha[1,2,3]

[1] Institute of Pervasive Computing, Johannes Kepler University,
Altenbergerstr. 69, 4040 Linz, Austria
{haslgruebler,ferscha}@pervasive.jku.at
[2] Research Studios Austria FG mbH, Studio Pervasive Computing Applications,
Thurngasse 8, 1090 Vienna, Austria
gollan@researchstudio.at
[3] Pro2Future GmbH, Altenbergerstr. 69, 4040 Linz, Austria

Abstract. With the availability of miniaturized low cost sensors and the general availability and easy applicability of algorithms for activity recognition, we investigate how various sensors can be deployed in a harsh environment, the industrial shop-floor. We review related work and provide an in-depth review of our own experiences were sensors wer used to enable recognition of activity, task progress and also mental and cognitive states of assembly workers. The recognition process is based on stationary (RGBD cameras, stereo vision depth sensors) and wearable devices (IMUs, GSR, ECG, mobile eye tracker). We describe in detail the used sensors, the challenges of fusing the data from these various sources together in real-time and how to interpret that data semantically.

Keywords: Sensor evaluation ·
Industrial application multi-sensor fusion · Stational sensors ·
Wearable sensors · Challenges

1 Introduction

The increasing digitalization in industrial production processes goes hand in hand with the increased application of all kinds of sensors, whereby the majority of these sensors are exploited for automated machine-to-machine communication only. However, in all human-in-the-loop processes which involve manual or semi-manual labor, physiological sensors are on the rise, assessing the behavioral and somatic states of the human workers as to deduce on activity or task analysis as well as the estimation of human cognitive states.

The observable revival of human labor as an opposing trend to the pre-dominant tendency of full automation [7] is associated with the requirements of industrial processes to become more and more adaptive to dynamically chang-ing product requirements. The combination of the strengths of both men and

© Springer Nature Switzerland AG 2019
A. Holzinger et al. (Eds.): PhyCS 2016–2018, LNCS 10057, pp. 158–179, 2019.
https://doi.org/10.1007/978-3-030-27950-9_9

machine working together yields the best possible outcome for industrial production, as humans provide their creativity, adaptability, and machines ensuring process constraints such as quality or security.

In the light of these changes towards men-machine collaboration, it is essential for machines or computers to have a fundamental understanding of their users - their ongoing activities, their workflow state, intentions, and attention distributions. The creation of such a high level of awareness requires not only (i) the selection of suitable sensors but as well needs to solve fundamental problems regarding (ii) handling the highly frequent and big volumes of data, (iii) the correct fusion of different sensor types as well as (iv) the adequate interpretation of complex psycho-physiological states.

This work will introduce the industrial application scenario of an aware assistance system for a semi-manual assembly task, introduce and evaluate the employed sensors and discuss the derived challenges from the associated multi-sensor fusion task.

1.1   Related Work

With the ever-increasing number of sensors, the fusion of the data from multiple, potentially heterogeneous sources is becoming a non-trivial task that directly impacts application performance. When addressing physiological data, such sensor collections are often referred to as Body Sensor Networks (BSNs) with applications in many domains [25]. Such physiological sensor networks usually cover wearable accelerometers, gyroscopes, pressure sensors for body movements and applied forces, skin/chest electrodes (for electrocardiogram (ECG), electromyogram (EMG), galvanic skin response (GSR), and electrical impedance plethysmography (EIP)), (PPG) sensors, microphones (for voice, ambient, and heart sounds) and scalp-placed electrodes for electroencephalogram (EEG) [25]. These wearable sensor types can also be enriched with infrastructural, remote sensor systems such as traditional (RGB) and depth cameras.

Sensor networks are investigated in and employed by industrial applications [37], specifically in domains such as the Automotive Industry [42,44], healthcare IOT [6,12] or food industry [33], in industrial use cases as welding [20] or CNC-machining [28].

1.2   Contribution of This Work

This work introduces an industrial assistance system which is based on the integration of various sensors which have been applied and evaluated regarding their applicability and suitability in an industrial application. In this context, this work presents an overview of related work in workflow recognition, a crucial part for building industrial assistance systems and recognition of cognitive state featuring reviews and experiences regarding sensors' data quality, reliability, etc. Furthermore, this work reports on the key challenges and opportunities which are

(i) handling of big and high-frequent amounts of data in real-time, (ii) ensuring interoperability between different systems, (iii) handling uncertainty of sensor data, and the general issues of (iv) multi-sensor fusion.

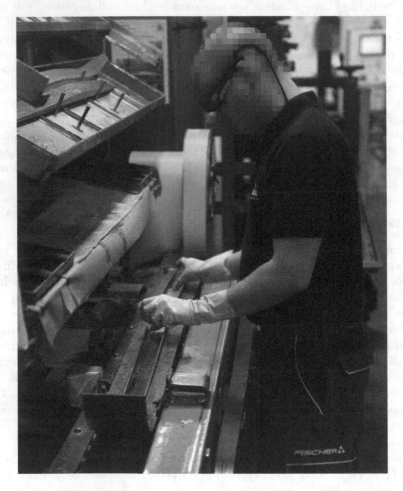

Fig. 1. Ski assembly procedure and environment [22].

While Sect. 2 describes the industrial application scenario, in Sects. 3 and 4 presents workflow and cognitive state recognition respectively both featuring an analysis of suitable sensors. Section 5 puts the focus on the discussions of challenges and opportunities and Sect. 6 provides a summary and addresses future work.

2   Industrial Application Scenario

The industrial application scenario (Fig. 1) is an industrial assistance system which is employed in a semi-manual industrial application of a complex assembly of premium alpine sports products, where it is supposed to ensure the high-quality requirements by providing adaptive worker support.

The work task consists of manually manipulating and arranging the multiple parts whereas errors can occur regarding workflow order, object orientation, or omission of parts. These errors express in unacceptable product quality differences regarding usage characteristics (e.g. stability, stiffness), thus increase rejects and inefficiency.

Full automation of the process is not feasible due to (i) required high flexibility (minimal lot sizes, changing production schedules), (ii) used material characteristics (highly sticky materials) and (iii) human-in-the-loop production principles enable the optimization of product quality and production processes.

In this context, the sensor-based assistance system is designed to enable the realization of an adaptive, sensitive assistance system as to provide guidance only if needed, thus minimizing obtrusiveness and enabling the assistance system to seamlessly disappear into the background. Furthermore, the adaptivity of the feedback design enables the education of novices in training-on-the-job scenarios, integrating novices directly into the production process during their one month training period without occupying productive specialists.

The assistance system is supposed to observe the task execution, identify the associated step in the workflow and identify errors or uncertainty (hesitation, deviation from work plan, etc.) to support the operator via different levels of assistance [27]. The selection of assistance depends on operator skill (i.e. day 1 trainee vs 30-year-in-the-company worker), cognitive load and perception capability to provide the best possible assistance with the least necessary disruption. Such supportive measures range from, laser-based markers for part placement or visual highlighting of upcoming work steps in case of uncertainty, to video snippets visualizing the correct execution of a task, in case of doubt.

3   Workflow Recognition

A key element for the industrial assistant system is to perform workflow recognition. For workflow recognition we classified related work into various properties, cf. Fig. 2:

Algorithm Type. The algorithm used for recognizing a pattern (i.e. classification) in a data stream is either based on supervised (training data comes with ground truth labels) or unsupervised learning (training data comes without labels).

Processing Paradigm. The raw data (collected by sensors) is either used directly for the overall classification or is per-processed or pre-classified (e.g. for sub/micro-activities).

Decision Data Quantity. The classification processes is done on data of a single point in time or from multi points in time, both either by data collected from a single or multiple sensors.

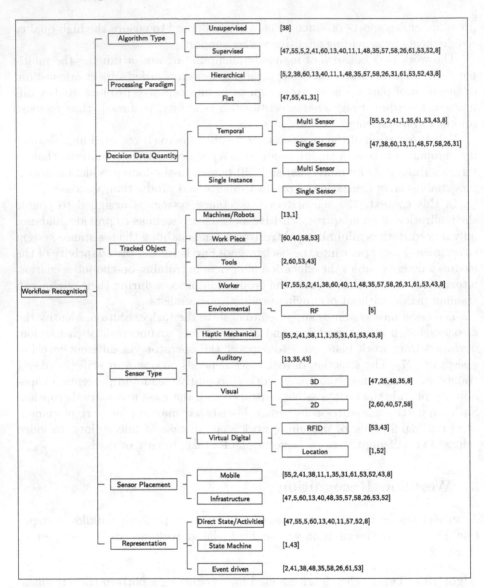

Fig. 2. An Ontology for workflow recognition in industrial environments.

Tracked Object. On the industrial shop floor various objects may need to be tracked to provide insight about the current state in a workflow such as machines/robots, tools, work pieces and the human workers.

Sensor Type. Various types of sensors have been used to recognize a workflow, prominently body worn devices such as IMUs (category haptic, mechanical) and visual sensors in form of rgb (2D) or depth cameras (3D). But also other types of sensors, such as environmental, auditory and virtual/digital, have been successfully deployed.

Sensor Placement. The sensors can be placed either into the infrastructure (e.g. observing a assembly station) or mobile (e.g. wearable on the worker or embedded into a power tool).

Representation. In order to perform workflow recognition successfully, algorithm have been trained to directly induce the state/activity or have used state machines or event driven models to not only model their workflow but also to reduce the decision complexity of recognition algorithms (to simple are we still in the current or already in the next work step).

3.1 Activity Sensing

The most common application of activity and behavior analysis in industrial applications is monitoring of task progress for documentation or assistance applications. The tracked objects can machines/robots, work pieces, tools and the workers. For the later, sensors and technologies that were previously exploited, cf. Fig. 2, are aiming for activity tracking based on (i) stationary (visual) sensors and (ii) wearable motion sensors. The different fields of application are introduced in the following, for an overview please refer to Table 1.

Skeleton Tracking. Mainly stationary visual sensors are employed to identify body joints and the resulting associated skeleton pose. Depending on the application, these sensors address the full skeleton or sub-selections of body joints.

Full Skeleton Tracking. **Sensor Description - Kinect v2.** The Microsoft Kinect v2 combines an infrared and an RGB camera to track up to six complete skeletons, each consisting of 26 joints. The Kinect uses an infrared time-of-flight technology to build a 3D map of the environment and the objects in view. Skeleton data is provided by the associated Microsoft SDK which is restricted to Microsoft Windows platforms.

In the described application scenario, two Kinect cameras have been installed on opposing sides of the work environment - as a frontal positioning was not possible - to avoid obstructions and enable an encompassing perception of the scene. Based on a manual calibration of the two sensors, the data is combined into a single skeleton representation via a multi-sensor fusion approach as described in Sect. 5.4. The calibration is achieved via a two-step process: (1) real-world measurement of the placement and orientation angle of the sensors in the application scenario, obtaining the viewpoints of the two sensors in a joint coordinate system and (2) fine adjustment based on skeleton joints that are observed at the same time, at different positions. For this purpose, the head joint was chosen as it represents the most stable joint of the Kinect tracking approach - according to our experience. The overall result of the calibration approach is the localization and orientation of the two sensors in a joint coordinate system, thus enabling the overlay and fusion of the respective sensor input data.

Evaluation. Kinect-like sensors provide unique opportunities of skeleton tracking, thus overcome many problems associated with professional motion tracking systems such as enabling (i) markerless tracking, (ii) fast and simple setup and (iii) low-cost tracking results. However, due to the infrared technology, the depth sensors do not perform well in outdoor settings with high infrared background noise. Furthermore, the cameras require good allocation of the scene, with a full view of the worker for best tracking results.

Overall, the application of Kinect sensors in industrial applications requires careful handling and substantial data post-processing. With the Kinect skeleton data showing large amounts of fluctuations, the Kinect represents a cheap, yet not per se reliable sensor for skeleton tracking.

Sub-Skeleton Tracking. **Sensor Description - Leap Motion.** Aiming only at tracking the hands of a user, specifically in Virtual Reality applications, the Leap Motion controller represents an infrared, stereo-vision-based gesture and position tracking system with sub-millimeter accuracy [59]. Suitable both for mobile and stationary application, it has been specifically developed to track hands and fingers in a close distance of up to 0.8 m, enabling highly accurate hand gesture control of interactive computer systems.

In the introduced industrial application scenario, the Leap Motion controllers are installed in the focus areas of the assembly tasks, trying to monitor the detailed hand movements.

Evaluation. The Leap Motion controller shows high accuracy and also high reliability. Yet, unfortunately, the sensor shows a high latency in the initial registration of hands (up to 1–2 s). In a highly dynamic application as in the presented use-case scenario, this latency prevented the applicability of the Leap Motion sensor, as the hands were often already leaving the area of interaction when they were detected. For this purpose, this highly accurate sensor could not be applied in the final assistance setup, yet they represent a very interesting sensor choice when addressing a very stationary industrial task.

Joint Tracking. Mobile, wearable sensors are used to extract the movement of single body joints, most commonly the wrists for inference on hand movement activity. The vast majority of these sensors are based on accelerometers and gyrometers to provide relative changes in motion and orientation for behavior analysis.

Sensor Description - Shimmer. The Shimmer sensors have already been validated for use in academic and industrial research applications [9,23,51] Also, Shimmer research offers the several tools and APIs for manipulation, integration and easy data access. Due to their small size and lightweight (28 g) wearable design, they can be worn on any body segment for the full range of motion during all types of tasks, without affecting the movement, techniques, or motion patterns. Built-in inertial measurement sensors are able to capture kinematic properties, such as movement in terms of (i) Acceleration, (ii) Rotation, (iii) Magnetic field.

The updated module boasts a 24 MHz CPU with a precision clock subsystem and provides the three-axis acceleration and gyrometer data. We applied a shimmer sensor on each of the worker's hands to obtain expressive manual activity data. The Shimmer sensors provide their data with a frame rate of 50 Hz. In the current scope of the implementation, hand activity data is parsed from respective text/csv-files in which the recorded data has been stored. This accumulates to 6 features per iteration per sensor (3x gyrometer, 3x accelerometer) every 20 ms.

Evaluation. Shimmer sensors provide reliable and accurate tracking data, also in rough industrial environments. The real-time analysis requires a smartphone as a transmission device, yet does work reliably. Overall, when aiming for raw accelerometer data, the Shimmer sensor platforms have proven their suitability.

Gesture Detection. The introduced Kinemic sensor is closely related to the previously described accelerometer sensors placed on the wrist of the worker. Yet, it does not provide access to the raw accelerometer data but directly provides only higher level gesture detections as result to the system. Due to this reason, the distinction between general joint tracking and hand gesture detection was made.

Sensor Description - Kinemic. The Kinemic wristband sensor for hand gesture detection is a new sensor for which almost no official information is available. It is based on - presumably - 3-axis accelerometer and gyrometer sensor and connected to a mobile computation platform (RaspberryPi) which carries out the gesture detection processes. Currently, 12 gestures are supported, with the goal to expand to customizable gestures, air writing, etc.

Evaluation. The sensors are easily initiated and integrated into a multi-sensor system. The recognition of the gestures works well for the majority of existing gestures. In summary, this sensor with the associated SDK provides a useful solution for people looking for high-level off-the-shelf gesture interaction, without requiring access to raw accelerometer data.

Behavior Analysis

Gaze-based Task Segmentation. The analysis of gaze behavior also provides interesting insights into the execution of activities, especially the segmentation of subsequent tasks in a work process. Recent work shows that the gaze feature *Nearest Neighbour Index* [10], which describes the spatial distribution of fixations in a dynamic environment [3]. Employing a wearable Pupil Labs eye tracker, this gaze behavior feature was capable of successfully segmenting and recognizing tasks. For the sensor discussion, please refer to Sect. 4.1.

4 Sensing of Cognitive States

4.1 Visual Attention

Generally, the human eye gaze represents the most efficient and fastest, consciously controlled form of information acquisition with the unique capability to bridge large distances. Intuitively, the human eye is mainly responsible for the positioning of eye gaze, thus represent an expression for stimulus selection, yet, fine details of gaze behavior also show connections to conscious and subconscious information processing mechanisms that allow inferences on internal attention processes.

Gaze Behavior

Sensor Description - Pupil Labs. The PupilLabs mobile eye tracker is realized as a modular and open source solution, providing direct access to all sensors and data streams (gaze position, gaze orientation, saccade analysis, pupil dilation, etc.), rendering the device as more suitable for academic research applications. The PupilLabs eye tracker enables direct access in real-time to all parameters and tracking results. The PupilLabs device provides the eye tracking data for each eye with a distinct timestamp, requiring additional synchronization of obtained data frames.

Evaluation. The PupilLabs eye tracker provides rather simple and encompassing access to basic data streams. As a consequence, the PupilLabs eye tracker is a suitable, low-cost device for ambitious developers that want to develop algorithms based on the raw sensor data. However, the sensor fails in outdoor environments when exposed to scattered infrared light. In the proposed application scenario, the PupilLabs eye tracker is employed for associating gaze orientation to objects in space (hands, task-relevant objects, etc.) via object recognition in the first person video. However, the achieved results are always situated in the user-specific coordinates, which, to be associated with an overall world space of the industrial shop floor requires a complex and detailed localization of the worker, regarding both head location and orientation.

Visual Focus of Attention. The general spatial allocation of attention can also be assessed on a less-fine-grained level via external, infrastructural sensors. The so-called visual focus of attention has found sustained application in human-computer-interaction applications. These differ in application and tracking technology but all use head orientation as the key information for attention orienting [4,36,50].

Sensor Description - Kinect v2. As described above, the Kinect provides a quite reliable skeleton information on a low-cost platform. It also provides joint orientation, yet not head orientation. To exploit the available data for the estimation of the visual focus of attention, an approximation of shoulder axis and neck-head axis can be employed.

Evaluation. The visual focus of attention data derived from this approach can only provide very rough information on the actually perceived objects and areas in space. However, it directly provides the spatial context, which misses in the assessment via wearable eye trackers, as described above. Hence, the combination of the two sensors, wearable and infrastructural, may help in providing substantial advances in the task of 3D-mapping of visual attention in industrial environments - a task which will be pursued in future work.

4.2 Arousal

In the literature, arousal is defined by Kahneman [29] as *general activation of mind*, or as *general operation of consciousness* by Thatcher and John [56].

Psychophysiological measures exploit these physical reactions of the human body in the preparation of, execution of, or as a reaction to cognitive activities. In contrast to self-reported or performance measures, psychophysiological indicators provide continuous data, thus allowing a better understanding of user-stimulus interactions as well as non-invasive and non-interruptive analysis, maybe even outside of the scope of the user's consciousness. Whereas these measures are objective representations of ongoing cognitive processes, they often are highly contaminated by reactions to other triggers, as e.g. physical workload or emotions.

Cognitive Load. Besides light incidence control, the pupil is also sensitive to psychological and cognitive activities and mechanisms, as the musculus dilatator pupillae is directly connected to the limbic system via sympathetic control [19], hence, the human eye also represents a promising indicator of cognitive state. Currently, existing analysis approaches towards analysis of cognitive load from pupil dilation - Task-Evoked Pupil Response (TEPR) [21] and Index of Cognitive Activity (ICA) [32] - both find application mainly in laboratory environments due to their sensitivity to changes in environment illumination.

Sensor Description - PupilLabs. The employed Pupil Labs mobile eye tracker provides pupil diameter as raw measurement data, both in relative (pixel size) as in absolute (mm) units due to the freely positionable IR eye cameras. The transformation is achieved via a 3D model of the eyeball and thus an adaptive scaling of the pixel values to absolute mm measurements.

Evaluation. The assessment of pupil dilation works as reliably as the gaze localization with the lack of official accuracy measures in comparative studies. Hence, it is difficult to evaluate the sensor regarding data quality. Overall, the assessment of pupil dilation with the mobile Pupil Labs eye tracker provides reliable data, for laboratory studies or field application. Erroneous data like blinks needs to be filtered in post-processing of the raw data.

Cardiac Indicators. The cardiac function, i.e. heart rate, represents another fundamental somatic indicator of arousal and thus of attentional activation as a direct physiological reaction to phasic changes in the autonomic nervous system [24]. Heart Rate Variability (HRV), heart rate response (HRR) or T-Wave amplitude analysis are the most expressive physiologic indicators of arousal [34,54].

The stationary and mobile assessment of cardiac data is very well established in medical as well as customer products via diverse realizations of ECG sensors. The different sensors are based on two main independent measurement approaches: (i) measuring the electric activity of the heart over time via electrodes that are placed directly on the skin and which detect minimal electrical changes from the heart muscle's electro-physiologic pattern of depolarizing during each heartbeat; and (ii) measuring the blood volume peak of each heartbeat via optical sensors (pulse oximeters) which illuminates the skin and measures the changes in light absorption to capture volumetric changes of the blood vessels (Photoplethysmography (PPG)).

Sensor Description - Shimmer. Shimmer sensors use a photoplethysmogram (PPG) which detects the change in volume by illuminating the skin with the light from a light-emitting diode (LED) and then measuring the amount of light transmitted or reflected towards a photodiode. From this volume changes an estimate of heart rate can be obtained.

Sensor Description - Empatica E4. The E4 wristband allows two modes of data collection: (i) in-memory recording and (ii) live streaming of data. Accessing in-memory recorded data requires a USB connection to a Mac or Windows PC running Empatica Manager Software for a posteriori analysis. Accessing streaming data for real-time analysis of somatic data, the Empatica Real-time App can be installed from the Apple App Store or Google Play Market onto a smartphone device via Bluetooth on which the data can be processed or forwarded. Additionally, a custom application can be implemented for Android and iOS systems.

Sensor Description - Microsoft Band 2. The Microsoft Band 2 is equipped with an optical PPG sensor for analysis of pulse. With the Microsoft Band representing an end-user product, the focus in the provided functionality is not set on providing most accessible interfaces for academic purposes, yet, still, the available SDK enables the access of raw sensor data in real-time. For data access, the sensor needs to be paired with a smartphone device and data can be transferred via a Bluetooth connection for either direct processing on the mobile device or further transmission to a general processing unit.

Evaluation. The Microsoft Band is highly restricted in sensor placement as the sensor is integrated into the wristband of the device and thus measures the skin response on the bottom surface of the wrist. In experiments, the Microsoft Band sensor showed large drops in measurement data, most probably due to a change of contact between the sensor and the skin during device shifts. In contrast, the

Shimmer Sensing Platform allows much more freedom in the placement of the sensor with the help of external sensing modules e.g. pre-shaped for mounting on fingers which show the most promising locations for reliable GSR measurements.

Accessing real-time data for the E4 wristband shows similar comfort levels as the Microsoft Band as the device needs to be paired with a smartphone device and data can be transferred via a Bluetooth connection for either direct processing on the mobile device or further transmission to a general processing unit. Being designed for research and academic purposes, the Shimmer platform provides easiest and fastest access via open and intuitive interfaces. Overall, the data from all devices can be accessed in real-time, yet the destinated applications of the products resemble in their applicability in research and development approaches.

Galvanic Skin Response. From the very early 1900s, the Galvanic Skin Response has been the focus of academic research. The skin is the only organ that is purely innervated by the sympathetic nervous system (and not affected by parasympathetic activation). The GSR analyzes the electrodermal activity (EDA) of the human skin which represents an automatic reflection of synaptic arousal as increased skin conductance shows significant correlations with neuronal activities [14,18]. Hence, Galvanic Skin Response (GSR) acts as an indicator of arousal and increases monotonically with attention in task execution [29].

Sensorial Assessment. The accessibility of the raw and real-time data depends on the respective development environment which is provided to support these sensors, ranging from a general limitation to statistical information to access of true real-time data.

The GSR can be assessed via mobile, wearable sensors worn on the bare skin, e.g., as integrated into activity trackers or smartwatches or scientific activity and acceleration sensors. These sensors measure the skin conductance, i.e. skin resistivity via small integrated electrodes. The skin conductance response is measured from the eccrine glands, which cover most of the body and are especially dense in the palms and soles of the feet. In the following, three wearable sensors are explored which provide the analysis of skin conductance response:

Evaluation

E4 Wristband is a hand wearable wireless devices designated for continuous, real-time data acquisition of daily life activities. It is specifically designed in an extremely lightweight (25 g) watch-like form factor that allows hassle-free unobtrusive monitoring in- or outside the lab. With the built-in 3-axis accelerometer sensor the device is able to capture motion-based activities. Additionally, the device is able to capture the following physiological features (i) Galvanic skin response (ii) Photoplethysmography (heart rate) (iii) Infrared thermophile (peripheral skin temperature). The employed Empatica E4 Wristband has already found application in various academic research applications and publications [15,17].

Table 1. Overview on introduced sensors [22], grouped according to their sensing category and analysis type, listing the associated technologies and sensor parameters.

Category		Type	Sensor Name	Technology	Accuracy/Range
Activity	Skeleton	Full Skeleton	Microsoft Kinect v2	Time-of-Flight Infrared	Depth: 512 × 424 @ 30 Hz FOV: 70° × 60° RGB: 1920 × 1080 @ 30 Hz FOV: 84° × 53° acc: 0.027 m, (SD: 0.018m) depth range: 4 m
		Sub-Skeleton	Leap Motion [46]	Stereo-Vision Infrared *hand tracking*	FOV: 150° × 120° avg error: < 0.0012 m [59] depth range: 0.8 m
		Joint Tracking (wrist)	Shimmer	3-axis accelerometer gyrometer	Range: ±16 g Sensitivity: 1000 LSB/g at ±2 g Resolution: 16 bit
	Gesture	Hand Gesture	Kinemic	3-axis accelerometer gyrometer	not available
	Behavior Analysis	Gaze Behavior	Pupil Labs [30]	Mobile Eyetracker *gaze feature analysis for task segmentation*	accuracy 91% [3]
Cognitive States	Visual Attention	Gaze Behavior	Pupil Labs [30]	Mobile Eyetracker *fixations, saccades, gaze features*	Gaze acc: 0.6° Sampling Rate: 120 Hz Scene Camera: 30 Hz @ 1080p 60 Hz @ 720p 120 Hz @ VGA Calibration: 5-point, 9 point
		Visual Focus of Attention	Microsoft Kinect v2	Head Orientation from Skeleton Tracking	not available
	Arousal	Cognitive Load	Pupil Labs	Mobile Eyetracker *pupil dilation*	pupil size in pixel or mm via 3D model acc. not available
		Heart Rate (HRV, HRR)	Microsoft Band 2	PPG	avg. error rate: 5.6% [49]
			Empatica E4 Wristband [45]	PPG	samping frequency: 64 Hz error rate: 2.14%
		Galvanic Skin Response	Microsoft Band 2		data rate: 0.2/5 Hz acc. not available
			Empatica Wristband	Empatica E3 EDA proprietary design	data rate: 4 Hz mean cor. to reference 0.93, $p < 0.0001$ [16]

Microsoft Band 2 offers an affordable mean for tracking a variety of parameters of daily living. Besides 11 advanced sensors for capturing movement kinematics, physical parameters and environmental factors the device also offers various channels for providing feedback. A 1.26 × 0.5-in. curved screen with a resolution of 320 × 128 pixels can be used to display visual messages. Additionally, a haptic vibration motor is capable of generating private vibration notifications.

Shimmer sensors have already been validated for use in biomedical-oriented research applications. Due to their small size and lightweight (28 g) wearable design, they can be worn on any body segment for the full range of motion during all types of tasks, without affecting the movement, techniques, for motion patterns. Built-in inertial measurement sensors are able to capture kinematic properties, such as movement in terms of (i) Acceleration, (ii) Rotation, (iii) Magnetic field.

5 Challenges and Opportunities

See Fig. 3.

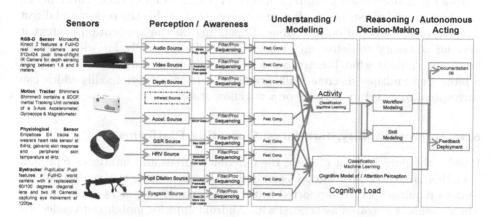

Fig. 3. Scheme of the introduced industrial multi-sensor assistance system [22] with the various level of abstractions: Perception, Understanding, Reasoning, Acting. Data from Sensors are processed individually and in aggregated form to perform activity, work-step, skill and cognitive recognition. Reasoning Models are then used to select appropriate assistance measure via different actors.

5.1 Summary

In the previous chapters, several sensors have been described regarding their underlying technology, access to sensor data and evaluation regarding suitability for academic or industrial exploitation. As an overview, a short fact summary of the information is collected in Table 1, including further numerical data regarding the accuracy and range of the sensors, if available.

5.2 Handling Amounts of Data

The first challenge in the analysis of multi-sensor applications is the handling of the amounts of data, usually with real-time requirements. This applies both the required levels of computational performance as well as to further hardware assets as BUS bandwidth or hard drive access speed.

But also the offline handling of the data may represent problems for the design of interactive systems as especially raw video data - when stored - quickly exceeds GigaBytes of data. These amounts of data need to be managed, if possible in suitable database structures to enable efficient further processing of recorded data.

Other than data transfer and storage, also human resources for post-processing of the data represents a substantial challenge. This implies checking, filtering data, extracting relevant segments of data, etc. Especially - when aiming for supervised machine learning tasks - the manual labeling of activities represents an effort which often substantially exceeds the actual time of collected data and needs to be considered in the application setup. If possible one should consider if unsupervised machine learning, cf. Fig. 2, is an option. This labeling can be improved via suitable software solutions that enable the review and direct labeling of multimodal data streams. Depending on the application context it may be necessary to define and label micro tasks especially for what workers are doing. This is what literature is also referring to as a discrete skill [39]. In a later step multiple discrete skills are used to form up serial skills which can correspond to a certain activity or a workflow state.

5.3   Interoperability, Interfaces, Operating Platforms

Besides the pure amount of data, the different sources and interfaces represent a further source of problems. Depending on the producer, the analysis of the sensors requires specific supported frameworks and development environments. Mobile sensors are often associated with Android apps for mobile data collection and transfer, or e.g. the Microsoft Kinect sensors require Microsoft Windows platforms for operation, etc.

Creating a multi-sensor industrial application requires the multi-platform capability of development staff and often the creation of distributed systems operating on different native platforms. In the presented industrial application, such a distributed set of platforms is employed, inter-connected with a cross-platform messaging solution, thus overcoming the interoperability issue.

Any technical solution should not only work on the major operating systems for developers but also be able to support the most common development languages according to the TIOBE Index (i.e. Java, Python, C/C++)[1].

5.4   Multi-sensor Fusion

In many industrial applications, no single sensor is suitable to cover the overall complexity of a situation. Furthermore, no sensor provides perfect data, so redundant sensor designs enable the compensation of sensor failure. However, the handling of parallel, multi-modal datastreams provides several issues regarding data processing and system design, as discussed in the following paragraphs.

---

[1] https://www.tiobe.com/tiobe-index/, Retrieved January 2019.

Synchronization and Subsampling. The synchronization of different sensor types represents a substantial problem, especially of non-visual sensors (accelerometers, etc.). It is advisable to introduce a synchronizing activity which is unambiguously identifiable in diverse data representations. In the introduced industrial application, a single hand clap has proved to provide useful data for synchronization as it shows explicit peaks in motions sensing and can precisely be timed also in visual and auditory sensors.

However, a single synchronization is usually not sufficient. Different sampling rates from the diverse sensor types require a sub-or re-sampling of data to combine single data snippets into collected data frames which are able to provide an overall representation of the scene over the various available sensors. Sometimes, when recording long sessions (>1 h), the differences in the internal clocks of the sensors may also cause significant shifts in the data, making re-synchronization in periodic time ranges advisable.

In addition, it can be crucial to not only synchronize the sensor streams in the time domain but to harmonize the data in various aspects, e.g. such as data normalization or to transform local sensor information into a global space, cf. Fig. 4, such as transforming skeleton sensor data from its sensors' local space into a global space, where e.g. others skeleton data also report into. This provides

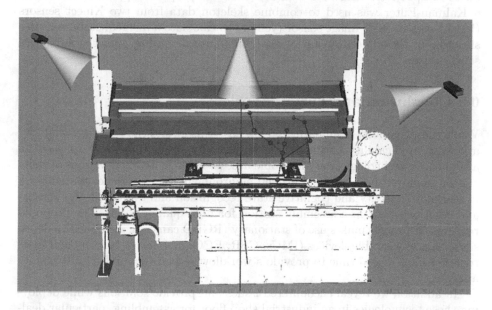

Fig. 4. It may not be enough to synchronize data in the time domain but also to merge local (sensor) data into a global space and provide a digital twin of the captured process for analysis and debugging of correct multi sensor fusion. Here skeleton tracking devices are positioned around a virtual assembly place, representing the real environment. Sensor Data (i.e. Skeletons) are transformed from their local coordinate space to the global coordinate space based on their placement in the virtual world. (Color figure online)

use with (i) the ability to create tracking beyond a single sensor space or (ii) be able to use the data redundantly either for fail-safe or for error mitigation.

Dealing with the Uncertainty of Sensor Data. One of the most critical and difficult aspects of multi-modal sensor applications is the evaluation of data quality as this directly affects fusion of different data types. Some sensors directly provide measures of confidence of sensor data, while others require hand-made post-processing for the evaluation of data quality. These can range from rule-based evaluation criteria as application-based plausibility checks (e.g. avoiding jitter in hand tracking data by limiting the maximal distance between consecutive data frames) to statistical measures (check if data lies in the standard value range) or comparison of actual data with predictions from previous frames.

Such evaluation of data quality is required to dynamically select the sensors with the currently best and most reliable sensor data, hence is the main prerequisite for the fusion of redundant sensor data.

Fusion of Redundant Data. Based on an evaluation of incoming sensor data quality, the different data types can be merged via different weights based on the respective sensor data confidence. In the proposed application-scenario, a Kalman-Filter was used to combine skeleton data from two Kinect sensors (black) and an RGB image sensor (yellow) to calculate a merged, stabilized user skeleton for the adjacent behavior analysis approach, cf. Fig. 4 for the respective sensor setup.

6   Conclusion and Future Work

While the availability of miniaturized low cost sensors and the general availability and easy applicability of algorithms for activity recognition have sparked an avalanche of technology ready for home use, we investigated how various of these can be deployed in a harsh industrial environment. We reviewed related work in workflow, activity and cognitive state recognition and evaluated how sensors and solutions work in a assembly station for high quality goods. The proposed recognition process makes use of stationary (RGBD cameras, stereo vision depth sensors) and wearable devices (IMUs, GSR, ECG, mobile eye tracker) and fuses together data in real time to provide a workflow recognition and cognitive state analysis.

In addition we reveal encountered issues and provide solutions while deploying these technologies in an industrial shop floor for assembling, particular dealing with for multi-sensor fusion or near real-time recognition.

For future work we plan to realize a truly opportunistic sensor framework which dynamically selects sensors based on a best fit between application demands, processing capabilities and available data sources.

Acknowledgements. This work was supported by the projects Attentive Machines (FFG, Contract No. 849976) and Attend2IT (FFG, Contract No. 856393) and Pro²Future (FFG, Contract No. 6112792). Part of this work appeared in [22]. Special thanks to team members Christian Thomay, Sabrina Amrouche, Michael Matscheko, Igor Pernek and Peter Fritz for their valuable contributions.

References

1. Akhavian, R., Behzadan, A.H.: Construction equipment activity recognition for simulation input modeling using mobile sensors and machine learning classifiers. Adv. Eng. Inform. **29**(4), 867–877 (2015). https://doi.org/10.1016/j.aei.2015.03. 001. http://www.sciencedirect.com/science/article/pii/S1474034615000282, collective Intelligence Modeling, Analysis, and Synthesis for Innovative Engineering Decision Making Special Issue of the 1st International Conference on Civil and Building Engineering Informatics
2. Al-Naser, M., et al.: Hierarchical model for zero-shot activity recognition using wearable sensors. In: Proceedings of the 10th International Conference on Agents and Artificial Intelligence - Volume 2: ICAART, pp. 478–485. INSTICC, SciTePress (2018). https://doi.org/10.5220/0006595204780485
3. Amrouche, S., Gollan, B., Ferscha, A., Heftberger, J.: Activity segmentation and identification based on eye gaze features. In: PErvasive Technologies Related to Assistive Environments (PETRA), Jun 2018. Accepted for publishing in June 2018
4. Asteriadis, S., Tzouveli, P., Karpouzis, K., Kollias, S.: Estimation of behavioral user state based on eye gaze and head pose—application in an e-learning environment. Multimed. Tools Appl. **41**(3), 469–493 (2009)
5. Avrahami, D., Patel, M., Yamaura, Y., Kratz, S.: Below the surface: unobtrusive activity recognition for work surfaces using RF-radar sensing. In: 23rd International Conference on Intelligent User Interfaces, IUI 2018, pp. 439–451. ACM, New York (2018). https://doi.org/10.1145/3172944.3172962, http://doi.acm.org/ 10.1145/3172944.3172962
6. Baloch, Z., Shaikh, F.K., Unar, M.A.: A context-aware data fusion approach for health-IoT. Int. J. Inf. Technol. **10**(3), 241–245 (2018)
7. Behrmann, E., Rauwald, C.: Mercedes boots robots from the production line (2016). Accessed Feb 01 2017
8. Bleser, G., et al.: Cognitive learning, monitoring and assistance of industrial workflows using egocentric sensor networks. PLoS ONE **10**(6), 0127769 (2015)
9. Burns, A., et al.: Shimmer™–a wireless sensor platform for noninvasive biomedical research. IEEE Sens. J. **10**(9), 1527–1534 (2010)
10. Camilli, M., Nacchia, R., Terenzi, M., Di Nocera, F.: ASTEF: a simple tool for examining fixations. Behav. Res. Methods **40**(2), 373–382 (2008)
11. Campbell, T., Harper, J., Hartmann, B., Paulos, E.: Towards digital apprenticeship: wearable activity recognition in the workshop setting. Technical report, University of California, Berkeley (2015)
12. Chen, M., Ma, Y., Li, Y., Wu, D., Zhang, Y., Youn, C.H.: Wearable 2.0: enabling human-cloud integration in next generation healthcare systems. IEEE Commun. Mag. **55**(1), 54–61 (2017)
13. Cheng, C.F., Rashidi, A., Davenport, M.A., Anderson, D.: Audio signal processing for activity recognition of construction heavy equipment. In: ISARC Proceedings of the International Symposium on Automation and Robotics in Construction, vol. 33, p. 1 (2016)

14. Critchley, H.D., Elliott, R., Mathias, C.J., Dolan, R.J.: Neural activity relating to generation and representation of galvanic skin conductance responses: a functional magnetic resonance imaging study. J. Neurosci. **20**(8), 3033–3040 (2000)
15. van Dooren, M., de Vries, J.J.G.G.J., Janssen, J.H.: Emotional sweating across the body: comparing 16 different skin conductance measurement locations. Physiol. Behav. **106**(2), 298–304 (2012). https://doi.org/10.1016/j.physbeh.2012.01.020
16. Empatica: comparison procomp vs empatica E3 skin conductance signal (2016). https://empatica.app.box.com/s/a53t8mnose4l3331529r1ma3fbzmxtcb
17. Fedor, S., Picard, R.W.: Ambulatory EDA: comparisons of bilateral forearm and calf locations, September 2014
18. Frith, C.D., Allen, H.A.: The skin conductance orienting response as an index of attention. Biol. Psychol. **17**(1), 27–39 (1983)
19. Gabay, S., Pertzov, Y., Henik, A.: Orienting of attention, pupil size, and the norepinephrine system. Atten. Percept. Psychophys. **73**(1), 123–129 (2011)
20. Gao, X., Sun, Y., You, D., Xiao, Z., Chen, X.: Multi-sensor information fusion for monitoring disk laser welding. Int. J. Adv. Manuf. Technol. **85**(5–8), 1167–1175 (2016)
21. Gollan, B., Ferscha, A.: Modeling pupil dilation as online input for estimation of cognitive load in non-laboratory attention-aware systems. In: COGNITIVE 2016-The Eighth International Conference on Advanced Cognitive Technologies and Applications (2016)
22. Gollan, B., Haslgrübler, M., Ferscha, A., Heftberger, J.: Making sense: Experiences with multi-sensor fusion in industrial assistance systems. In: Proceedings of the 5th International Conference on Physiological Computing Systems, PhyCS 2018, Seville, Spain, 19–21 September 2018, pp. 64–74 (2018). https://doi.org/10.5220/0007227600640074
23. Gradl, S., Kugler, P., Lohmüller, C., Eskofier, B.: Real-time ECG monitoring and arrhythmia detection using android-based mobile devices. In: 2012 Annual International Conference of the IEEE Engineering in Medicine and Biology Society (EMBC), pp. 2452–2455. IEEE (2012)
24. Graham, F.K.: Attention: the heartbeat, the blink, and the brain. Int. J. Adv. Manuf. Technol. **8**, 3–29 (1992)
25. Gravina, R., Alinia, P., Ghasemzadeh, H., Fortino, G.: Multi-sensor fusion in body sensor networks: state-of-the-art and research challenges. Inf. Fusion **35**, 68–80 (2017)
26. Hahn, M., Krüger, L., Wöhler, C., Kummert, F.: 3D action recognition in an industrial environment: cognition, interaction, technology. In: Ritter, H., Sagerer, G., Dillmann, R., Buss, M. (eds.) Human Centered Robot Systems. Cognitive Systems Monographs, vol. 6, pp. 141–150. Springer, Heidelberg (2009). https://doi.org/10.1007/978-3-642-10403-9_15
27. Haslgrübler, M., Fritz, P., Gollan, B., Ferscha, A.: Getting through: modality selection in a multi-sensor-actuator industrial IoT environment. In: Proceedings of the Seventh International Conference on the Internet of Things. ACM (2017)
28. Jovic, S., Anicic, O., Jovanovic, M.: Adaptive neuro-fuzzy fusion of multi-sensor data for monitoring of CNC machining. Sens. Rev. **37**(1), 78–81 (2017)
29. Kahneman, D.: Attention and Effort, vol. 1063. Prentice-Hall Enlegwood Cliffs, Upper Saddle River (1973)
30. Kassner, M., Patera, W., Bulling, A.: Pupil: an open source platform for pervasive eye tracking and mobile gaze-based interaction. In: Proceedings of the 2014 ACM International Joint Conference on Pervasive and Ubiquitous Computing: Adjunct Publication, pp. 1151–1160. ACM (2014)

31. Koskimaki, H., Huikari, V., Siirtola, P., Laurinen, P., Roning, J.: Activity recognition using a wrist-worn inertial measurement unit: a case study for industrial assembly lines. In: 2009 17th Mediterranean Conference on Control and Automation, pp. 401–405, June 2009. https://doi.org/10.1109/MED.2009.5164574
32. Kramer, A.F.: Physiological metrics of mental workload: a review of recent progress. In: Multiple-Task Performance, pp. 279–328 (1991)
33. Kröger, M., Sauer-Greff, W., Urbansky, R., Lorang, M., Siegrist, M.: Performance evaluation on contour extraction using hough transform and RANSAC for multi-sensor data fusion applications in industrial food inspection. In: Signal Processing: Algorithms, Architectures, Arrangements, and Applications (SPA), 2016, pp. 234–237. IEEE (2016)
34. Lacey, J.I.: Somatic response patterning and stress: some revisions of activation theory. In: Appley, M.H., Trumbull, R. (eds.) Psychological Stress: Some Issues in Research, Appleton-Century-Crofts, New York (1967)
35. Lenz, C., et al.: Human workflow analysis using 3D occupancy grid hand tracking in a human-robot collaboration scenario. In: 2011 IEEE/RSJ International Conference on Intelligent Robots and Systems, pp. 3375–3380, September 2011. https://doi.org/10.1109/IROS.2011.6094570
36. Leykin, A., Hammoud, R.: Real-time estimation of human attention field in LWIR and color surveillance videos. In: IEEE Computer Society Conference on Computer Vision and Pattern Recognition Workshops, CVPRW 2008, pp. 1–6. IEEE (2008)
37. Li, X., Li, D., Wan, J., Vasilakos, A.V., Lai, C.F., Wang, S.: A review of industrial wireless networks in the context of industry 4.0. Wirel. Netw. **23**(1), 23–41 (2017)
38. Maekawa, T., Nakai, D., Ohara, K., Namioka, Y.: Toward practical factory activity recognition: unsupervised understanding of repetitive assembly work in a factory. In: Proceedings of the 2016 ACM International Joint Conference on Pervasive and Ubiquitous Computing, UbiComp 2016, pp. 1088–1099. ACM, New York (2016). https://doi.org/10.1145/2971648.2971721, http://doi.acm.org/10.1145/2971648.2971721
39. Magill, R.A., Hall, K.G.: A review of the contextual interference effect in motor skill acquisition. Hum. Mov. Sci. **9**(3), 241–289 (1990)
40. Makantasis, K., Doulamis, A., Doulamis, N., Psychas, K.: Deep learning based human behavior recognition in industrial workflows. In: 2016 IEEE International Conference on Image Processing (ICIP), pp. 1609–1613, September 2016. https://doi.org/10.1109/ICIP.2016.7532630
41. Malaisé, A., Maurice, P., Colas, F., Charpillet, F.c., Ivaldi, S.: Activity recognition with multiple wearable sensors for industrial applications. In: ACHI 2018 - Eleventh International Conference on Advances in Computer-Human Interactions, Rome, Italy, March 2018. https://hal.archives-ouvertes.fr/hal-01701996
42. Marabelli, M., Hansen, S., Newell, S., Frigerio, C.: The light and dark side of the black box: sensor-based technology in the automotive industry. CAIS **40**, 16 (2017)
43. Maurtua, I., Kirisci, P.T., Stiefmeier, T., Sbodio, M.L., Witt, H.: A wearable computing prototype for supporting training activities in automotive production. In: 4th International Forum on Applied Wearable Computing 2007, pp. 1–12, March 2007
44. Otto, M.M., Agethen, P., Geiselhart, F., Rietzler, M., Gaisbauer, F., Rukzio, E.: Presenting a holistic framework for scalable, marker-less motion capturing: skeletal tracking performance analysis, sensor fusion algorithms and usage in automotive industry. J. Virtual R. Broadcast. **13**(3) (2016)
45. Poh, M.Z., et al.: Convulsive seizure detection using a wrist-worn electrodermal activity and accelerometry biosensor. Epilepsia **53**(5), e93–e97 (2012). https://doi.org/10.1111/j.1528-1167.2012.03444.x

46. Potter, L.E., Araullo, J., Carter, L.: The leap motion controller: a view on sign language. In: Proceedings of the 25th Australian Computer-Human Interaction Conference: Augmentation, Application, Innovation, Collaboration, pp. 175–178. ACM (2013)
47. Reining, C., Schlangen, M., Hissmann, L., ten Hompel, M., Moya, F., Fink, G.A.: Attribute representation for human activity recognition of manual order picking activities. In: Proceedings of the 5th International Workshop on Sensor-Based Activity Recognition and Interaction, iWOAR 2018, pp. 10–1. ACM, New York (2018). https://doi.org/10.1145/3266157.3266214, http://doi.acm.org/10.1145/3266157.3266214
48. Rude, D.J., Adams, S., Beling, P.A.: A benchmark dataset for depth sensor based activity recognition in a manufacturing process. IFAC-PapersOnLine **48**(3), 668–674 (2015). https://doi.org/10.1016/j.ifacol.2015.06.159. http://www.sciencedirect.com/science/article/pii/S2405896315003985, 15th IFAC Symposium onInformation Control Problems inManufacturing
49. Shcherbina, A.: Accuracy in wrist-worn, sensor-based measurements of heart rate and energy expenditure in a diverse cohort. J. Pers. Med. **7**(2), 3 (2017)
50. Smith, K.C., Ba, S.O., Odobez, J.M., Gatica-Perez, D.: Tracking attention for multiple people: wandering visual focus of attention estimation. Tech. rep., IDIAP (2006)
51. Srbinovska, M., Gavrovski, C., Dimcev, V., Krkoleva, A., Borozan, V.: Environmental parameters monitoring in precision agriculture using wireless sensor networks. J. Clean. Prod. **88**, 297–307 (2015)
52. Stiefmeier, T., Ogris, G., Junker, H., Lukowicz, P., Troster, G.: Combining motion sensors and ultrasonic hands tracking for continuous activity recognition in a maintenance scenario. In: 2006 10th IEEE International Symposium on Wearable Computers, pp. 97–104, October 2006. https://doi.org/10.1109/ISWC.2006.286350
53. Stiefmeier, T., Roggen, D., Ogris, G., Lukowicz, P., Tröster, G.: Wearable activity tracking in car manufacturing. IEEE Pervasive Comput. **7**(2) (2008). https://doi.org/10.1109/MPRV.2008.40
54. Suriya-Prakash, M., John-Preetham, G., Sharma, R.: Is heart rate variability related to cognitive performance in visuospatial working memory? PeerJ PrePrints (2015)
55. Tao, W., Lai, Z.H., Leu, M.C., Yin, Z.: Worker activity recognition in smart manufacturing using IMU and semg signals with convolutional neural networks. Procedia Manuf. **26**, 1159–1166 (2018). https://doi.org/10.1016/j.promfg.2018.07.152. http://www.sciencedirect.com/science/article/pii/S235197891830828X, 46th SME North American Manufacturing Research Conference, NAMRC 46, Texas, USA
56. Thatcher, R.W., John, E.R.: Functional neuroscience: I. Foundations of cognitive processes. Lawrence Erlbaum (1977)
57. Veres, G., Grabner, H., Middleton, L., Van Gool, L.: Automatic workflow monitoring in industrial environments. In: Kimmel, R., Klette, R., Sugimoto, A. (eds.) ACCV 2010. LNCS, vol. 6492, pp. 200–213. Springer, Heidelberg (2011). https://doi.org/10.1007/978-3-642-19315-6_16
58. Voulodimos, A., Grabner, H., Kosmopoulos, D., Van Gool, L., Varvarigou, T.: Robust workflow recognition using holistic features and outlier-tolerant fused hidden markov models. In: Diamantaras, K., Duch, W., Iliadis, L.S. (eds.) ICANN 2010. LNCS, vol. 6352, pp. 551–560. Springer, Heidelberg (2010). https://doi.org/10.1007/978-3-642-15819-3_71
59. Weichert, F., Bachmann, D., Rudak, B., Fisseler, D.: Analysis of the accuracy and robustness of the leap motion controller. Sensors **13**(5), 6380–6393 (2013)

60. Yang, J., Shi, Z., Wu, Z.: Vision-based action recognition of construction workers using dense trajectories. Adv. Eng. Inform. **30**(3), 327–336 (2016). https://doi.org/10.1016/j.aei.2016.04.009. http://www.sciencedirect.com/science/article/pii/S1474034616300842
61. Zappi, P., et al.: Activity recognition from on-body sensors: accuracy-power trade-off by dynamic sensor selection. In: Verdone, R. (ed.) EWSN 2008. LNCS, vol. 4913, pp. 17–33. Springer, Heidelberg (2008). https://doi.org/10.1007/978-3-540-77690-1_2

Hand Gesture Recognition Based on EMG Data: A Convolutional Neural Network Approach

Panagiotis Tsinganos[1,2]([✉]), Bruno Cornelis[2], Jan Cornelis[2], Bart Jansen[2,3], and Athanassios Skodras[1]

[1] Department of Electrical and Computer Engineering, University of Patras, 26504 Patras, Greece
{panagiotis.tsinganos,skodras}@ece.upatras.gr
[2] Department of Electronics and Informatics, Vrije Universiteit Brussel, 1050 Brussels, Belgium
ptsingan@etrovub.be, {bcorneli,jpcorneli,bjansen}@etrovub.be
[3] imec, Kapeldreef 75, 3001 Leuven, Belgium

Abstract. Deep learning (DL) has transformed the field of data analysis by dramatically improving the state of the art in various classification and prediction tasks. Especially in the area of computer vision and speech processing, DL has recently demonstrated better performance and generalisation properties, compared to classical machine learning approaches, which are based on the extraction of hand-crafted model-based features followed by classification. Hand gestures and speech constitute two of the most important modalities in human-to-human communication and man-machine interaction. In biomedical engineering, a lot of new work is directed towards electromyography-based gesture recognition. In this paper, we present a brief overview of DL methods for electromyography-based hand gesture recognition and then we select from literature a simple model based on Convolutional Neural Networks that we consider as the baseline model. The proposed modifications to the baseline model yield a 3% classification improvement. In the current paper, we concentrate on the explanatory analysis of this performance improvement. An ablation study identifies which modifications are the most important ones, and label smoothing is investigated to verify if the results can be improved by reducing a priori bias. The analysis helps in understanding the limitations of the model and exploring new ways to improve the performance.

Keywords: Deep learning · CNN · Biomedical engineering · sEMG hand gesture recognition · Label smoothing · Ablation study

This work was supported by the VUB-UPatras International Joint Research Group (IJRG) on ICT.

© Springer Nature Switzerland AG 2019
A. Holzinger et al. (Eds.): PhyCS 2016–2018, LNCS 10057, pp. 180–197, 2019.
https://doi.org/10.1007/978-3-030-27950-9_10

1   Introduction

Hand gestures constitute one of the most important modalities in human-to-human communication. Also for human-computer interaction (HCI), there has been a particular interest in (hand) gesture recognition. This finds many applications, including sign language recognition, robotic equipment control, virtual reality gaming, and prosthetics control [7]. Among the various sensor modalities that have been used to capture hand gesture information, electromyography (EMG) is considered more appropriate since it captures the muscle's electrical activity; the physical phenomenon that results in hand gestures. EMG data can be recorded either in an invasive or a non-invasive manner. Surface electromyography (sEMG) is a non-invasive technique that measures muscle's action potential from the surface of the skin, contrary to invasive methods that penetrate the skin to reach the muscle directly.

A popular approach to sEMG-based gesture recognition consists of using pattern recognition methods derived from Machine Learning (ML) [28]. Conventional ML pipelines include the following sequential stages: data acquisition, feature extraction, model definition and inference. Acquisition of sEMG signals involves one or more electrodes attached around the target muscle group. The features used for classification are usually hand-crafted by human experts and capture the temporal and frequency characteristics of the data. Typical features that have been used for sEMG pattern classification are listed in Table 1. These extracted features serve as the input to ML classifiers, such as k-Nearest Neighbors (kNN), Support Vector Machines (SVM), Multi-Layered Perceptron (MLP), Linear Discriminant Analysis (LDA), Random Forests (RF), and Hidden Markov Models (HMM), where the classifier's parameters are adjusted towards accurate classification.

Deep Learning (DL) is a class of ML algorithms that has revolutionized many fields of data analysis [16]. For example, Convolutional Neural Networks (CNNs) and Recurrent Neural Networks (RNNs) were successfully deployed for image classification and speech recognition tasks, respectively. DL methods differ from conventional ML approaches in that feature extraction is part of the model definition, therefore obviating the need for hand-crafted features. Although these methods are not new [16], they recently gained more attention due to the increased availability of abundant data and vast improvements in computing hardware allowing these computationally demanding methods to be executed in less time.

Motivated by the progress of DL methods we provide an overview of the use of DL methods for sEMG pattern classification problems and propose modifications to a simple CNN model [1]. The comparison with the state of the art and the analysis of the results sheds light on how this architecture performs and allows for improvements to be made.

The remainder of the paper is organized as follows. In Sect. 2, we provide an overview of ML- and DL-based gesture recognition approaches. Section 3 gives a detailed description of the proposed CNN architecture. The experiments performed for the evaluation of the model are presented in Sect. 4, while the results

Table 1. Typical sEMG features [34].

Feature	Domain	Reference
Root mean square	time	[5]
Variance	time	[20]
Mean absolute value	time	[2, 11, 18, 20]
Zero crossings	time	[2, 11, 18]
Slope sign changes	time	[2, 11, 18]
Waveform length	time	[2, 11, 18, 20]
Histogram	time	[2, 11, 18, 20]
Short time fourier transform	frequency	[12, 20]
Cepstral coefficients	frequency	[20]
Marginal discrete wavelet transform	time-frequency	[2, 20]

and a brief discussion are given in Sect. 5. Finally, in Sect. 6 we conclude the paper and outline future work.

2   Related Work

There exists a great body of literature on the problem of sEMG-based hand gesture recognition. One can discriminate between approaches that use conventional ML techniques and studies based on DL methods.

The most significant study on sEMG classification with traditional ML techniques is described in [18]. For every 200 ms segment of 2 channel sEMG signals, 5 time-domain features are extracted and fed to an MLP classifier, achieving an accuracy of 91.2% on the classification of 4 hand gestures. Later approaches based on this work improve the classification performance by either using more features or different classifiers. In [11], the same set of features is extracted from 4 channel sEMG signals and fed to an LDA classifier. The average accuracy obtained is greater than 90% and is further improved by applying a majority vote window to the predictions of the classifier. The work presented in [5] achieves a 97.14% accuracy on the task of classifying 3 types of grasp motions using the RMS value from 7 electrodes as the input to an SVM classifier. In [20], a set of time- and frequency- domain features is extracted from 8 channel myoelectric signals and evaluated with various classifiers. This experiment is considered the first successful approach for the classification of a large number of hand gestures, since they achieve high accuracy (70–80%) on a set of 52 hand gestures (Ninapro dataset [3]) using any of the proposed features and an SVM classifier with RBF kernel. This work was further improved in [2] by considering linear combination of features and using a RF classifier, resulting in an average accuracy of 75.32%. In [14], different kernel classifiers were evaluated jointly on EMG and acceleration signals, improving the classification accuracy by 5%. Most recently, in [26] an HMM-based model along with an EMG channel selection method shows significant improvement in the classification accuracy of 18 gestures from the Ninapro dataset compared to using all available channels.

Given the many successes of DL methods in the fields of image processing and speech recognition, many works have investigated their application to EMG-based hand gesture recognition. In [31] and [30], the authors propose a Deep Belief Network (DBN) classifier as a more effective model compared to a shallow MLP network trained with back-propagation. Time-domain features are extracted from segments of 2 channel EMG signals that are used to train the model in a layer-by-layer fashion, either with a greedy approach or using genetic algorithms, achieving an accuracy of 88.59% and 89.29% respectively on a set of 5 movements.

The first end-to-end DL architecture, however, was proposed in [23]. The authors built a CNN-based model for the classification of 6 common hand movements resulting in a better classification accuracy compared to SVM. In [1], a simple CNN architecture based on 5 blocks of convolutional and pooling layers is used to classify a large number of gestures. The classification accuracy is comparable to those obtained with classical methods, though not higher than the best performance achieved on the same problem using a RF classifier. The works described in [13] and [35] improve the results across various datasets incorporating dropout [32] and batch normalization [29] techniques in their methodology. Apart from choosing different model architectures, a difference to previous works consists of using a high-density electrode array to capture EMG data. Using instantaneous EMG images, i.e. images generated from the instant values of the sEMG grid, [13] achieves a 89.3% accuracy on a set of 8 movements, going up to 99.0% when using majority voting over 40 ms windows. In [35], the observation is made that a small group of muscles play a significant role in some movements. Therefore, a multi-stream CNN architecture is employed, where the input is divided into smaller images that are separately processed by convolutional layers before being merged with fully connected layers. With this model the reported accuracy on the Ninapro dataset is improved by 7.2% (from 77.8% to 85%). In a similar fashion, the work of [9] supports the idea that EMG signals of each channel should be first processed independently (with 1D convolutions), before being jointly analysed (with 2D convolutions) in order to eliminate possible errors due to premature fusion. In addition, their model uses two different sizes for the 1D filters which are applied in parallel. This architecture results in an average accuracy of 78.86% on 18 gestures of the Ninapro dataset.

Later works deal with the problem of inter-subject classification, i.e. where the train and test data come from different subjects, either with recalibration ([36]) or model adaptation ([8,10]). The performance of the network proposed in [36], which takes as input downsampled spectrograms of EMG segments, is improved by updating the network weights using the predictions of previous sessions corrected by majority voting. In [10] it is assumed that the weights of each layer of the network contain information that allows for differentiation between gestures, while the mean and variance of the batch normalization layers correspond to discriminating between sessions/subjects. Therefore, they apply adaptive batch normalization (AdaBN) [22], where only the normalization statistics are updated for each subject using a few unlabeled data. The results show improved performance compared to a model without adaptation. The authors of [8] use transfer learning techniques to exploit inter-subject data learned by a pre-trained source network. In their architecture, for each subject a new network is instantiated with weighted connections to the source network. Through this technique, which achieves an accuracy of 98.31% on 7 movements, predictions for a new subject are based both on previously learned information and subject-specific data.

Lately, new model architectures have been applied to the problem of EMG-based gesture recognition. In [6], the final fully connected layer on top of CNN's is replaced by an SVM. The proposed architecture outperforms both an SVM classifier based on hand-crafted features and a CNN model with a fully connected layers classifier on the problems of inter-session (i.e. where train and test data come from the same subject but different recording sessions, therefore a different electrode position is induced) and inter-subject classification. The work of [17] presents a compact CNN that adjusts the 'Fire module' of the SqueezeNet model [19] by performing temporal convolutions. Using less than 6 K parameters it achieves higher intra-subject accuracy than the models proposed in [1] and [13] with sizes of 100 K and 600 K parameters, respectively. Although both networks in [6] and [17] introduce models that perform well, they tackle the classification of a rather small set of gestures (10 and 15 gestures respectively). Finally, the authors of [27] investigate the application of RNN models with Long Short-Term Memory (LSTM) and Gated Recurrent Units (GRU). Among various configurations evaluated on the Ninapro dataset, a bidirectional RNN with LSTM units and an attention mechanism [25] obtains an intra-subject accuracy of 86.7% on the classification problem of 18 gestures.

3   Model Architecture

The problem of sEMG-based hand gesture recognition can be formulated as an image classification problem using CNNs, where the input sEMG image has a size of $H \times W \times 1$ (height × width × depth). Various approaches have been employed to construct an sEMG image. For example, in the works of [13,35], and [10], the instantaneous sEMG signals from a high density electrode array have been used; the width and the height of the array match the dimensions of the image. In addition, sEMG images can be constructed with segments of sEMG signals using (overlapping) time-windows, in which case the width matches the number of electrodes and the height is equal to the window length [1]. Another approach is based on spectrograms using the Short Time Fourier Transform (STFT) of sEMG segments, where for each channel of the EMG a spectrogram is created resulting in an image of size frequency × time-bins × channels [8,36].

In this work, we adhere to the approach of [1] and generate sEMG images with sliding windows. These images are created using a window length of 150 ms and an overlap of 60%, i.e. 90 ms, in order to make fair comparisons with previous works in the literature that use similar time-windows. Therefore, the input

EMG image has a size of 15×10 (height $\times$ width), where the height dimension corresponds to the window length (i.e. 150 ms sampled at 100 Hz) and the width equals the number of electrodes. An example of an image created with this method is shown in Fig. 1.

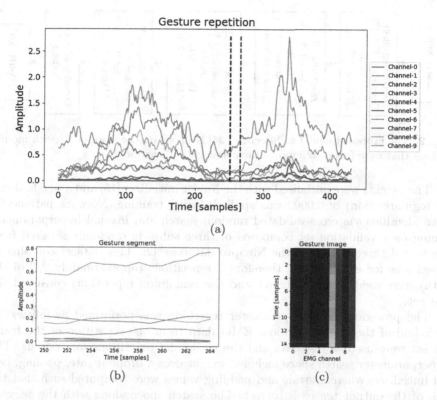

Fig. 1. Based on the work of [1], the creation of EMG images consists of segmenting the EMG signals and stacking them into an image. (a) Initial multi-channel rectified EMG signal with 150 ms segment denoted with dotted lines, (b) The 150 ms EMG window, and (c) The EMG signal represented as an image.

The proposed CNN (depicted in Fig. 2 [34]) is based on the architecture introduced in [1]. However, substantial modifications have been made to increase the model's classification accuracy. The main adjustments in the architecture are the introduction of dropout [32] layers and the use of max pooling instead of average pooling, while the number of trainable parameters remains the same.

The CNN architecture has 4 hidden convolutional layers and 1 output layer. The first two hidden layers consist of 32 filters of size 1×10 and 3×3. The third layer consists of 64 filters of size 5×5. The fourth layer contains 64 filters of 5×1 size, whereas the last one is a G-way convolutional layer with 1×1 filters, where G is the number of gestures to be classified. Zero padding is applied before the convolutions of the hidden layers, which are followed by rectified linear unit

(ReLU) non-linearities and dropout layer with a probability of 0.15 for zeroing the output of a hidden unit. In addition, a subsampling layer performs max pooling over a 3×3 window after the dropout of the second and third layers. Finally, the last convolutional layer is followed by a softmax activation function.

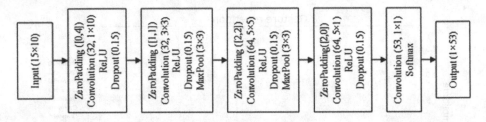

Fig. 2. The proposed model architecture [34] is based on the work of [1] with modifications that were found to improve the classification accuracy.

The weights were initialized with the Xavier initializer [15] and a weight decay (l_2 regularization) of 0.0002 was applied during training. Network parameters were identified via cross-validated random search and manual hyperparameter tuning on a validation set composed of three subjects randomly selected from the first dataset (DB-1) of the Ninapro database [2]. This dataset contains 10 repetitions for each gesture, therefore 7 repetitions (approximately 2/3 of the data) were used as the train set and the remaining repetitions consisted the test set.

The procedure of hyperparameter searching was performed as follows. In each fold of the cross-validation, EMG data from one repetition of the training set were used as test data and the remaining repetitions for training. The hyperparameter search space included weight decay, dropout rate, pooling, kernel initializer, whereas stride and padding values were computed such that the size of the output tensor is correct. The search space along with the selected values are listed in Table 2 [34]. Additionally, the proper optimizer parameters were found in the same fashion for each evaluation method.

Table 2. Hyperparameter tuning [34].

Parameter	Search space	Selected value
Weight decay	[0.0001, 0.001]	0.0002
Dropout	[0, 0.333]	0.15
Pooling method	'max', 'average'	'max'
Kernel initializer	'glorot', 'he', 'normal', 'uniform'	'glorot'
Optimizer	'SGD', 'Adam'	'SGD'
Learning rate	[0.001, 0.1]	0.05
Learning schedule	'constant', 'step decay', 'exponential decay'	'step decay'
Epochs	[30,150]	100
Batch size	32, 64, 128, 256, 512, 1024	512

The preprocessing of EMG signals is described next. Firstly, a 1st order 1 Hz low-pass Butterworth filter is applied as in previous studies on Ninapro database ([1,13]). Then, training data are augmented by duplicating the signals of each repetition and adding Gaussian noise with a signal to noise ratio (SNR) equal to 25 dB, where the amount of noise was calculated separately for each EMG channel. Finally, both for training and testing, the EMG signals are segmented into overlapping windows of 150 ms length and 90 ms overlap, which can be considered as a form of data augmentation similar to image shifting.

Due to the recording process followed in the Ninapro database, each gesture repetition is followed by a resting phase, meaning that the majority of the images correspond to the 'rest' gesture. In addition, there are variations in the duration of the gesture repetitions, which affects the number of generated images. Therefore, accounting for the fact that gestures are not equally represented in the dataset, two steps are taken to deal with the imbalance problem. First, the EMG data of the 'rest' gesture are subsampled, such that the same number of repetitions is shared between all gestures. Secondly, during training the loss function is weighted such that the network pays more attention to under-represented gestures.

4   Experiments

The proposed CNN architecture is evaluated on data from the Ninapro database that includes sEMG data related to 53 hand movements of 78 subjects (11 transradial amputees, 67 intact subjects) divided into three datasets. The Ninapro DB-1 includes data acquisitions of 27 intact subjects (7 females, 20 males; 2 left handed, 25 right handed; age 28 ± 3.4 years). The second dataset includes data acquisitions of 40 intact subjects (12 females, 28 males; 6 left handed, 34 right handed; age 29.9 ± 3.9 years). The third dataset includes data acquisitions of 11 transradial amputees (11 males; 1 left handed, 10 right handed; age 42.36 ± 11.96 years). More details about the database and the acquisition procedure can be found in [1], and [2]. Tables 3 and 4 summarize the information about the Ninapro database [34].

Table 3. The Ninapro dataset [34].

Dataset	Subjects	Movements	Electrodes	Sampling (Hz)
Dataset 1 (DB 1)	27	53	10	100
Dataset 2 (DB-2)	40	53	12	2000
Dataset 3 (DB-3)	11	53	12	2000

All the evaluations of the model were carried out on the Ninapro DB-1 using all the data available. This dataset is comprised of sEMG signals captured from 27 subjects using 10 electrodes, of which 8 are placed around the forearm and the other 2 are placed on the main activity spots of the large flexor and extensor muscles of the forearm [2]. For a fair comparison with current literature, the data were split into train and test datasets following the approach described in [1], i.e. repetitions 2, 5, and 7 were used for testing and the rest for training. Hyperparameter tuning was performed using cross-validation on the training set.

Table 4. Gestures label/number as in [2].

Label	Gesture
0	Rest
1–12	Individual finger extension/flexion
13–20	Isometric/isotonic configurations
20–29	Wrist movements
30–52	Grasps and functional movements

The models were trained on a workstation with an Intel Xeon, 2.40 GHz (E5-2630v3) processor, 16 GB RAM and an Nvidia GTX1080, 8 GB GPU.

4.1 Evaluation

The model is evaluated by means of two experiments. The first one adheres to the evaluation procedure described in [1], while the second uses the setting of [13]. As performance metrics, we use the average accuracies on the train and test sets, the average of the top-3 test accuracies (i.e. the accuracy when any of the 3 highest output probabilities match the expected gesture) and the test accuracy after majority voting on each gesture repetition (i.e. the repetition segment of a specific gesture is assigned the majority gesture label of the sEMG images that correspond to that repetition). Additionally, the model performance is further evaluated by analyzing misclassifications per class, provided by a confusion matrix, and the accuracy over the gesture duration normalized time as in [3].

In accordance with [1], a model was trained using 7 repetitions and tested with the remaining 3 for each of the 27 subjects in the dataset. Each model is initialized with randomized weights and trained using stochastic gradient descent (SGD) for 100 epochs with 0.05 initial learning rate and a batch size of 512. The learning rate was reduced every 15th epoch by a factor of 50%.

The second experiment follows the set up of [13], which differs from the procedure of [1] in that a pre-trained network is created using all the training data of all subjects and then a fine-tuned model is generated for each subject. The first model is initialized with randomized weights and trained using SGD for 100 epochs with 0.05 learning rate, and a batch size of 512. The learning rate was reduced every 15 epochs by a factor of 50%. The subject-specific models were initialized with the pre-trained network and the last two convolutional layers were fine-tuned using SGD optimizer for 30 epochs with a learning rate of 0.01 halved every 10th epoch, and a batch size of 128.

4.2   Ablation Study

In ML, an ablation study typically refers to the procedure that removes some 'feature' or component of the model, and measures how that affects performance compared to the model that includes all the components of the study. In this work, an ablation study was conducted investigating the impact of the model components shown in Table 5. Specifically, each parameter was in turn set to the values proposed in the initial paper of [1] and the performance, as in the first evaluation experiment, was recorded for 10 subjects.

Pooling: All pooling layers use the 'average' method as in [1] while the rest of the parameters remain as in Table 2 [34].

Dropout: Early experiments showed that the model might suffer from over-fitting, thus dropout layers were used as regularizers. In this case, the network is trained without dropout ($dropout = 0$).

Weight decay: The value of the l_2 regularization is set to 0.0005 as described in the original paper.

Regularization: We examine the impact of both the dropout and the weight decay by setting each one to their original values ($dropout = 0, l_2 = 0.0005$).

Optimizer: The parameters of the optimizer (i.e. the learning rate, the batch size and the number of epochs) are reverted to their initial values while retaining the remaining parameters of the model.

Table 5. Hyperparameter values for the experiments of ablation study.

Affected component	Pooling	Dropout	L_2	Learning rate	Batch size	Epochs
Default	'max'	0.15	0.0002	0.05, 'step'	512	100
Pooling	'average'	0.15	0.0002	0.05, 'step'	512	100
Dropout	'max'	0.0	0.0002	0.05, 'step'	512	100
Weight decay	'max'	0.15	0.0005	0.05, 'step'	512	100
Regularization	'max'	0.0	0.0005	0.05, 'step'	512	100
Optimizer	'max'	0.15	0.0002	0.001, 'fixed'	256	30

4.3   Label Smoothing

Label smoothing is a regularization method that was first described in [33]. It consists of redistributing the ground-truth softmax probabilities of the training examples using a distribution function. This function can be any distribution such as the uniform [33] or even another neural network [4,24]. Adding noise to the labels acts as a regularizer since it prevents the model from becoming too confident about its predictions therefore encouraging generalization.

In these experiments, three label smoothing methods are investigated:

(a) Smoothing with the uniform distribution where the one-hot ground-truth label $q(k) = \delta_{k,y}$ is replaced by

$$q'(k) = (1 - \epsilon)\delta_{k,y} + \epsilon g(k) \tag{1}$$

where $k, y \in [0, 52]$, $\delta_{k,y}$ is a Dirac delta, which equals 1 for $k = y$ and 0 otherwise, $g(k) = \mathcal{U}\{0, 52\}$ the uniform distribution and ϵ is a smoothing factor.

(b) Uniform smoothing conditioned on the general group type of the gesture. The gesture groups as defined in the Ninapro dataset are shown in Table 4. Therefore, $g(k)$ in Eq. 1 becomes

$$
\begin{aligned}
g(k|y = 0) &= \mathcal{U}\{0, 52\} \\
g(k|y \in [1, 12]) &= \begin{cases} 1/13 \text{ for } k \leq 12 \\ 0 \quad \text{elsewhere} \end{cases} \\
g(k|y \in [13, 20]) &= \begin{cases} 1/9 \text{ for } k = 0 \text{ or } k \in [13, 20] \\ 0 \quad \text{elsewhere} \end{cases} \\
g(k|y \in [21, 29]) &= \begin{cases} 1/10 \text{ for } k = 0 \text{ or } k \in [21, 29] \\ 0 \quad \text{elsewhere} \end{cases} \\
g(k|y \in [30, 52]) &= \begin{cases} 1/24 \text{ for } k = 0 \text{ or } k \in [30, 52] \\ 0 \quad \text{elsewhere} \end{cases}
\end{aligned} \tag{2}
$$

(c) A refinery network $f_r()$ [4] is initially trained with the ground-truth labels of the training examples $\{X_{train}, Y_{train}\}$, while a second network is trained with the predictions of the refinery model on the training data $\{X_{train}, f_r(X_{train})\}$. The network architectures can be the same or different, and both are randomly initialized.

The parameters of the smoothing methods that were used are as follows. For the uniform and group-based distributions the smoothing factor is set to $\epsilon = 0.1$, as in other works in the literature [33], while in the case of the refinery network, both models have the same architecture and they are trained with the same parameters as in Table 2 [34]. The performance is measured as in the first evaluation experiment.

5   Results and Discussion

This paper presents an overview of DL approaches, based on convolutional layers and learning methods that were successful in other application domains, applied to the problem of hand gesture recognition. The results of the model evaluation are summarized in Table 6. Compared to similar works evaluated on the same dataset, the proposed model outperforms the original network of [1], while it is inferior to the more complex approaches of [13] and [35]. Table 7 [34] shows the comparison between these works under the same evaluation that was used in each paper. The model of [13] uses as input the instantaneous EMG images,

Table 6. Evaluation results for two different configurations [34].

Setting	Train accuracy	Test accuracy	Top-3 accuracy	Vote accuracy
[1]	0.8303	0.7048	0.8706	0.9231
[13]	0.8121	0.7206	0.8806	0.9306

Table 7. Accuracy comparisons. In [13], the value in parentheses is the accuracy over a majority window of 200 ms [34].

Setting	This work	[1]	[13]	[35]
[1]	0.7048	0.6659	-	-
[13]	0.7206	-	0.7610 (0.7780)	0.85

i.e. 1 × 10 for the Ninapro DB-1, so the majority vote over 200 ms is shown in parentheses, whereas the input image in the network of [35] is 20 × 10 pixels.

Apart from differences in the input, there are more model architecture dissimilarities. Both [13] and [35] incorporate batch normalization [29] that allows for faster convergence, and fully connected layers that offer increased network capacity due to more trainable weights. In addition, the approach of [35] adopts a multi-stream pipeline where a number of EMG electrodes are processed separately and are then merged with fully connected layers. This split-and-merge approach enables learning the correlation between individual muscles and specific gestures leading to state-of-the-art accuracy of 85% on the Ninapro DB-1. However, we explicitly chose not to follow similar approaches in this paper in order to develop a better understanding of how DL methods can be applied to sEMG data through a simpler network.

The proposed network is further evaluated through loss graphs and an error analysis. Figure 3 shows the loss graphs during training on the train and test sets. It can be observed that decaying the learning rate helps the network parameters converge to a better optimum. When comparing the loss between the train and

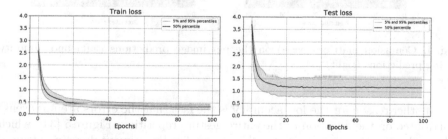

Fig. 3. Loss value after each training epoch calculated on train set (left) and test set (right). The solid line is the median value across subjects while the shaded area corresponds to the 5% and 95% percentiles.

test sets, it is obvious that there is some degree of overfitting. However, applying more regularization (e.g. dropout, weight decay) does not decrease the test
loss. Therefore, a different pipeline (e.g. preprocessing steps, data augmentation,
different filter sizes) may reduce the generalization error of the network.

An error analysis was performed to better understand the performance of our
model. The confusion matrix is calculated for each subject evaluation and the
average is shown in Fig. 4 [34]. Most misclassifications occur around the main
diagonal and according to the class labels (Table 4) mostly similar movements
are falsely categorized. That is expected considering the location of the EMG
electrodes and the muscles that participate in each movement. For example,
gesture labels '9', '11' represent the adduction and flexion of the thumb that are
coordinated by the same forearm muscles. In addition, there is a concentration
of errors in the low-right corner that corresponds to grasps and functional hand
gestures that involve more muscles. Taking into account that each EMG image
is a 150 ms segment and the gesture repetition lasts 5 s, we may conclude that
for a given misclassification a proportion of the images will be similar between
the two gestures. A possible explanation is that some groups of movements
can be broken down into the same smaller movements. It is only when the full
sequence of images is available that the network can decide correctly which
gesture is performed. Comparing the confusion matrices before and after the
majority voting we see that most errors around the diagonal are reduced.

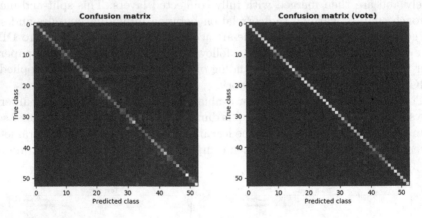

Fig. 4. Confusion matrices based on the per image predictions (left) and majority
voting predictions (right) [34].

Another reason for the low accuracy is the fact that the errors are not evenly
distributed on the duration of the entire gesture repetition. Figure 5 [34], which
relates classification errors with the time-normalized movement duration, demon-
strates that misclassifications are primarily concentrated in the beginning and at
the completion of the movement. The reason is that during the recording session
there is a gradual transition between rest, gesture and rest, in contrast to the

discrete changes of the gesture labels. Consequently, accuracy is lower during these transition periods where the change in movement is not yet clearly evident from the input EMG signal [3].

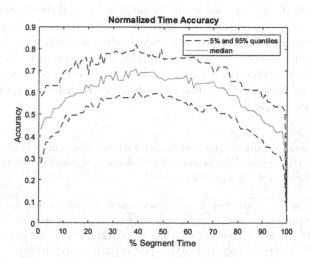

Fig. 5. Plot of prediction accuracy against normalized time duration. It can be seen that at the start and completion of the gesture repetition the accuracy is lower [34].

The results of the ablation study are presented next. Each row in Table 8 shows the difference in the average accuracy (train, test and majority voting) of ten subjects between the baseline model and the corresponding ablated model. It is obvious that between the two modifications made to the architecture of [1], the type of pooling method has huge impact on the model performance (9% on the test set). The dropout and the weight decay affect the accuracy by about 2.5%, which means that the model can be effectively regularized using only data augmentation methods. In addition, modifications to the optimizer parameters were observed to be essential to achieve an accuracy similar to the one reported in [1].

Table 8. Difference in accuracy between the control model and the parameters of the ablation study. The values in parentheses are the standard deviations.

	Train accuracy	Test accuracy	Vote accuracy
Pooling	−0.2315 (0.0346)	−0.0905 (0.0391)	−0.0423 (0.0389)
Dropout	+0.1095 (0.0051)	−0.0255 (0.0534)	−0.0114 (0.0472)
Weight decay	−0.0249 (0.0287)	+0.0011 (0.0462)	+0.0040 (0.0368)
Regularization	+0.0954 (0.0099)	−0.0173 (0.0443)	−0.0077 (0.0437)
Optimizer	−0.6782 (0.0751)	−0.4272 (0.0868)	−0.4540 (0.1276)

Additional experiments examined the regularization effect of label smoothing. The purpose of this method is to improve the ability of the model to generalize to unseen data, thus reducing the loss on the test data. The results of these experiments, as well as a comparison to the baseline model without label smoothing (Table 6 [34]), are shown in Table 9. Statistical significance is assessed with the Wilcoxon signed-rank test and an '*' denotes a significant difference between the baseline model and the corresponding smoothing method at a significance level of 5%. We see that the loss value during training is increased in all cases, while the expected decrease in the test loss is observed only for the label refinery method. However, this difference does not translate to an improvement on the accuracy metric.

Table 9. Loss and accuracy values with and without label smoothing. The values in parentheses are the standard deviations. An '*' denotes significant difference compared to the 'Base' model at a 5% significance level.

	Train loss	Test loss	Train accuracy	Test accuracy	Vote accuracy
Base	0.3337 (0.0679)	1.1947 (0.2795)	0.8303 (0.0410)	0.7048 (0.0626)	0.9231 (0.0340)
Uniform	0.8891* (0.0799)	1.3352* (0.1933)	0.8150* (0.0429)	0.7057* (0.0602)	0.9162 (0.0343)
Group	0.7638* (0.0722)	1.2595* (0.2060)	0.8195* (0.0423)	0.7033 (0.0604)	0.9143 (0.0298)
Refinery	0.5378* (0.1059)	1.1109* (0.2407)	0.8192* (0.0365)	0.6957* (0.0613)	0.9234 (0.0354)

Overall, it is shown that a simple CNN architecture can be successful at the task of sEMG hand gesture recognition, taking into account accuracy of a model that performs at random when classifying 53 gestures. Small modifications to the model parameters and the training process can boost the performance, whereas deeper and more complex networks yield the best performance. The inability of the proposed model to generalize well to unseen data needs to be addressed to facilitate further improvement. Finally, the use of small EMG segments accounts for much of the classification error as there is a significant amount of overlap happens between EMG signals of similar gesture groups, especially during their transitive periods. Therefore, majority voting over these small EMG segments provides a better evaluation metric.

6   Conclusions

This paper presents an overview of recent advances in the use of DL methods for sEMG hand gesture classification, while improvements to existing architectures are discussed. The proposed modified CNN model extends the basic model described in [1] and is compared to the state of the art. It improves on the selected baseline model by 3%, yet the works of [13] and [35] outperform it under the same evaluation settings, but at the cost of models with much higher complexity. Our analysis shows that among the proposed modifications, the use of max pooling has the greatest effect on the model accuracy. Label smoothing was applied in order to verify if the classification performance is hampered by a priori bias, but no significant performance improvement has been measured.

In future work, we plan to investigate the utilization of time-frequency representations (e.g. Wavelet and Fourier transforms) as a preprocessing step. By treating the EMG signals as images, temporal causality is ignored in the EMG data, and hence more complex architectures based on RNNs and Temporal Convolutional Networks Networks [21] will be developed to benefit from the temporal information in the data.

The implementation code is available at https://github.com/DSIP-UPatras/PhyCS2018_paper.

References

1. Atzori, M., Cognolato, M., Müller, H.: Deep learning with convolutional neural networks applied to electromyography data: a resource for the classification of movements for prosthetic hands. Front. Neurorobot. **10**, 9 (2016). https://doi.org/10.3389/fnbot.2016.00009. http://journal.frontiersin.org/Article/10.3389/fnbot.2016.00009/abstract
2. Atzori, M., et al.: Electromyography data for non-invasive naturally-controlled robotic hand prostheses. Sci. Data **1**, 140053 (2014). https://doi.org/10.1038/sdata.2014.53. http://www.nature.com/articles/sdata201453
3. Atzori, M., et al.: Characterization of a benchmark database for myoelectric movement classification. IEEE Trans. Neural Syst. Rehabil. Eng. **23**(1), 73–83 (2015). https://doi.org/10.1109/TNSRE.2014.2328495. http://ieeexplore.ieee.org/document/6825822/
4. Bagherinezhad, H., Horton, M., Rastegari, M., Farhadi, A.: Label refinery: improving ImageNet classification through label progression. ArXiv e-prints (May 2018). http://arxiv.org/abs/1805.02641
5. Castellini, C., Fiorilla, A., Sandini, G.: Multi-subject/daily-life activity EMG-based control of mechanical hands. J. Neuroeng. Rehabil. **6**, 41 (2009). https://doi.org/10.1186/1743-0003-6-41. www.pubmedcentral.nih.gov/articlerender.fcgi?artid=PMC2784470, http://www.ncbi.nlm.nih.gov/pubmed/19919710
6. Chen, H., Tong, R., Chen, M., Fang, Y., Liu, H.: A hybrid CNN-SVM classifier for hand gesture recognition with surface EMG signals. In: 2018 International Conference on Machine Learning and Cybernetics (ICMLC), pp. 619–624. IEEE, July 2018. https://doi.org/10.1109/ICMLC.2018.8526976, https://ieeexplore.ieee.org/document/8526976/
7. Cheok, M., Omar, Z., Jaward, M.: A review of hand gesture and sign language recognition techniques. Int. J. Mach. Learn. Cybern. **10**, 1–3 (2017). https://doi.org/10.1007/s13042-017-0705-5
8. Côté-Allard, U., et al.: Deep learning for electromyographic hand gesture signal classification by leveraging transfer learning. ArXiv e-prints (Jan 2018). http://arxiv.org/abs/1801.07756
9. Ding, Z., Yang, C., Tian, Z., Yi, C., Fu, Y., Jiang, F.: sEMG-based gesture recognition with convolution neural networks. Sustainability **10**(6), 1865 (2018). https://doi.org/10.3390/su10061865. http://www.mdpi.com/2071-1050/10/6/1865
10. Du, Y., Jin, W., Wei, W., Hu, Y., Geng, W.: Surface EMG-based inter-session gesture recognition enhanced by deep domain adaptation. Sensors **17**(3), 458 (2017). https://doi.org/10.3390/s17030458. http://www.mdpi.com/1424-8220/17/3/458

11. Englehart, K., Hudgins, B.: A robust, real-time control scheme for multifunction myoelectric control. IEEE Trans. Biomed. Eng. **50**(7), 848–854 (2003). https://doi. org/10.1109/TBME.2003.813539. http://ieeexplore.ieee.org/document/1206493/
12. Englehart, K., Hudgins, B., Parker, P., Stevenson, M.: Classification of the myoelectric signal using time-frequency based representations. Med. Eng. Phys. **21**(6), 431–438 (1999). https://doi.org/10.1016/S1350-4533(99)00066-1. http://www.sciencedirect.com/science/article/pii/S1350453399000661
13. Geng, W., Du, Y., Jin, W., Wei, W., Hu, Y., Li, J.: Gesture recognition by instantaneous surface EMG images. Sci. Rep. **6**, 36571 (2016). https://doi.org/10.1038/srep36571
14. Gijsberts, A., Atzori, M., Castellini, C., Müller, H., Caputo, B.: Movement error rate for evaluation of machine learning methods for sEMG-based hand movement classification. IEEE Trans. Neural Syst. Rehabil. Eng. **22**(4), 735–744 (2014). https://doi.org/10.1109/TNSRE.2014.2303394
15. Glorot, X., Bengio, Y.: Understanding the difficulty of training deep feedforward Neural Networks. In: Proceedings of the 13th International Conference on Artificial Intelligence and Statistics (AISTATS). Sardinia, Italy (2010). http://proceedings. mlr.press/v9/glorot10a/glorot10a.pdf
16. Goodfellow, I., Bengio, Y., Courville, A.: Deep Learning. MIT Press, Cambridge (2016). www.deeplearningbook.org
17. Hartwell, A., Kadirkamanathan, V., Anderson, S.R.: Compact deep neural networks for computationally efficient gesture classification from electromyography signals. In: 2018 7th IEEE International Conference on Biomedical Robotics and Biomechatronics (Biorob), pp. 891–896. IEEE, August 2018. https://doi.org/10. 1109/BIOROB.2018.8487853, https://ieeexplore.ieee.org/document/8487853/
18. Hudgins, B., Parker, P., Scott, R.: A new strategy for multifunction myoelectric control. IEEE Trans. Biomed. Eng. **40**(1), 82–94 (1993). https://doi.org/10.1109/ 10.204774. http://ieeexplore.ieee.org/document/204774/
19. Iandola, F.N., Han, S., Moskewicz, M.W., Ashraf, K., Dally, W.J., Keutzer, K.: SqueezeNet: AlexNet-level accuracy with 50x fewer parameters and <0.5MB model size. ArXiv e-prints (Feb 2016). http://arxiv.org/abs/1602.07360
20. Kuzborskij, I., Gijsberts, A., Caputo, B.: On the challenge of classifying 52 hand movements from surface electromyography. In: 2012 Annual International Conference of the IEEE Engineering in Medicine and Biology Society, pp. 4931–4937. IEEE, August 2012. https://doi.org/10.1109/EMBC.2012.6347099, http:// ieeexplore.ieee.org/document/6347099/
21. Lea, C., Flynn, M., Vidal, R., Reiter, A., Hager, G.: Temporal convolutional networks for action segmentation and detection. In: 2017 IEEE Conference on Computer Vision and Pattern Recognition (CVPR), pp. 1003–1012. IEEE, July 2017. https://doi.org/10.1109/CVPR.2017.113, http://ieeexplore.ieee.org/ document/8099596/
22. Li, Y., Wang, N., Shi, J., Liu, J., Hou, X.: Revisiting Batch Normalization for practical domain adaptation. ArXiv e-prints (Mar 2016). https://arxiv.org/abs/ 1603.04779
23. Park, K., Lee, S.: Movement intention decoding based on deep learning for multiuser myoelectric interfaces. In: 2016 4th International Winter Conference on Brain-Computer Interface (BCI), pp. 1–2. IEEE, Febuary 2016. https://doi.org/ 10.1109/IWW-BCI.2016.7457459, http://ieeexplore.ieee.org/document/7457459/
24. Pereyra, G., Tucker, G., Chorowski, J., Kaiser, Ł., Hinton, G.: Regularizing Neural Networks by penalizing confident output distributions. ArXiv e-prints (Jan 2017). http://arxiv.org/abs/1701.06548

25. Raffel, C., Ellis, D.P.W.: Feed-forward networks with attention can solve some long-term memory problems. ArXiv e-prints (Dec 2015). http://arxiv.org/abs/1512.08756

26. Samadani, A.: EMG channel selection for improved hand gesture classification. In: 2018 40th Annual International Conference of the IEEE Engineering in Medicine and Biology Society (EMBC), pp. 4297–4300. IEEE, July 2018. https://doi.org/10.1109/EMBC.2018.8513395, https://ieeexplore.ieee.org/document/8513395/

27. Samadani, A.: Gated recurrent neural networks for EMG-based hand gesture classification. a comparative study. In: 2018 40th Annual International Conference of the IEEE Engineering in Medicine and Biology Society (EMBC), pp. 1–4. IEEE, July 2018. https://doi.org/10.1109/EMBC.2018.8512531, https://ieeexplore.ieee.org/document/8512531/

28. Scheme, E., Englehart, K.: Electromyogram pattern recognition for control of powered upper-limb prostheses: state of the art and challenges for clinical use. J. Rehabil. Res. Dev. 48(6), 643–659 (2011). https://doi.org/10.1682/JRRD.2010.09.0177. http://www.rehab.research.va.gov/jour/11/486/pdf/scheme486.pdf

29. Sergey, I., Szegedy, C.: Batch Normalization: Accelerating Deep Network training by reducing internal covariate shift. ArXiv e-prints (Feb 2015). https://arxiv.org/abs/1502.03167

30. Shim, H., An, H., Lee, S., Lee, E., Min, H., Lee, S.: EMG pattern classification by split and merge deep belief network. Symmetry 8(12), 148 (2016). https://doi.org/10.3390/sym8120148. http://www.mdpi.com/2073-8994/8/12/148

31. Shim, H., Lee, S.: Multi-channel electromyography pattern classification using deep belief networks for enhanced user experience. J. Cent. South Univ. 22(5), 1801–1808 (2015). https://doi.org/10.1007/s11771-015-2698-0. http://link.springer.com/10.1007/s11771-015-2698-0

32. Srivastava, N., Hinton, G., Krizhevsky, A., Sutskever, I., Salakhutdinov, R.: Dropout: a simple way to prevent neural networks from overfitting. J. Mach. Learn. Res. 15, 1929–1958 (2014)

33. Szegedy, C., Vanhoucke, V., Ioffe, S., Shlens, J., Wojna, Z.: Rethinking the inception architecture for computer vision. In: 2016 IEEE Conference on Computer Vision and Pattern Recognition (CVPR), pp. 2818–2826. IEEE, June 2016. https://doi.org/10.1109/CVPR.2016.308, http://ieeexplore.ieee.org/document/7780677/

34. Tsinganos, P., Cornelis, B., Cornelis, J., Jansen, B., Skodras, A.: Deep learning in EMG-based gesture recognition. In: Proceedings of the 5th International Conference on Physiological Computing Systems, pp. 107–114. SCITEPRESS - Science and Technology Publications, Seville, Spain (2018). https://doi.org/10.5220/0006960201070114, http://www.scitepress.org/DigitalLibrary/Link.aspx?doi=10.5220/0006960201070114

35. Wei, W., Wong, Y., Du, Y., Hu, Y., Kankanhalli, M., Geng, W.: A multistream convolutional neural network for sEMG-based gesture recognition in muscle-computer interface. Pattern Recogn. Lett. (2017). https://doi.org/10.1016/j.patrec.2017.12.005

36. Zhai, X., Jelfs, B., Chan, R., Tin, C.: Self-recalibrating surface EMG pattern recognition for neuroprosthesis control based on convolutional neural network. Front. Neurosci. 11, 379–390 (2017). https://doi.org/10.3389/fnins.2017.00379. http://journal.frontiersin.org/article/10.3389/fnins.2017.00379/full

Heart Rhythm Qualitative Analysis Using Low-Cost and Open Source Electrocardiography: A Study Based on Atrial Fibrillation Detection

Hélio B. M. Lourenço[1]([✉])[iD], Víctor Sanfins[3][iD], Fernando Torgal[3][iD], Sílvia Ala[4,5,6], Manuel J. C. S. Reis[2,9][iD], Hugo P. Silva[7,8][iD], and Francisco Barros[2,5]

[1] Ace Centre, Oxford OX14 1RG, UK
helourenco@outlook.pt
[2] University of Trás-os-Montes and Alto Douro, Quinta de Prados, 5000-801 Vila Real, Portugal
{mcabral,flbarros}@utad.pt
[3] Laboratório de Arritmologia, Pacing e Electrofisiologia, Hospital de Guimarães, Serviço de Cardiologia, Guimarães, Portugal
vsanfins@hotmail.com, fernandotorgal64@gmail.com
[4] Departamento de Ciências Sociais e Gerontologia, Instituto Politécnico de Bragança, Bragança, Portugal
silvia.ala@ipb.pt
[5] Instituto de Investigación Sanitaria Galicia Sur—Grupo de Investigación en Neurociencia y Enfermedades Psiquiátricas, Vigo, Spain
[6] Neurosciences and Clinical Psychology, University of Vigo, Vigo, Spain
[7] IT—Instituto de Telecomunicações, Lisbon, Portugal
hsilva@lx.it.pt
[8] Escola Superior de Tecnologia do Instituto Politécnico de Setúbal, Setúbal, Portugal
[9] Department of Engineering, IEETA—The Institute of Electronics and Informatics Engineering of Aveiro, Aveiro, Portugal

Abstract. In the current digital era, cardiovascular activity analysis is becoming ubiquitous with the increasing availability of embedded systems, and, in some cases, these systems are even endowed with the capabilities of detecting health risk factors identified through electrocardiographic (ECG) markers. Aligned with this trend, and inspired by the results from our pilot study, we focus this research on exploring the potential of a low-cost and open source device for heart rhythm analysis, with emphasis on Atrial Fibrillation (AF). AF is the most common cardiac arrhythmia, defined as a complex cardiac disease which is highly correlated to stroke and heart failure, and its prevalence is especially high in elderly population. Given the importance and impact of such cardiovascular disease, we performed ECG acquisitions in a hospital setting to evaluate the potential of this device to identify heart rhythms. These ECG acquisitions were performed in 10 patients, accomplished simultaneously with the low-cost

© Springer Nature Switzerland AG 2019
A. Holzinger et al. (Eds.): PhyCS 2016–2018, LNCS 10057, pp. 198–217, 2019.
https://doi.org/10.1007/978-3-030-27950-9_11

device and the gold standard devices used in the clinical routine of the hospital. The data collected from the low-cost device was analysed by the cardiologist specialized in rhythmology, along with the conventional ECG exam analysis, whom suggested 100% accuracy of the low-cost device in differentiating a sinus rhythm from AF. The results also present great accuracy in the detection of atypical cardiac events through ECG analysis, as well as a good agreement for the corroboration of the numerical data from the devices used for this study, as the RR intervals and QTc intervals values suggest.

Keywords: Electrocardiography · Atrial fibrillation · Low-cost · Open source · Cardiovascular disease · Heart rhythm · QTc

1 Introduction

Bio-signal analysis with open source and low-cost devices has increasingly gained popularity in the past decade, as its applications are being recognized and extensively explored by research and industrial engineering fields. The convergence of synergies between diverse communities has allowed significant advances in research and development activities, due to the opportunity for experimentation given by the low-cost, versatility and accuracy of the current Do-it-Yourself (DIY) devices. More importantly, the development of proof of concept methodologies or prototypes for bio-signal applications can represent significant cost and development time reduction when compared to more standardized medical devices. They can even be further enhanced when allied with other areas sharing the same philosophy (i.e., spreading the opportunity to gain knowledge and experiment), such as 3D printing.

Within DIY and open source devices for biomedical applications, BITalino[1] has been described as a viable choice [2]. This platform presents a wide range of sensors, as well as a high level of hardware configurability, due to its developmental ideological nature. There are a comprehensive range of software resources allowing deeper physiological data exploitation, within which particular attention has been given to the ECG [10,13,15].

In our previous research [7], we have presented an empirical corroboration of the data acquired with BITalino and a medical-grade ECG device, acquired at rest from a control group of 21 subjects, by analysing the QTc interval for the heart rate and the segmented heartbeat waveform. The results have shown a good agreement between the numerical data acquired from the gold standard and the low-cost device. We have also included the results of the Heart Rate Variability (HRV) numerical data analysis for this control group. Beyond this main control group, we have also tested ECG acquisition with the low-cost device in static and dynamic conditions, as well as further HRV analysis for both acquisition conditions, which revealed a great performance for rhythmical ECG analysis. Also, by analysing the data from our preliminary study and the control group, promising

---

[1] http://bitalino.com/en/.

results regarding BITalino's potentiality for cardiomyopathy pre-screening were found. In particular, ECG abnormalities in two volunteers were detected by BITalino and confirmed with the results from the gold standard devices.

Inspired by the results from our previous research, we focused this study on exploring BITalino's reliability for cardiomyopathy pre-screening with real patients, in a hospital setting – mostly in the Cardiology Department. In this case study-based article, we are exploring the low-cost device's accuracy in detecting arrhythmias, namely, Atrial Fibrillation (AF). The main gold standard device used was an ELI^{TM} 280 12-lead Resting ECG, hereinafter referred to as ELI. In case study 10, a different gold standard device was used – Philips PageWriter Trim III – as this patient was monitored in the Emergency Department, where this is the device available. For this study, we were able to record the ECG signal with both devices recording simultaneously. The ECG acquisition was performed by the medical team with the hospital patients, along with their conventional ECG diagnostic exams.

The data collected from the low-cost device was analysed by the cardiologist specialized in rhythmology, along with the conventional ECG exam analysis. With this analysis we aimed to verify BITalino's reliability in detecting pathologic cardiac rhythms. The enrolled patients are usually referred for ECG analysis by routine hospital appointments as, usually, they present typical symptoms of cardiac disease. A total of 10 patients were monitored: two of them have shown sinus rhythm, and the remaining patients were diagnosed with AF. In addition to the rhythmic analysis, we performed the waveform morphology analysis, as well as the numerical data analysis – corrected QT interval for the heart rate (QTc). The QTc interval is an important marker for the rhythmic disease, as it represents the depolarization and repolarization of the ventricles and it can give important information in situations where there is the risk of sudden death. The finding of this study suggests that BITalino demonstrated precise signal quality for rhythmical analysis and ECG waveform segments analysis, and it was possible to detect healthy and pathological rhythms with 100% accuracy. The results also show great accuracy for abnormal events detection (i.e., extrasystoles), as well as heart's electrical conduction blocks. Also, the corroborated numerical data obtained from BITalino and the medical grade devices present good agreement.

2   Motivation

The current digital era is surrounding us with technology that has vastly increased its capabilities on tracking vital signs, specifically, cardiovascular markers. Such devices allow proactive monitoring and can be present in daily wearables that are evolving in the direction of diagnostic supporting tools. Apple Watch is an example of such technology. However, this device is still in working progress to achieve accurate cardiac disease detection [19]. Such devices are also being deftly empowered through Artificial Intelligence (i.e., Heartsense[2]), improving their ability to detect cardiac pathology. The portability of such devices can make the difference in their ease of use and range of applications, being the e-textile applications an example of such portability and ubiquitous use [14,17].

These technologies have been paving the way for continuous and more pervasive ECG data acquisition, which can become crucial in supporting patients with cardiovascular diseases to track their health status or benefit from preventive interventions. However, such technology is still yet to be accessible for a wide range of users due to its cost. For example, due to the limited infrastructures, access to technology, as well as access to health services, developing countries and remote communities can face insufficient primary care; and DIY and low-cost devices have been used to develop solutions for ECG acquisition, in an attempt to promote access to health in such cases [4,12,21].

The World Health Organization reported, in 2017, that cardiovascular diseases continue to be the main cause of death globally.[3] Within cardiovascular diseases, AF is the most common cardiac arrhythmia and its prevalence in developed countries range from 1.5% to 2% of the general population [18]. A study conducted by Marini et al. revealed that, in the United States (US) only, 17% of the deaths from their cohort were attributed to the presence of AF in patients with ischemic stroke [8]. The US population projections by the US Census Bureau estimates that the cases of AF will increase to 12 million until 2050 [9].

The prevalence of AF increases with ageing, and its episodes increase in frequency and duration, which makes its early detection pivotal to increase the possibility of using reversible and less invasive interventions. AF can be a chronic condition where electrocardiographic diagnosis is easy, it can be paroxysmal, which makes its electrocardiographic documentation more difficult and dependent on prolonged electrocardiographic monitoring techniques.

In the presence of AF, the myocardium shows uncoordinated and ineffective atrial contractions, which can result in hemodynamic instability. Such disorganized atrial activity consequently causes irregular ventricular rate, and it can be detected through ECG analysis, once its main characteristics are the irregularity of RR intervals and the absence of P-waves [6,18,20].

This work aims at finding the potential of using a low-cost device for arrhythmias pre-screening, in particular AF, due to its importance and prevalence in the general elderly population. We aim to take a step further in expanding the evidence that can sustain the use of BITalino for a broader range of applications, and to influence the research and educational communities to direct their attention to such significant matter in public health.

Previous researches found that BITalino presents high similarity on the results for ECG acquisition by benchmarking with gold standard devices. Multiple studies, with non-pathologic volunteers, have explored the potentiality of this low-cost device through the analysis of Signal-to-Noise Ratio (SNR), Root Mean Square Error (RMSE), morphological analysis and R-peak detection for

---

[2] http://www.cambridgeheartwear.com.

[3] https://www.who.int/en/news-room/fact-sheets/detail/cardiovascular-diseases-(cvds).

segmentation [1,2,16]. Silva et al. [16] presented a correlation of ECG data, acquired from 38 volunteers at rest, between a medical device (Philips PageWriter Trim III series) and the first version of BITalino, aiming to validate the signal acquisition accuracy for "off-the-person" applications. The medical device used a setup that included the classical 12-lead ECG placement system, whilst BITalino used a single lead, in a setup with two dry electrodes placed at the index fingers. The comparative tests showed that the "off-the-person" ECG data had a precision for R-peak detection above 98% when compared to the corresponding lead in the gold standard device. Additionally, the segmentation performance and morphological waveform analysis showed a strong correlation between the real-world empirical data assessed for both devices, reinforcing the potential of low-cost devices.

3   Materials and Methods

3.1   Volunteers

The data was collected in a hospital setting from 10 patients aged 80.5 ± 6.06 years old where 4 are male and 6 are female. These patients were referred for the 12-lead ECG, at rest, for evaluation of palpitations, a symptom that suggests the presence of arrhythmias.

The medical team accomplished the ECG acquisitions with BITalino along with the conventional 12-lead ECG acquisition, following the same clinical procedures for ECG acquisition.

In order to proceed with the experimental part of the study, we had the approval of the hospital to conduct the ECG acquisition with BITalino as well as to use the data collected from the medical ECG devices. The consent of the volunteers who have participated in this study was also obtained. Data acquisition was performed in accordance with the existing institutional rules and regulations.

3.2   Methodology

Building upon our previous work [7], we performed an empirical corroboration of the ECG data acquired from BITalino and with the gold standard devices, focusing on determining the accuracy of the low-cost device to detect arrhythmias, specifically, AF. In addition to the traditional ECG screening exam using the conventional 12-lead ECG, acquired at rest and supine position, the medical team of the Cardiology Department added the modified bipolar leads CM_5 and Lead II, suggested by [3,5], to be used with BITalino.

In relation to our previous study, we have modified the experimental protocol by changing the previously used Conventional Lead (CL) for the Modified Lead II, both suggested by the same author [3], as these leads have an approximate configuration and electrical vector, as well as similar signal output. Also, the modified Lead II can give us an approximate waveform pattern to the standard Lead II used in the conventional 12-lead ECG. Although the signal output from the bipolar Modified Lead II and the conventional Lead II have the best waveform pattern similarity, within the leads that were used, it is still differentiated due to the characteristic electrode placement configuration of each lead.

The ECG data acquisition carried out with the ELI device was recorded with 25 mm/s of speed and 10 mm/mV in amplitude. The ECG machine automatically selects the 10 best seconds of recording to obtain the ECG tracings. The data obtained with BITalino was made correspondent to the data obtained with the gold standard devices. The devices features for ECG acquisition are described in Table 1.

The data from the conventional 12-lead ECGs were provided in portable document format (PDF), and we were able to further perform the signal synchronization between this data and BITalino's data, through ECG traces observation. To support the synchronization process, the ECG acquisitions performed with the low-cost device had a time frame ranging from 0:41 to 2:36 min, and the ECG acquisitions using the medical devices were performed simultaneously, so the moment of the data collected by the medical devices could be contained in the former acquisition. The initial and final moment of the ECG acquisition with the gold standard device was recorded on BITalino, by triggering an input signal to mark the recording instant, using a pushbutton.

Once the data was collected, BITalino's raw data was post-processed so the signal filtering and feature extraction could be performed (see Sect. 3.4). Therefore, once the post-processing was accomplished, BITalino's ECG tracings resulting from the synchronization with the 12-lead ECGs were analysed by the cardiologist. The data analysed is presented in Sect. 4.

3.3   Acquisition Setup

Hardware. Adding to the hardware used in our previous work [7], where we used the BITalino (r)evolution Core BT with two ECG sensors, and respective 3-lead cables, we included the pushbutton sensor for event annotation. To house each of the components we used 3D printed enclosures. Another modification developed for this study was reducing the number of cable connections by removing the UC-E6 connectors and soldering the cables directly on the sensors in order to improve usability, which also resulted in a *poka-yoke* procedure for the medical team when handling the BITalino hardware system (see Fig. 1).

The BITalino main board was powered by a 500 mAh capacity and 3.7 V output LiPo battery and data transmission performed by Bluetooth to our base station—a laptop with Windows operating system. Pre-gelled Ag/AgCl electrodes were used to interface the electrode leads with the subject body.

Table 1 presents the BITalino ECG sensors and the ELI^{TM} 280[4] hardware specifications. Note that the features from the ELI device presented are the same used for this study, as this device presents different features.

---

[4] https://www.welchallyn.com/content/dam/welchallyn/documents/sap-documents/
MRC/80022/80022538MRCPDF.pdf.

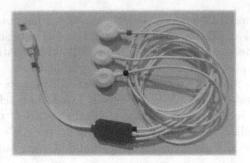

Fig. 1. BITalino ECG sensor adapted with the UC-E6 cable connector and 3-lead cable soldered.

Table 1. BITalino (r)evolution ECG and ELI^{TM} 280 specifications.

Feature	BITalino	ELI
Sampling rate	1000 Hz	1000 Hz
ADC resolution	10 bit	20 bit
Gain	1100	n.a.
Range	±1.5 mV (VCC = 3.3 V)	Meets or exceeds the requirements of ANSI/AAMI EC11
Bandwidth	0.5–40 Hz	0.05–300 Hz
Input voltage range	±1.65 V	Universal AC power supply (100–240 VAC at 50/60 Hz) 110 VA
Input impedance	7.5 GΩ	Meets or exceeds the requirements of ANSI/AAMI EC11
CMRR	86 dB	Meets or exceeds the requirements of ANSI/AAMI EC11

Software. For data acquisition with BITalino we used the OpenSignals software; the recorded data was acquired using 1000 Hz sampling rate. The ELI device was set up for 1000 Hz and had digital filters incorporated in the hardware, namely high-performance baseline filter, AC interference filter 50/60 Hz, band-pass filter [0,05–40] Hz.

The feature extraction and automatic ECG analysis for ELI^{TM} 280 are integrated into the ECG device hardware.

3.4   Data Post-processing

Although the ELI^{TM} 280 already provides the ECG signal filtered, BITalino mostly performs raw data acquisition, reason why data post-processing was needed. For raw data conversion to the correct physical units - millivolt -, the transfer functions suggested in BITalino's manuals[5] were implemented. Equation 1 converts the raw data into Volts units, and Eq. 2 converts the data obtained from the former equation into millivolts.

$$ECG(V) = \frac{\left(\frac{ADC}{2^n} - \frac{1}{2}\right) \cdot VCC}{G_{ECG}} \tag{1}$$

$$ECG(mV) = ECG(V) \cdot 1000 \tag{2}$$

Further feature extraction was performed using the BioSPPy[6] toolbox, a set of open source and Python-based routines for biomedical signal analysis, that includes modules for ECG filtering, R-peak detection, HR plot, waveform template.

The BioSPPy toolbox original band-pass filter of [3–45] Hz was modified to [0.05–40] Hz so it could correspond to the filter used by the ELI device. The toolbox was adapted to obtain the standard ECG trace grid for 25 mm/s recording speed and 10 mm/mV amplitude for our previous study and improved for this work. This grid allows rhythmical and morphological ECG trace analysis by observation. For each subject, we have extracted ECG traces for 10 s, for both ECG bipolar leads.

Once accomplished the signal post-processing procedure, the corrected QT interval was collected. The values for the classic 12-lead ECG were obtained through the automatic extraction features from the gold standard devices, whilst the values for BITalino were obtained through ECG trace scalar measurement (QT interval and QTc interval). QT interval variation is inverse to the heart rate, and, for this reason, multiple expressions were suggested to adjust it to the heart rate. Bazett formulae [11] is one of the most popular calculation methods and it was the selected method for this study. The data for the classic 12-lead ECG was obtained through the feature extraction provided by the ELI, whereas the values for BITalino were obtained through ECG trace scalar measurement (QT and QTc intervals).

The statistical parameters of RR intervals were extracted through the OpenSignals's Heart Rate Variability (HRV) add-on, from the raw data.

4   Results

4.1   General Considerations

The results are presented in a case study structure and are individually analysed. There are a total of 10 case studies, where the case studies 1 and 2 represent

---

[5] http://bitalino.com/datasheets/REVOLUTION_ECG_Sensor_Datasheet.pdf.
[6] http://biosppy.readthedocs.io/en/stable/.

sinus rhythm and the remaining were diagnosed with AF. The AF case studies share two distinctive characteristics: irregular RR intervals and P wave absence. The ECG acquisitions for subjects 1 to 9 were synchronized by visual observation.

Even though this analysis consists in a rhythmical analysis, some morphological aspects of the ECG tracings were further analysed and described on the results. For this reason, the case studies are presented individually. Case studies (CS) 3, 4 and 5 are presented altogether as they exhibit similar characteristics.

The RR intervals, QT interval and QTc interval were obtained for all volunteers, through the ECG traces obtained from both devices. Table 2 presents these values.

The OpenSignals add-on used to obtain the RR intervals is restricted by the minimum number intervals needed to extract these parameters, which corresponds to 11 QRS complexes. For this reason, we used the RR intervals average duration within the whole monitoring. Case studies 4 and 9 are exceptions, as they present a higher heart rate, and it complies with the minimum number of RR peaks needed.

4.2   Case Study 1—Sinus Rhythm with Extrasystoles

The subject presented in CS1, designated as S1, is a 73 years old male and presents a sinus rhythm. However, during the screening exam, two supraventricular extrasystoles were detected. These events were detected by both the ELI and BITalino, as represented in Figs. 2 and 3, respectively.

Table 2. QTc values obtained for the 10 subjects, with respective QT and RR intervals, as well as the average and standard deviation for the overall values for both devices. AVG - Average; STD - Standard Deviation.

Subject	BITalino (r)evolution					ELI^{TM} 280		
	Min RR (ms)	Max RR (ms)	AVG RR (ms)	QT (ms)	QTc (ms)	AVG RR (ms)	QT (ms)	QTc (ms)
S1	555	2157	1075	440	424	1021	409	404
S2	406	1814	925	520	540	964	416	423
S3	657	1788	954	420	430	1023	411	406
S4	484	1184	775 (787*)	440	499	786	362	408
S5	914	1804	1008	520	500	1182	426	391
S6	684	1732	1057	500	486	1007	475	473
S7	713	1445	944	540	555	954	447	457
S8	455	2028	994	520	521	1027	431	425
S9	253	1149	757 (770*)	480	551	770	439	500
S10	564	1171	740	540	627	659	368	453
AVG	559	1760	949	510	511	986	421	424
SD	184.871	366.778	131.064	44.422	60.373	155.068	34.209	35.242

* Shows the values extracted automatically through OpenSignals add-on

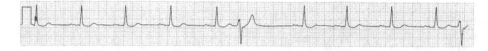

Fig. 2. CS1 – ECG trace from Lead II extracted with ELI, representing the sinus rhythm with two supraventricular extrasystoles during the signal acquisition.

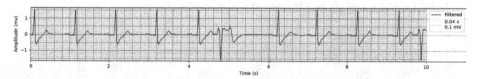

Fig. 3. CS1 – ECG trace from Modified Lead II extracted with BITalino, representing the sinus rhythm with two supraventricular extrasystoles.

4.3 Case Study 2—Sinus Rhythm with Supraventricular Extrasystole

In this case study, an ECG tracing from an 83 years old female, who presents a sinus rhythm, is analysed. Although this subject presents a non-pathological cardiac rhythm, this subject presents a supraventricular extrasystole that was detected by both devices, represented in Figs. 4 and 5.

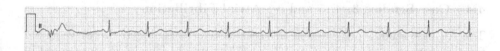

Fig. 4. CS2 – ECG trace from Lead II extracted with the ELI, showing the sinus rhythm and the supraventricular extrasystole.

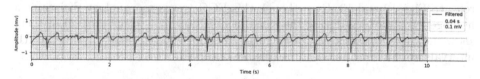

Fig. 5. CS2 – ECG trace recorded from Modified Lead II with BITalino, showing the sinus rhythm and the supraventricular extrasystole.

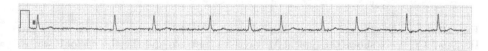

Fig. 6. CS3 – 12-lead ECG trace extracted with ELI device. The irregular RR intervals and P wave absence are the only factors that can be observed during this ECG acquisition.

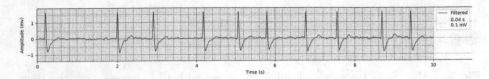

Fig. 7. CS3 – ECG trace from the bipolar Modified Lead II obtained with BITalino. The irregular RR intervals and P wave absence can be observed.

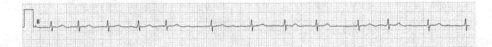

Fig. 8. CS4 – ECG trace from Lead II extracted with the ELI device. The RR intervals irregularity and P waves absence present on this cardiac rhythm can be observed.

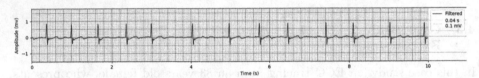

Fig. 9. CS4 – ECG acquisition from the bipolar Modified Lead II obtained with BITalino. Irregular RR intervals and the absence of P waves can be observed.

4.4   Case Studies 3, 4, 5 and 6—Atrial Fibrillation

The AF case studies presented in this section refer to: subjects S3 (81 years old female), represented in Figs. 6 and 7; S4 (77 years old female) is represented in Figs. 8 and 9 – these ECG tracings recorded with BITalino show high morphological similarity to the classic Lead II from the 12-lead ECG; S5 (87 years old male) is represented in Figs. 10 and 11; and S6 (76 years old female), results refer to Figs. 12 and 13. Even though this ECG traces morphology maintains a homogeneous pattern during the signal acquisition, it is clear that all of them show the characteristics that distinguish AF from another heart rhythm: all RR intervals are different and no P waves are observed.

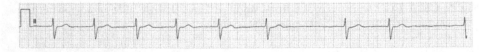

Fig. 10. CS5 – ECG acquisition accomplished with the ELI device, recorded from Lead II. This ECG trace shows the typical AF rhythmic pattern and the absence of P waves.

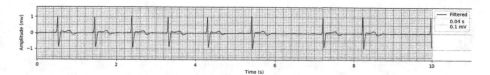

Fig. 11. CS5 – ECG acquisition accomplished with BITalino from Modified Lead II. The arrythmic AF rhythm can be recognized, as well as the absence of P waves.

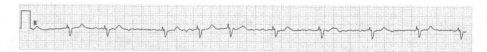

Fig. 12. CS6 – This ECG trace was generated by the ELI device, recorded from Lead II. The typical characteristics of AF are recognised.

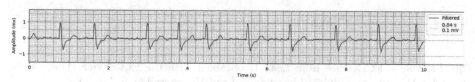

Fig. 13. CS6 – This ECG acquisition was recorded with BITalino, from Modified Lead II. The IBIs irregularity and P waves absence can be observed on this ECG trace.

4.5 Case Study 7—AF with Undulated Baseline

CS7 is a 67 years old female and presents AF. This arrhythmia was detected by the medical device (Fig. 14) and by BITalino (Fig. 15). Beyond the classic AF characteristics shown, this ECG presents undulated baseline that can be recognized in Lead V_1, and also V_2, on the 12-lead ECG obtained with the ELI device. This chaotic baseline is also present in the signal extracted with BITalino, particularly in Modified Lead II. The Lead CM_5 also shows these events in the waveform morphology (Fig. 16), although they are clearer in Modified Lead II.

During the analysis of BITalino's complete monitoring, wide and bizarre QRS complexes were detected in multiple moments of the acquisition, on both leads. Figure 16 shows one of those moments.

4.6 Case Study 8—AF with Atypical QRS Complex

CS8 is based on the rhythmic analysis of an ECG record from an 81 years old female, who was diagnosed with AF. This 10 s ECG trace present the RR intervals irregularly, and the P wave absence is detected. The synchronization of both ECG acquisitions was possible to accomplish by visual observation, due to the extrasystole found in the 12-Lead ECG (Fig. 17) – Lead II, and also affecting the morphology of the QRS complex on Lead V_1 –, as well as in both bipolar leads acquired with BITalino (Fig. 18).

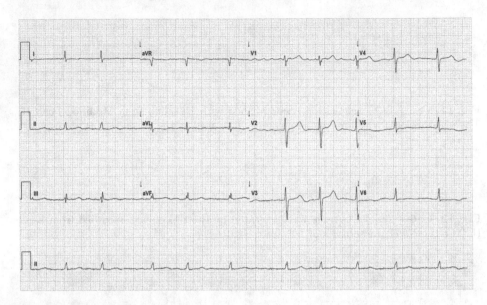

Fig. 14. CS7 – ECG trace from Lead II obtained with the ELI device. The results show the AF and the undulated baseline in Lead V_1, as well as in Lead V_2.

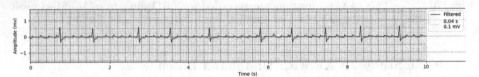

Fig. 15. CS7 – ECG trace recorded from Modified Lead II with BITalino, synchronized with the ECG trace obtained from the ELI device. The irregular cardiac rhythm and undulated baseline can be recognised.

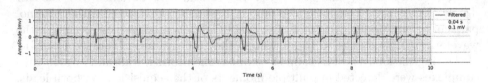

Fig. 16. CS7 – ECG trace recorded from Modified Lead II with BITalino. The AF characteristics are explicit, as well as the two wide QRS complexes. This ECG trace was obtained during the long signal acquisition performed with BITalino.

4.7   Case Study 9—AF with Atypical QRS-T

Case study 9 is made from the ECG acquisition from a 86 years old male. This person was diagnosed with AF by the medical team as the ECG traces clearly shows the irregular RR intervals and absence of P waves.

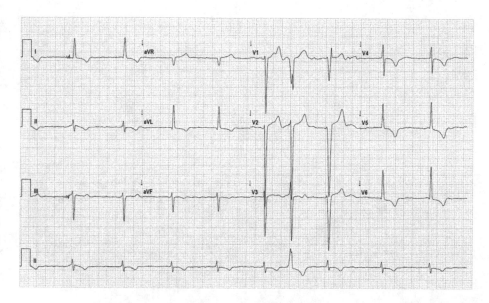

Fig. 17. CS8 – 12-lead ECG representing the extrasystole in Lead II and atypical QRS complex in Lead V₁ at the same instant, as well as the T wave inverted polarity. The RR intervals irregularity and P wave absence that characterize AF can be observed.

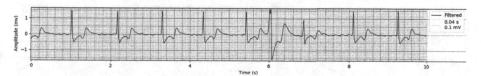

Fig. 18. CS8 – ECG tracing recorded from Modified Lead II using BITalino. AF can be detected in this strip, as well as the extrasystole that yields a peculiar QRS complex morphology.

In terms of morphological analysis, an extrasystole was detected during the ECG acquisition, through which the ECG tracing from BITalino (Figs. 20 and 21) were synchronized with the ECG tracing recorded with the gold standard (Fig. 19). This event was detected with all the leads that have recorded that moment. Looking at the ECG tracings recorded with BITalino, this event is more pronounced in Lead CM₅, as in Modified Lead II this change in wave morphology is subtle, even though the amplitude in S wave is higher, and its duration is shorter than the pattern of the remaining S waves.

4.8 Case Study 10—AF, Anterior Fascicular Block and Right Bundle Branch Block

This case study consists of an analysis of an ECG exam from an 80 years old male. This subject's ECG strip reveals that this person has AF. Beyond the

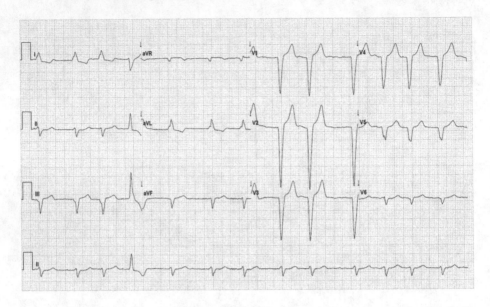

Fig. 19. CS9 – 12-lead ECG obtained with ELI. This ECG represents the IBIs irregularity, as well as the P wave absence. The extrasystole can be observed in Leads I, II and III, which were recorded at the same moment.

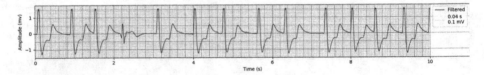

Fig. 20. CS9 – ECG tracing from Lead CM₅, obtained with BITalino. The extrasystole is detected, as well as the AF characteristics.

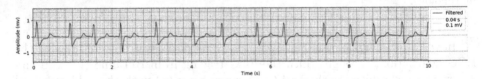

Fig. 21. CS9 – ECG trace obtained from Modified Lead II, recorded with BITalino. This ECG tracing shows the RR intervals irregularly and absence of P waves. However, the extrasystole is less evident than in Lead CM₅.

arrhythmia, the ECG shows evidences that suggests left anterior fascicle block, and right bundle branch block – the effects of these conduction blocks on the 12-lead ECG are represented by markers such as tall R waves, wide QRS complexes, left axis deviation and ST depression in Leads V_1 and V_2.

The 12-lead ECG is represented in Fig. 22. Note that this ECG was recorded with a different ECG machine than the one used with the remaining case studies presented, as this patient was monitored in the Emergency Department, while the remaining patients were monitored in the Cardiology Department. The medical device used with this patient was a Philips PageWriter Trim III – the recording speed and signal amplitude represented was accomplished at the same standards used with ELI, but different filters are applied by this ECG machine: baseline correction filter 35 Hz and AC interference filter 50 Hz.

The markers found with the medical grade device were also detected on the ECG traces recorded with BITalino, as Fig. 23 represents.

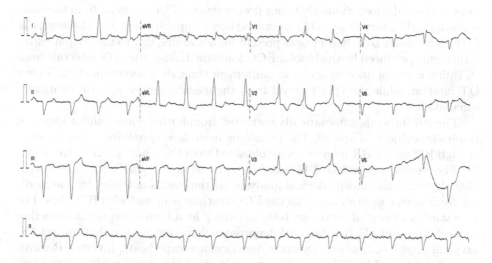

Fig. 22. CS10 – complete 12-lead ECG obtained with Philips PageWriter Trim III that represents AF, left anterior fascicle block, and right bundle branch block.

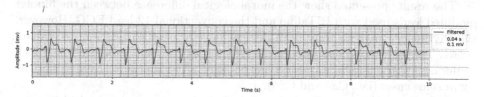

Fig. 23. Subject 10 – ECG trace from Modified Lead II, obtained with BITalino. This ECG represents the evidences for AF, left anterior fascicle block, and right bundle branch block for this subject.

5   Discussion

Since this study is focused on the detection of AF, the case studies presented were selected from a broader sample of volunteers. A requirement for this selection was the fact that the ECG traces could be synchronized by observation so the ECG recordings could be properly matched up. Case study 10 was an exception, as the process of synchronization by observation has limited this action. The fact that the gold standard devices automatically select the best 10 s of the recording, where the signal is less affected by noise, causes some disparity on the recording moment registered in each device. The selected case studies have evident morphology patterns that can be recognized by observation, which highly contributed to their selection.

Even though the main objective of this work is to determine BITalino's reliability for arrythmia detection, we have also analysed morphological aspects of the ECG waveform, as well as the comparison of the RR intervals and QTc interval between both devices. Similarly to our previous work [7], the results from the comparison of RR intervals and QTc intervals show comparable results. However, the QTc intervals for BITalino's traces present higher values, due to the output waveform signal produced by the bipolar ECG leads used. Also, the QTc intervals from BITalino were obtained by scalar measurement through observation of the longer QT interval, while the QTc interval from the medical device was automatically calculated.

The RR intervals automatically extracted from both devices exhibit identical results for subject S4 and S9. The remaining ones show approximate results even though BITalino's RR intervals were obtained from the whole ECG monitoring.

The results suggest that BITalino has a precise signal quality that allows reliable rhythmic and morphological analysis, as the events detected by the medical grade device were all found on the ECG tracings acquired with BITalino. The case studies presented represent 100% accuracy by a human expert in detecting sinus rhythm and AF. Besides the differentiated detection of sinus rhythm and AF, atypical events such as extrasystoles, ventricular escape beats, inverted P waves were also detected by BITalino, demonstrating that the signal quality allows correct identification of each event and the origin of these events in the heart's electrical conductive system and myocardium.

The results presented show the morphological difference between the bipolar modified leads used with BITalino and the conventional 12-lead ECG. However, the rhythmical analysis from both devices have a great correlation, as Table 2 shows. This morphological difference is affected by the lead configuration, which confer on a characteristic waveform morphology, although there is a high similarity in some cases (i.e., CS4 and CS5).

CS9 reveals that some atypical morphological events can be masked to some ECG leads, as the atypical QRS-T segment detected by both BITalino's ECG leads shows (Figs. 20 and 21). CS8 represents a similar situation, but in this case, the extrasystole is masked in some of the leads of the conventional ECG trace (Fig. 17).

The fact that we only had access to the data in PDF format has limited the feature extraction from the 12-lead ECGs. We have selected a group of case studies, from a broader sample, which allowed us to synchronize the ECG strips from both devices for rhythmic and morphological analysis. Case study 10 was the exception, as the task of synchronizing the ECG strips by observation needs clear reference points (i.e., IBIs clear pattern; extrasystoles; among others). Even without a synchronized ECG tracing, and considering the fact that this subject was monitored with a different ECG machine, which slightly differs from our experimental protocol, we decided to include this case study as it presents a range of cardiac pathologies that were detected by both devices, even considering that there are only two leads available from BITalino.

6 Conclusions and Future Work

In the sequence of our previous study, we present an evaluation of the potential of a low-cost and DIY device for detection of cardiac disease, namely, Atrial Fibrillation, in an empirical corroboration of the data with gold standard devices. The results from the 10 case studies described have demonstrated that the signal quality allows reliable ECG acquisition at rest, for further rhythmic analysis, using the bipolar leads sensor configuration that we propose. BITalino could clearly identify a sinus rhythm from a rhythm where Atrial Fibrillation is present. Atrial fibrillation is a very complex and relevant clinical pathology and its identification and electrocardiographic documentation has a high clinical significance, given the therapeutic implications that this pathology implies.

There were also found promising results that suggest that the use of this low-cost device can support ECG morphological analysis in the prevention and diagnosis of other cardiac disorders, such as conduction blocks and its origins.

QTc interval can vary with age and gender of the subject, and it is generally estimated to be higher in women than in man [11]. The cut-off values found in the state-of-art are defined for the classic 12-lead ECG. For these reasons, further investigation needs to be carried to define appropriate cut-off values for modified bipolar leads, due to its inherent morphological characteristics. The fact that we have a reduced number of ECG leads can be a limitation for an appropriate estimation of this important electrocardiographic marker, although the use of the QTc interval is still very useful in certain clinical situations (i.e., patients that take medication which can affect the duration of the ventricular systole and diastole).

The possibility of performing longer ECG acquisitions with BITalino, through which a broader and richer set of data can be collected, allied with its accuracy and low-cost, are additional arguments for its use in future investigation with people with cardiovascular disease.

Acknowledgements. Our team would like to thank to all the anonymous volunteers that agreed to collaborate with this study and also to Hospital da Senhora da Oliveira Guimarães, namely, the Cardiology Department that supported with the data acquisition process.

References

1. Alves, A.P., Martins, J., Silva, H.P., Lourenço, A., Fred, A., Ferreira, H.: Paper-based inkjet electrodes. In: Silva, H.P., Holzinger, A., Fairclough, S., Majoe, D. (eds.) PhyCS 2014. LNCS, vol. 8908, pp. 59–70. Springer, Heidelberg (2014). https://doi.org/10.1007/978-3-662-45686-6_4
2. Batista, D., da Silva, H.P., Fred, A., Moreira, C., Reis, M., Ferreira, H.: Benchmarking of the BITalino biomedical toolkit against an established gold standard. Healthc. Technol. Lett. **6**, 32–36 (2019)
3. Dubin, D.: Rapid Interpretation of an Interactive Course, 6th edn. Cover Pub. Co, Tampa (2000)
4. Ertola, J.P., Figueira, S., Carlsen, M., Palaniappan, U., Rondini, K.: Low-cost electrocardiogram device for preventive health care in rural populations of developing countries. In: IEEE Global Humanitarian Technology Conference (GHTC), pp. 646–655 (2016)
5. Francis, J.: ECG monitoring leads and special leads. Indian Pacing Electrophysiol. J. **16**(3), 92–95 (2016)
6. January, C.T., et al.: 2014 AHA/ACC/HRS guideline for the management of patients with atrial fibrillation: executive summary. Circulation **130**(23), 2071–2104 (2014)
7. Lourenço, H.B.M., Sanfins, V., Ala, S., Barros, F., Silva, H.P., Reis, M.J.C.S.: Empirical evaluation of the potential of low-cost and open source "on-the-person" ECG for cardiopathy pre-screening. In: Proceedings of the 5th International Conference on Physiological Computing Systems (PhyCS), pp. 115–122 (2018)
8. Marini, C., et al.: Contribution of atrial fibrillation to incidence and outcome of ischemic stroke. Stroke **36**(6), 1115–1119 (2005)
9. Miyasaka, Y., et al.: Secular trends in incidence of atrial fibrillation in Olmsted County, Minnesota, 1980 to 2000, and implications on the projections for future prevalence. Circulation **114**(2), 119–125 (2006)
10. Němcová, A., Maršánová, L., Smisek, R., Vitek, M., Kolářová, J.: Recommendations for ECG acquisition using BITalino. In: EEICT Conference, pp. 543–547 (2016)
11. Postema, P.G., Wilde, A.A.: The measurement of the QT interval. Curr. Cardiol. Rev. **10**(3), 287–294 (2014)
12. Queiroz, J.A., Borralho, A.G.S., Barros, A.K.: Low cost electrocardiogram and easy manipulation. Biomed. J. Sci. Tech. Res. **42**, 371–377 (2018)
13. Silva, H., Lourenço, A., Fred, A.L.N., Martins, R.C.M.: BIT: biosignal igniter toolkit. Comput. Methods Programs Biomed. **115**(1), 20–32 (2014)
14. Silva, H., Lourenço, A., Lourenço, R., Leite, P., Coutinho, D., Fred, A.: Study and evaluation of a single differential sensor design based on electro-textile electrodes for ECG biometrics applications. In: IEEE Sensors Conference, pp. 1764–1767 (2011)
15. Silva, H., Lourenço, A., Paz, N.: Real-time biosignal acquisition and telemedicine platform for AAL based on Android OS. In: International Living Usability Lab Workshop on AAL Latest Solutions, Trends and Applications (2011)
16. Silva, H.P., Carreiras, C., Lourenço, A., Fred, A., Neves, R.C., Ferreira, R.: Off-the-person electrocardiography: performance assessment and clinical correlation. Health Technol. **4**(4), 309–318 (2015)
17. Tong, W., Kan, C., Yang, H.: Sensitivity analysis of wearable textiles for ECG sensing. In: Proceedings of International Conference on IEEE EMBS on Biomedical Health Informatics (BHI), pp. 157–160 (2018)

18. Torbicki, A., et al., Authors/Task Force Members and Document Reviewers and ESC Committee for Practice Guidelines (CPG): 2012 focused update of the ESC Guidelines for the management of atrial fibrillation: an update of the 2010 ESC Guidelines for the management of atrial fibrillation. Developed with the special contribution of the European Heart Rhythm Association. Eur. Heart J. **33**(21), 2719–2747 (2012)

19. Turakhia, M.P., et al.: Rationale and design of a large-scale, app-based study to identify cardiac arrhythmias using a smartwatch: the apple heart study. Am. Heart J. **207**, 66–75 (2019)

20. Violi, F., Soliman, E.Z., Pignatelli, P., Pastori, D.: Atrial fibrillation and myocardial infarction: a systematic review and appraisal of pathophysiologic mechanisms. J. Am. Heart Assoc. **5**(5) (2016)

21. Walker, B.A., Khandoker, A.H., Black, J.: Low cost ECG monitor for developing countries. In: 2009 International Conference on Intelligent Sensors, Sensor Networks and Information Processing (ISSNIP), pp. 195–199 (2009)

Integrating Biocybernetic Adaptation in Virtual Reality Training Concentration and Calmness in Target Shooting

John E. Muñoz[1](✉), Alan T. Pope[2], and Luis E. Velez[3]

[1] System Design and Engineering Department, University of Waterloo,
Waterloo, Canada
john.munoz.hci@uwaterloo.ca
[2] NASA Langley Research Center, Hampton, USA
alan.t.pope@nasa.gov
[3] Department of Computer and Systems Sciences at Stockholm University,
Stockholm, Sweden
levelezq@gmail.com

Abstract. Training military readiness can significantly reduce potentially avoidable mistakes in real life situations. Virtual Reality (VR) has been widely used to provide a controlled and immersive medium for training both trainees' physical and cognitive skills. Despite the tremendous advances in VR-based training for military personnel, the attention has been mainly paid on improving simulation's realism through hardware tools and enhancing graphics and data input paradigms, rather than augmenting the human-computer interaction. Biocybernetic adaptation is a technique from the physiological computing field that allows creating real-time modulations based on detected human states indicated by psychophysiological responses. Although very sophisticated, the creation of biocybernetic loops has been mainly confined to research laboratories and very complex and invasive setups. Moreover, the combination of VR applications and biocybernetic adaptation has rarely been pursued beyond exploratory experiments. The Biocyber Physical System (*BioPhyS*) for military training in VR constitutes the first fully integrated, distributed and replicable VR simulator that is biocybernetically modulated. *BioPhyS* uses neurophysiological and cardiovascular measurements recorded from wearable sensors to detect calmness and cognitive readiness states to create dynamic changes in a VR target shooting simulator. The design process, psychophysiological modeling, and biocybernetic loop technology integration are shown, describing a pilot study carried out with a group of non-military participants. We highlight the software elements used for the VR-biocybernetic integration, and the psychophysiological model created for the real-time system as well as the timeline used to develop the functional prototype. We conclude this paper with a set of guidelines for developing meaningful physiological adaptations in VR applications.

Keywords: Biocybernetic loop · Virtual reality · Military training ·
Virtual simulator · Target shooting · Neurophysiological · Cardiovascular ·
Cognitive readiness · Physiological adaptation · Psychophysiology

A. Holzinger et al. (Eds.): PhyCS 2016–2018, LNCS 10057, pp. 218–237, 2019.
https://doi.org/10.1007/978-3-030-27950-9_12

1 Background

Novel virtual reality (VR) technologies have been booming in the last five years, providing substantial evidence of the role that virtual simulations and immersive games will play in our modern society [1]. The widespread use of VR in education, health and training applications has been mainly driven by the need to improve particular user experience aspects such as *immersivity*, presence, and vividness through modern computationally generated graphics, visualization techniques and interactive sensors [2]. In this race to provide complementary technologies that will enhance the already realistic and highly engaging VR experiences, the physiological computing field has been illustrating how, via integrating human body signals into the virtual environments, users can extend the conventional human-computer communication pathways [3–5]. A more sophisticated way to use the physiological signals is by allowing the VR application to be aware of important users' psychophysiological states, such as stress or concentration levels, and to provide real-time adaptations accordingly. This physiological intelligence layer is known as the Biocybernetic Loop (BL) construct, and it employs adaptation strategies from control theory that places the human-in-the-loop to create more *humanized* systems [6]. In other words, BLs have the potential to augment VR applications by allowing the virtual elements to be modulated or paced by detected human states [7]. While research has been widely carried out in detecting human psychophysiological states through numerous computational techniques [8], it is the case that a lot less has been done towards using those states to intelligently and programmatically adapt the system [6, 9]. In response to this obvious and overlooked aspect in the marriage between VR and physiologically intelligent systems, we have conducted research that embraces both theoretical and practical notions and experiences for integrating biocybernetic adaptation in a VR simulator aimed at improving the self-regulation capabilities of military personnel. We document the process from the design to the implementation stages, and summarize our learnings in a set of guidelines that constitutes an effort towards disseminating biocybernetic technologies applied in VR simulations and games.

1.1 Military Training in VR and the *BioPhyS* Approach

The military sector has understood the importance of simulation and constant training for decades. Modern simulators nowadays have successfully integrated flexible, upgradeable, realistic and less expensive software and hardware elements that provide a very vivid representation of real-life scenarios for military training [10–12]. The capabilities of VR technologies to meet military applications were nicely summarized in human factors and man-machine systems meetings carried out in the US [11], featuring exciting projects covering applications for dismounted combatants, mission rehearsal for special operations, telerobotics, military training, and medical procedures. Examples of the use of VR simulators and applications can be found in all branches of the military industry: army, navy, air force and more [10]. Scientific validation of VR simulations used in clinical scenarios has been found in studies that employ very sophisticated technologies to provide exposure therapies for Post-Traumatic Stress Disorder patients [13]. The same approach, where very controlled, flexible and realistic simulations are used as rehabilitation and assessment tools, can be used for preventing avoidable mistakes in real-life scenarios with healthy participants by leveraging novel wearable, multimodal and cost-effective physiological sensing technologies, able to identify covert human states (e.g. stress, anxiety, mental workload) and react accordingly [14–16]. All in all, although the development of virtual simulators for military training has been widely explored, attention has been mostly paid to the machine side, trying to improve the realism and *immersivity* of the simulations, and little attention has been paid to system adaptation to users' needs and responses [10, 17].

Based on licensed patents from Pope and colleagues at NASA Langley [18–21], the Biocyber Physical System (*BioPhyS*) approach aims at creating an intelligent system that uses sophisticated biofeedback technologies to enhance cognitive skills in virtual military training. The *BioPhyS* system was initially conceived in the J&F Alliance Group (US Company) headquarters, in a close collaboration between physiological computing researchers, US veterans, VR developers and industry partners. The system integrates novel VR and biocybernetic technologies to deliver highly adaptive scenarios, aimed at boosting the training of critical cognitive skills in military personnel. The conceptualization of the *BioPhyS* system was the result of a brainstorming process carried out by the team wherein different potential applications and scenarios of biocybernetic systems were explored. After matching the company's clients and interests with the feasibility of using BLs as an adaptation mechanism, we came out with the idea of creating a virtual simulator for military training. In particular, we started exploring marksmanship training in target-shooting by developing a VR-based simulator. The *BioPhyS* approach has been designed for training two important human states: concentration and calmness, which have been found to be particularly relevant to promote cognitive readiness in shooting scenarios [16, 22]. By using both cardiovascular and neurophysiological measurements, calmness and concentration levels of trainees can be computed and used in real time to adapt the content in the VR target-shooting simulator dynamically. This paper shows the first effort carried out to deliver a functional and demonstrable prototype of the combined use of these technologies and it constitutes an initial step towards more complex and robust physiologically aware systems in the military industry.

1.2 The Biocybernetic Loop Engine Software Tool

To aid the integration process of BLs in the virtual target-shooting simulator, we used a previously developed engine that has been used to provide physiological intelligence in videogames[1]. The Biocybernetic Loop Engine (BL Engine) is an integrative software tool created to design, prototype, iterate and evaluate BLs in videogames and interactive applications made in Unity3D (Unity Technologies, San Francisco, USA) [23]. The BL Engine targets both users with and without expertise in game programming or physiological computing, since it can be fully operated through graphical user interfaces and it uses a streamlined method to integrate physiological parameters, adaptive rules, and game variables. The BL Engine includes signal acquisition, signal processing, and

---

[1] https://sites.google.com/view/physio2games.

feature extraction stages as well as a dedicated tool to create heuristic rules for the real-time adaptation (more details about the software design can be seen in [23]).

The BL Engine builds on top of past physiologically adaptive systems evaluated in games and virtual simulations [6, 24], as well as a robust theoretical framework in physiological computing systems [9, 25], and proposes a practical paradigm that can be used by both experts and technology enthusiasts. The BL Engine uses external clients to provide access to the sensors' services and make them available for further processing. The clients are developed in different programming languages such as C++, C#, and Java and they stream data from sensors through User Datagram Protocol (UDP) following the Reh@Net communication protocol [26]. For the *BioPhyS* approach, we used the cardiac panel that allows the communication with wearable and inexpensive chest strap sensors for heart rate such as the Polar (H7 and H10). Moreover, the concentration part of the system was designed to be measured by wearable brain-computer interface (BCI) devices supported in the BL Engine such as the Muse BCI[2].

2 Procedures and Tools

In this section, we describe our efforts towards designing and developing a physiologically adaptive system for target shooting using VR. There are three main stages: the virtual simulator design, the physiological characterization of the user's responses while interacting with the system and a final BL implementation in the virtual simulator.

2.1 *BioPhyS* Virtual Simulator

Why Use Biocybernetic Adaptation? After conceptualizing the *BioPhyS* system, we investigated the physiological responses associated with the desired human target state: concentrated and calm. Following marksmanship training guidelines [22], we learned that a crucial factor that has to be trained in overall marksmanship scenarios is shooting during the natural respiratory pause. Since the lack of oxygen might affect the performance of cognitive skills and reduce the visual acuity, training what is called *autogenic* breathing (autonomic self-regulation training [27]) aimed at relaxing the body and keeping a natural breathing pattern has been defined as a major component of firearms training [28]. Via providing proper brain oxygenation through an optimal respiration pace, peripheral responses such as heart rate (HR) and heart rate variability (HRV) will be controlled in an attempt to maintain both body and mind collected. Therefore, the BL construct seems to provide an ideal strategy for enhancing shooting performance by adapting the virtual elements that define the simulation difficulty to the users' concentration and relaxation levels (so-called calm, concentrated or cool, and collected state). To improve their scores in the shooting scenarios, users would have to use self-regulation strategies (e.g. respiration, sustained attention) that will keep them

---

[2] http://developer.choosemuse.com/tools/mac-tools/muselab.

calm and focused, thus increasing the likelihood of avoiding mistakes in real life scenarios [16].

Simulator Features and VR Implementation. An initial target-shooting scenario was developed for the *BioPhyS* approach, which simulates a training field with twenty horizontal tracks for the targets' positioning. Visually, the scenario includes conventional elements of an outdoor target shooting range such as cable reels, wooden tables, tents, barricades, weapons and water towers (see Fig. 1 left). Three weapons are used for training: The Pistols M1911 and SIG Sauer P250, and the Reichsrevolver M1879 (see Fig. 1 right), each with different impact strength on the targets.

A configuration console called Wizard of Oz (*Woz*) panel was implemented to allow trainers modify the simulation variables both before and during the interaction, providing a more controlled scenario for studying participants' responses and behavior once exposed to different stressors. The target-shooting simulator has a number of variables that were defined to carry out the physiological modulation. Variables were grouped considering their final effector as showed in Table 1:

Table 1. List of simulation variables carefully defined to create the physiological modulation in the BioPhyS simulator.

Simulation effect	Simulation variable	Range
Targets	Number of targets	3–20 (targets)
	Target Size	0.3–3 (units)
	Target Speed (horizontal)	0–5 (m/s)
	Target hardness	1–20 (units)
Simulation Environment	Day light	0–10 (units)
	Rain Intensity	0–1 (units)

The simulation can use both the wireless controllers and an air pistol gun adapted with the HTC Vive tracker to handle and shoot with the weapon. By using the wireless controllers, users can use the teleportation option to move freely in the virtual environment. The lateral buttons are used to grab the virtual gun, while the trigger is used for shooting (see Fig. 1, right).

2.2   Users' Physiological and Behavioral Characterization

After implementing an initial version of the system with the *Woz* panel and data logging, we carried out a first characterization study to better understand the cardiovascular and neurophysiological responses during different setups of the VR target-shooting training. For that, we used a repeated measures design in order to quantify the responses of users to different scenarios and difficulties.

System Setup. To provide a more immersive experience, we used the room-scale tracking system of the HTC Vive pro VR headset. Users can freely walk in an area of up to 12 m^2 (max 5 m between both tracking cameras), and the wireless HTC Vive controllers are used to provide manual interaction inside the virtual environment.

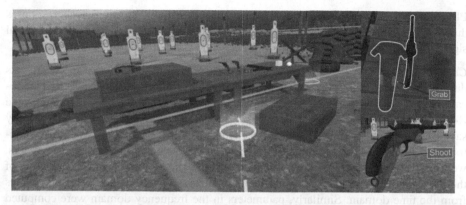

Fig. 1. Screenshots of the BioPhyS virtual simulator created in VR. Left: the shooting field with the targets placed randomly and a table with the guns. Right: the instructions for grabbing and shooting the Reichsrevolver gun.

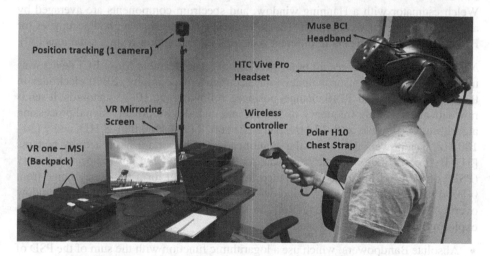

Fig. 2. System setup describing the elements used for the experiment.

For this particular characterization study, only one camera was used, since users were not required to teleport and were placed in front of the targets. We used the VR One MSI backpack computer to run the simulation, and an extra screen was used to configure the scenarios and to mirror the VR simulation (see Fig. 2).

Participants. 10 male users (ages 19–32) were voluntarily recruited for this experiment. Seven users had past experience with target shooting, six with virtual training and eight were right-handed. Before starting, users were informed about the details of the experiment which was promoted as a VR playtest, and an informed consent was individually signed.

Physiological Measurements. To measure participants' physiological responses during the interaction with the virtual simulator, cardiovascular and neurophysiological signals were synchronously recorded in a separate computer during the interaction.

Cardiovascular. The Polar H10 chest strap sensor was used to record the heartbeats during the interaction. The sensor includes onboard algorithms to compute electro-cardiography (ECG) parameters needed for the HRV analysis. Mainly, it computes the R-to-R intervals (RRI) with units of $1/1024$ s[3]. HR and RRIs are streamed and locally saved through a personalized Bluetooth client developed based on a Windows Bluetooth Low Energy API. To compute both time and frequency domain HRV parameters, we used the PhysioLab toolbox [29] which allows extracting the standard deviation of the RRIs (SDNN) and the root mean square of successive differences (RMSSD) values from the time domain. Similarly, parameters in the frequency domain were computed as follows: the high frequency - HF (0.15–0.40 Hz), low frequency – LF (0.04–0.15 Hz) and very low frequency – VLF (0.0033–0.04 Hz) were extracted from the Power Spectrum Density (PSD) of the RRI signal. The PSD is computed by using a Welch estimator with a Hanning window, and spectrum components are averaged by an area-under-the-curve approach. The polar chest strap has shown good accuracies for HR and RRI measurements in different scenarios including non-resting situations [30].

Neurophysiological. To record brainwave activity, the wearable Muse BCI device was used. The headband sensor includes four electroencephalography (EEG) electrodes in the TP9, Fp1, Fp2 and TP10 channel positions following the 10-20 standards. It sends raw data at a sampling frequency of 500 Hz and includes proprietary signal processing algorithms to compute α (8–12 Hz), β (12–30 Hz), ∂ (1–4 Hz), θ (4–8 Hz), and γ (30–100 Hz) bandpowers that allow the quantification of important brain activity patterns [31]. By means of a proprietary software tool (Muse Lab[4]), the power spectral density (PSD) of the EEG raw data is computed for each channel for a frequency range from 0 Hz–110 Hz. The Hamming windowing technique is used with a 90% window overlapping with a window-length of 256 samples. We were particularly interested in exploring the following EEG metrics:

- Absolute Bandpowers: which use a logarithmic function with the sum of the PSD of the EEG data in a specific frequency range. The absolute α, β, ∂, θ, and γ bandpowers were computed for the frontal electrodes of the Muse BCI sensor.
- EEG indexes: three different indexes were explored considering past investigations [32–34]. First, the Engagement index was computed by using the ratio of Beta to Alpha + Theta. The frontal asymmetry index was computed by subtracting the Alpha in Fp2 (right hemisphere) with the Alpha in Fp1 (left hemisphere). Finally, the Theta to Beta ratio was also computed to see the neurophysiological responses in those two bandpowers.

---

[3] https://developer.polar.com/wiki/H6,_H7,_H10_and_OH1_Heart_rate_sensors.

[4] http://developer.choosemuse.com/tools/available-data.

Questionnaires:

Perceived Task Difficulty. To measure the participants' perceived difficulty levels, we designed a 7-point Likert-type scale which will score the task difficulty as follows: 1 – extremely easy, 2 – easy, 3 – somewhat easy, 4 – moderate, 5 – somewhat hard, 6 – hard and 7 – extremely hard.

Motion Sickness. The Simulator Sickness Questionnaire was used to evaluate the level of motion sickness produced during the interaction with the VR system [35]. It evaluates two main components of the motion sickness called nausea (discomfort, salivation, sweating, dizziness, vertigo, stomach awareness, and burping) and oculomotor (fatigue, headache, eyestrain, focusing, concentration, fullness of head, vision).

Simulation Data Logging. Data from the VR simulation was recorded to compute participants' performance while shooting the virtual targets. Three main measurements were established: the total amount of shot bullets, number of destroyed targets, headshots. A shooting performance metric was considered as the ratio between the number of destroyed targets and the shot bullets.

Experimental Protocol and Data Analysis. To carry out an initial physiological characterization study in the target-shooting simulator, we designed three different scenarios that aimed at eliciting participants' responses to different difficulty levels.

Simulation Scenarios. Three difficulty modes were established during the training protocol: easy, medium and hard; each of them lasting 3 min. The *easy* configuration was set up as follows: 10 static targets randomly distributed in the ten first horizontal tracks (one target per horizontal track) of the training scenario. The *medium* configuration uses 10 moving targets at 0.5 units/s speed. Finally, the *hard* scenario used 20 moving targets at 1 units/s speed (double speed than in the *medium* difficulty). Both the target size and hardness were maintained constant across the difficulty levels, and the same Reichsrevolver was always used. The revolver was configured to have a shooting power equivalent to the target hardness, thus allowing destroying them in one shot. An initial *baseline* was also used wherein the participants' physiological signals were recorded during a passive stand-up situation, wearing the VR headset and physiological sensors, while holding the weapon without shooting or interacting with it.

Procedure. Participants were invited to interact with the system within a period lasting around 40 min (questionnaires, connections, interaction). Users were informed about the experiment details with an informed consent that was signed before starting. Then participants filled out a small demographics form and the perceived task difficulty scale was explained. The physiological sensors were next connected as well as the VR headset, and participants were instructed to grab the weapon and shoot targets to ensure they understood the process. The baseline measurements were taken during three minutes after explaining to participants the need to avoid exaggerated facial expressions, speaking or closing one of the eyes while aiming. Participants were then instructed to shoot in the *easy-medium-hard* scenarios, which were each manually set up by the researcher. A two minutes resting period was used between each scenario during which participants were asked to rate the difficulty by telling a number between one and seven. Finally, users were invited to fill out the Perceived Task Difficulty and the Simulator Sickness Questionnaire, as well as to briefly comment about the experience to finish their participation. Some sessions were video recorded to be later analyzed.

Data Analysis. Physiological data collected was processed offline using MatLab (v2013b). Individual cardiovascular and neurophysiological parameters were computed and averaged for the statistical analysis. Physiological data from one user was discarded due to human error. For the EEG bandpower and indexes analysis, we first explored the frontal Fp1 and Fp2 electrodes separately. The brainwave activity in the frontal lobe was finally weighted by averaging the contribution of both Fp1 and Fp2 electrodes. Data normality was checked by the Kolmogorov Smirnoff tests. Data with normal distributions were statistically analyzed with parametric tests while non-parametric tests were used for the non-normal distributions to determine the influence of the simulation difficulty as main effect.

2.3   Physiological and Behavioral Characterization Study Results

Perceived Difficulty and Simulation Performance. The perceived levels of difficulty were significantly affected by the pre-established simulation difficulty, $\chi^2(2) = 17.9$, $p < 0.05$. The simulation performance, $\chi^2(2) = 14.6$, $p < 0.05$ was also affected. Figure 3 shows the trends of both perceived difficulty and simulation performance across the three different simulation difficulties (values were normalized to get percentages). Notice that while the trend in the perceived difficulty is towards increasing while the simulation difficulty is increasing from easy to hard, the performance reflects an inverse relationship.

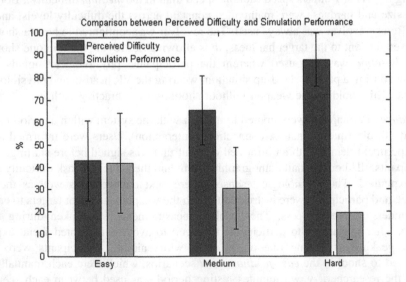

Fig. 3. Comparison between the perceived difficulty and simulation performance described in percentage.

Cardiovascular Responses. Cardiac regulation responses were quantified by means of HR and HRV parameters. Simulation difficulty significantly affected the HR levels of participants, $\chi^2(3) = 20.73$, $p < 0.05$, and the RMSSD values of the time domain HRV branch, $\chi^2(3) = 20.73$, $p < 0.05$, as shown in Fig. 4.

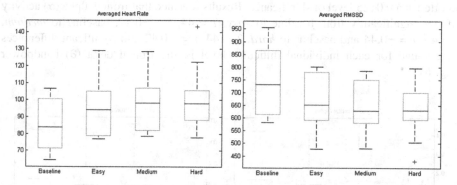

Fig. 4. HR and time-domain HRV parameters that were significantly affected by the simulation difficulty (baseline, easy, medium, hard).

The HRV frequency domain also revealed a significant effect of the simulation difficulty for the HF, $\chi^2(3) = 11.36$, $p < 0.05$, and VLF, $\chi^2(3) = 24.51$, $p < 0.05$, components. Figure 5 shows boxplots representing the differences found.

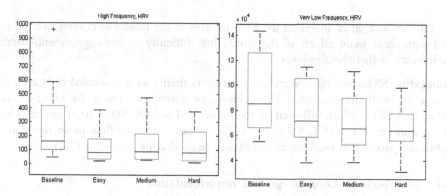

Fig. 5. Frequency-domain HRV parameters that were significantly affected by the simulation difficulty (baseline, easy, medium, hard).

Wilcoxon tests were used to follow up these findings. A Bonferroni correction was applied, so all effects are reported at a 0.0125 level of significance. Baseline HR levels, RMSSD, and VLF differed significantly from the *easy*, *medium* and *hard* simulation difficulties, T = 45, $r = -0.44$, while for the HF only the comparison between baseline and *easy* was significantly different, T = 45, $r = -0.44$.

Brain Activity Patterns. Brain activity measured in the frontal lobe using the Fp1 and Fp2 electrodes revealed significant findings for the absolute bandpowers analysis. The frontal alpha (α), $\chi^2(3) = 12.33$, $p < 0.05$, and frontal delta (∂), $\chi^2(3) = 8.73$, $p < 0.05$, were significantly affected by the simulation difficulty. Wilcoxon tests were used to follow up these findings. A Bonferroni correction was applied, so all effects are reported at a 0.0125 level of significance. Results revealed that frontal alpha (α) activity differed significantly from baseline to *easy*, $T = 44$, $r = -0.42$, baseline to *medium*, $T = 45$, $r = -0.44$ and baseline to *hard*, $T = 44$, $r = -0.42$. No significant differences were found for each individual difficulty level in the frontal delta (∂) bandpower (Fig. 6).

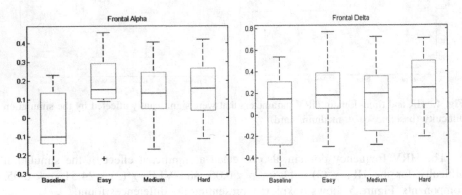

Fig. 6. Brainwave patterns significantly affected by the simulation difficulty factor.

Furthermore, after analyzing the EEG indexes in the frontal electrodes, we did not find significant main effects of the simulation difficulty in the engagement, frontal asymmetry or theta/beta indexes.

Simulation Sickness. Nausea and oculomotor domains were evaluated right after the interaction with the simulator. The oculomotor domain exhibited the highest score (M = 27.3, SD = 17.2), followed by the nausea (M = 23.8, SD = 10.3) and disorientation domains (M = 18.1, SD = 22.7). The values are lower than those reported in published papers that used virtual simulators (e.g., driving simulator [36]).

2.4   Biocybernetic Loop Design and Implementation

After processing both the qualitative and quantitative data in a complementary way, we started the design process of the BL that will be used to modulate the simulation variables automatically, based on the human states detected. Our design process was based on the methodology proposed by Fairclough and Gilleade [34], and the implementation was carried out using the BLE framework aforementioned [23]. Our BL was designed to promote optimal concentration and calmness levels during the target shooting simulation. In psychology, this can be associated with the state called *flow* or *engagement* [37] (colloquially, being "in the zone"), a state of total and optimal immersion in an activity that might optimize the users' performance. Flow state has been previously defined regarding the bio-behavioral (psychophysiological) correlates that clearly defined the cognitive and cardiovascular descriptors of an optimal experience [38]. In our experiment, we defined three difficulty modes to investigate participants' responses to simple, moderate and frustrating shooting scenarios.

We observed that frontal alpha and delta brainwaves as well as HR and HRV (time and frequency) domain features were significantly affected by the simulation difficulty effect. We chose frontal alpha and averaged HR levels as potential features to create the real-time system, since they showed the highest levels of statistical significance in our characterization study. Figure 7 shows the designed psychophysiological model for the state of calm, concentrated and collected during the target shooting in VR. The Target Zone was defined with the physiological responses that matched the *medium* simulation difficulty scenario, where we found the highest headshots (*easy*: 5.5, *medium*: 7.4, *hard*: 4.1) and the highest performance with moving targets (*medium*: 30%, *hard*: 19%). After defining the generic formulation of our psychophysiological model, we moved to the implementation of the system's physiological intelligence layer (the BL).

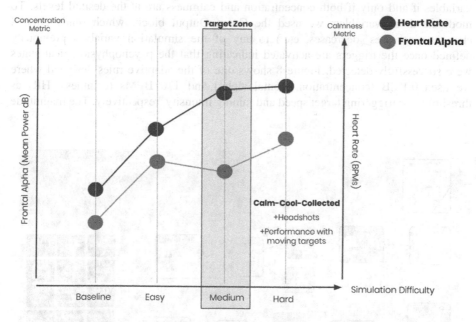

Fig. 7. Psychophysiological model for the state of Calm-Concentrated (or cool) and Collected of the target-shooting simulator in VR. Cardiovascular and neurophysiological measurements are used to compute the concentration (frontal alpha) and the calmness (heart rate) levels. The BL should persuade participants to get into a targeted zone that is where the performance of the simulator could be maximized (e.g., more headshots and better performance with moving targets).

First, the integration of the BLE was carried out via adding the game connector scripts in the target-shooting system, which allowed us to stream the simulation variables (Table 1) from the simulator to the BLE, and the physiological metrics and decisions in the adaptive rules from the BLE to the simulator. This bi-directional communication allows a more fluent exchange of data inside the game engine, reducing the risk of losing or delaying important information for the real-time BL. Multiple adaptive rules were designed and tested by means of using the BL console, a drag-and-drop programming environment incorporated in the BLE [23]. The adaptive rules can be defined by receivers, math operators and game outputs. The receivers are blocks that allow getting the physiological variables in real time from integrated sensor clients (e.g., real-time HR from the Polar H10) or from external applications (e.g., frontal alpha from Muse Lab). We defined individual adaptive rules for each of the desirable human states: calm and concentration. For those, we created array buffers of 10 s of real-time data (HR and frontal alpha EEG) that are averaged and compared against constant thresholds. Although changeable, the thresholds can be defined by seeing the frontal alpha and HR plots (Figs. 4 and 6) of the characterization study. It is worth noting that the thresholds are specifically for this virtual simulator and population. Finally, we used a logic operator block that allows the modulation of the simulation variables if and only if both concentration and calmness are at the desired levels. To modulate those variables, we used the Game Output block, which sends gradual changes (increases, decreases, etc.) to any of the simulation variables previously defined once the triggers are activated indicating that the psychophysiological states were successfully detected. Figure 8 shows one of the adaptive rules designed where we used 0.1 dB (concentration, frontal alpha) and 110 BPMs (calmness, HR) as thresholds for triggering target speed and raining intensity, respectively. The magnitude

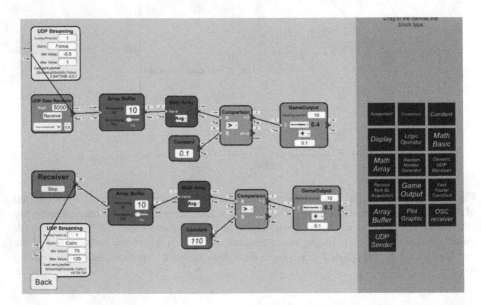

Fig. 8. Physiologically adaptive rules created in the BLE for experimentation. The adaptive rules can be seen as functional pipelines of processed data that triggers the modulation in the VR simulator.

of the change was defined as 0.1 for each simulation variable. The modulations are carried out in windows of 10 s allowing participants to improve or sustain their self-regulation strategies while shooting.

Figure 8 illustrates one of the multiple adaptive rules that can be created for training concentration and calmness in the *BioPhyS* simulator. Changes can be made on the fly, allowing a dynamic modification of thresholds values, simulation variables to be modulated, processing window's lengths, and others. Thus, the final integrated system can be used for testing multiple versions of the BLs which will allow a fast convergence to a stable physiologically adaptive system that maximizes training outcomes.

3   Guidelines for Biocybernetic Adaptation in Virtual Reality

After our initial conceptualization and development process of a biocybernetic system able to promote both concentration and calmness levels in the target-shooting simulator, we reflected on a set of relevant learnings that can be crucial in the integration of biocybernetic adaptation in VR applications. Although not extensive, we hope they can be used as a first milestone towards more widespread use of physiological intelligence in novel immersive media.

- **Before Starting, Answer the WHY of using BLs into Your VR Application.**
  Although there is much enthusiasm in regards of using physiological intelligence to enhance VR experiences, it might be important to take some time to analyze with the research/development team to know whether or not the BL is the most appropriate framework to approach. In our initial brainstorming process, we realized that some of the closed loop ideas might be transformed into potential products just by using simple biofeedback methods as a way to visualize user's inner states instead of having to go through the complete collection-analysis-translation model of BLs. In our case, there are very specific and already established guidelines that correlate psychophysiological states with improvements in shooting performance [22, 39, 40].
- **Define a Psychophysiological Model with Real Data before Moving to the Real-time System Implementation.** Carrying out a controlled experiment with physiological sensing in VR can be a very demanding task (e.g. sensor intrusiveness, VR system preparation, users recruitment, etc.). Nevertheless, this turns out to be a crucial preliminary step to better understand psychophysiological responses of users during immersive experiences in VR. Several assumptions can be wrongly used to drive the BL design process, producing very disappointing and confusing closed loop systems. In our case, we briefly entertained the idea that the optimal performance state in a stressful shooting scenario would simply be a low arousal state. This belief was empirically refuted by observation of the actual psychophysiological responses shown to correspond to effective shooting performance. Our psychophysiological model (see Fig. 7) allowed us a streamlined construction of the adaptive rule in the biocybernetic console of the BLE, including threshold values, windows for signal processing and math operators needed for a steady functioning of the real-time system.

- **Delimit the Adaptation Strategy and the Expected Benefits of the BL.** Although several projects have explored the use of physiological computing technologies to bring unique immersive VR experiences, attention has been mostly paid to either mirroring the signals to be displayed in the VR environment (conventional biofeedback) or using the physiological signals as control input [4, 24, 41]. Bio-cybernetic adaptation constitutes a more sophisticated use of interpreted psychophysiological states, and it must be interpreted as an adaptation layer of the VR application. That means that the VR application should be able to work independently without the BL. Theoretically, once integrated, the BL might have the potential to enhance the user's performance on pre-defined tasks by promoting physiological self-regulation skills (see BL evaluation stage [34]). In the *BioPhyS* simulator, we aimed at improving concentration and calmness during shooting scenarios via controlled respiration that will help at regulating cardiovascular responses and increase the frontal alpha activity.
- **Clearly Define the VR Game/Simulation Variables and Value Ranges to Be Modulated by Means of the BL.** Although there are endless variables that can be used for the physiological modulation in a VR application, a previous and clear definition of specific variables and ranges for testing different prototypes of the BL will ensure that you are not simply picking up the first and most evident of the virtual modulation parameters. In the integration with the BLE, it is recommended to let the software know the particular ranges within each simulation variable can be modulated in order to avoid redundancies or possible miscommunications between the entities (BLE and VR application). In our design process, we brainstormed and initially considered several variables that are not included in Table 1 (e.g., time manipulation, distractors, power-ups). In the implementation, due to time constraints, we decided to prioritize those simulation variables that allowed us to create comprehensible and intuitive metaphors (e.g., calmness and raining, concentration and target speed).
- **Avoid Generalizations.** As described before, each population should be modeled regarding the context and the specificities of the VR application. There are no generalizable psychophysiological models that can be transversally used from one population to the other in different contexts [42]. Additionally, VR raises very particular challenges regarding biocybernetic adaptation research since psychophysiological correlates have been inadequately explored with novel and highly immersive state-of-the-art VR hardware [38, 43–45].

4 Discussion and Future Work

After an intense and structured process of integrating VR and biocybernetic adaptation technologies in a functional prototype for a military-oriented company, we demonstrated how it is possible to create replicable physiologically adaptive systems by using state-of-the-art knowledge and tools. First, developing VR simulations is nowadays a very streamlined process where many 3D assets and tools for interaction design can speed up the prototyping process. Additionally, the use of such a very specialized and integrative software tool as the BL Engine aided in the incorporation of biocybernetic adaptation through an efficient and straightforward methodology. This tool streamlines the process of integrating the physiological signals into the game engine and extracting the features needed for the real-time modulation, enabling system designers to devote more time and effort to designing adaptations based upon detection of the human states and to how this information can be used to influence end-users.

The BL Engine tool automates the construction of algorithms that determine what and how physiological changes are reinforced by task adaptation changes. Stephens and colleagues [46] introduce the idea that, in addition to driving real-time adaptations that reward learning of self-regulation skill, the adaptation algorithms themselves could be periodically modified (e.g., higher thresholds) based upon longer time course changes that reflect a trainee's emerging ability to voluntarily control physiological parameters. In the *BioPhyS* project, the *Woz* configuration console implements a manual version of this capability by enabling trainers to modify the simulation variables during the interaction. Without this capability, the physiological modulation method would not take into account the likelihood that the physiological self-regulation behavior and skill of a trainee changes as training progresses. Fuchs and Schwarz [47] identify a method without this capability as a "hard-coded" adaptation strategy, where the system triggers a predetermined adaptation strategy.

From a psychophysiological point of view, the results of our characterization study revealed significant evidence of how users respond to VR shooting simulators. Past experiences using immersive virtual environments have found changes in Alpha oscillatory activity during aiming that are associated with better performance while shooting [48]. In our experiment, we found the frontal Alpha activity (as well as the Delta) to be a brainwave pattern that clearly allows the differentiation between baseline and active shooting states in our VR simulator. Furthermore, increases of Alpha EEG activity have also been associated with subjects who performed well in spatial navigation tasks in a VR environment [49]. Past research also suggested how to use Alpha-related activity to create modulations in a BCI version of the popular World of Warcraft videogame [50]. In summary, Alpha oscillatory activity resulted in a sensitive bio-marker to create real-time adaptations that accurately reflected users' concentration levels during target shooting tasks in the *BioPhyS* simulator.

Autonomic cardiac regulation has also been studied in VR experiences demonstrating how VR simulations can shape the cardiovascular responses of users. Significant difference in HR values was found during 5-min long interactions with a VR experience that required users to perform simple manual tasks involving the arrangement of virtual elements with multiple shapes [51]. Similarly to our easy-medium-hard difficulty levels, an experiment with a VR first person shooter experience showed non-significant differences for the main effect condition (boredom-flow-frustration) on the users' heart rate [43]. We believe that the novel room-size VR tracking used for the *BioPhyS* simulator may significantly affect the cardiovascular responses in VR experiences. Additionally, after exchanging information with professional police officers' trainers, we learned that some specific sympathetic responses are desired during military fighting situations that can be used as target states to create the BLs (e.g., 100–115 BPMs for HR levels) [52]. A similar concept was used to persuade older users to exert in targeted cardiac zones via biocybernetic adaptation strategies integrated during exercise-based videogames also called Exergames [53].

For future work, we are planning to compare the initial results found with the young male population assessed against a group of trained police officers. We have recorded police officers who went through the same data collection protocol, and now we are building a psychophysiological model for this population. Our initial hypothesis proposes a more controlled cardiac regulation behavior as well as different brainwave activation patterns. A very detailed description of the project design and development can be found at https://sites.google.com/view/johnhci/simulators/biophys.

5 Conclusion

Biocybernetic adaptation technologies are poised to exploit the very fast adoption of VR technologies that are now ubiquitous and accessible. With novel physiologically aware systems, the training process of any skill in a virtual environment can benefit from a more personalized and informed content delivery that has the potential to maximize the learning outcomes. The *BioPhyS* approach here presented, evidences how biocybernetic technologies can be meaningfully integrated with VR military training simulators to produce physiologically intelligent systems able to sharpen trainees' self-regulation capabilities. Those skills might impact the performance of daily worklife tasks (such as firing in the case of police officers), helping users to respond in a more controlled and physiologically regulated way to external stressors. We conclude our project, highlighting the potential of using biocybernetic adaptation in various VR scenarios that are now booming such as virtual rehabilitation, wellbeing promotion, pain treatment, and education. Moreover, we emphasize the benefits of this VR-biocybernetics symbiosis, which aids the creation of more adaptive VR systems and promotes a less tedious training process of physiological regulation skills.

Acknowledgments. Authors would like to thank: (i) the J&F Alliance Group who financially supported the internship and VR development process, (ii) the National Institute of Aerospace (NIA) that supported the convergence of the stakeholders for this project, (iii) the PRISM team from NASA Langley for his very supportive feedback throughout the project development and (iv) Zeltech employees at Hampton facilities. Special thanks to personnel from the Hampton Police Department who participated actively in our studies; and Jeremy Sklute and Mike Priddy from J&F Alliance who helped in improving the system's realism.

Contributions. JEM and ATP designed and defined the *BioPhyS* approach and the biocybernetic adaptation strategies. LEV developed the VR simulation and carried out the integration with the BL Engine. All authors revised and approved the current version of the manuscript.

References

1. Anthes, C., García-Hernández, R.J., Wiedemann, M., Kranzlmüller, D.: State of the art of virtual reality technology (2016)

2. Jerald, J.: The VR Book: Human-Centered Design for Virtual Reality. Morgan & Claypool, New York (2015)
3. Kosunen, I., Salminen, M., Järvelä, S., Ruonala, A., Ravaja, N., Jacucci, G.: RelaWorld: neuroadaptive and immersive virtual reality meditation system. In: Proceedings of the 21st International Conference on Intelligent User Interfaces, pp. 208–217. ACM (2016)
4. Sra, M., Xu, X., Maes, P.: BreathVR: leveraging breathing as a directly controlled interface for virtual reality games. In: Proceedings of the 2018 CHI Conference on Human Factors in Computing Systems, p. 340. ACM (2018)
5. Muñoz, J.E., Paulino, T., Vasanth, H., Baras, K.: PhysioVR: a novel mobile virtual reality framework for physiological computing. In: 2016 IEEE 18th International Conference on e-Health Networking, Applications and Services (Healthcom), pp. 1–6. IEEE (2016)
6. Pope, A.T., Stephens, C.L., Gilleade, K.: Biocybernetic adaptation as biofeedback training method. In: Fairclough, S.H., Gilleade, K. (eds.) Advances in Physiological Computing. HIS, pp. 91–115. Springer, London (2014). https://doi.org/10.1007/978-1-4471-6392-3_5
7. Fairclough, S.H.: Fundamentals of physiological computing. Interact. Comput. 21, 133–145 (2009)
8. Novak, D., Mihelj, M., Munih, M.: A survey of methods for data fusion and system adaptation using autonomic nervous system responses in physiological computing. Interact. Comput. 24, 154–172 (2012)
9. Fairclough, S.H.: Physiological computing and intelligent adaptation. In: Emotions and Affect in Human Factors and Human-Computer Interaction, pp. 539–556. Elsevier (2017)
10. Burdea, G.C., Coiffet, P.: Virtual Reality technology. Wiley, Hoboken (2003)
11. Kennedy, R.S., Stanney, K.M., Lawson, B.D.: Capability of virtual environments to meet military requirements. Essex Corp., Orlando, FL (2000)
12. Mead, C.: War Play: Video Games and the Future of Armed Conflict. Houghton Mifflin Harcourt, Boston (2013)
13. Roy, M.J., Rizzo, A., Difede, J., Rothbaum, B.O.: Virtual reality exposure therapy for PTSD. In: Complementary and Alternative Medicine for PTSD, p. 271 (2016)
14. Wood, D.P., et al.: Cost effectiveness of virtual reality graded exposure therapy with physiological monitoring for the treatment of combat related post traumatic stress disorder. Stud. Health Technol. Inform. 144, 223–229 (2009)
15. Ćosić, K., Popović, S., Kukolja, D., Horvat, M., Dropuljić, B.: Physiology-driven adaptive virtual reality stimulation for prevention and treatment of stress related disorders. Cyberpsychology Behav. Soc. Netw. 13, 73–78 (2010)
16. Blacker, K.J., Hamilton, J., Roush, G. et al.: Cognitive training for military application: a review of the literature and practical guide. J. Cogn. Enhanc. 3, 30 (2019). https://doi.org/10.1007/s41465-018-0076-1
17. Lele, A.: Virtual reality and its military utility. J. Ambient. Intell. Hum. Comput. 4, 17–26 (2013)
18. Palsson, O.S., Harris Sr, R.L., Pope, A.T.: Method and apparatus for encouraging physiological self-regulation through modulation of an operator's control input to a video game or training simulator (2002)
19. Prinzel III, L.J., Pope, A.T., Palsson, O.S., Turner, M.J.: Method and apparatus for performance optimization through physical perturbation of task elements (2014)
20. Pope, A.T., Stephens, C.L., Jones, C.A.: Method and system for physiologically modulating action role-playing open world video games and simulations which use gesture and body image sensing control input devices. Google Patents (2015)
21. Pope, A.T., Stephens, C.L., Blanson, N.M.: Physiologically modulating videogames or simulations which use motion-sensing input devices (2014)

22. Sajnog, C.: How to Shoot Like a Navy Seal: Combat Marksmanship Fundamentals. Center Mass Group, LLC (2013)
23. Muñoz, J.E., Rubio, E., Cameirao, M., Bermúdez, S.: The biocybernetic loop engine: an integrated tool for creating physiologically adaptive videogames. In: 4th International Conference in Physiological Computing Systems, Madrid, España (2017)
24. Bontchev, B.: Adaptation in affective video games: a literature review. Cybern. Inf. Technol. **16**, 3–34 (2016)
25. Jacucci, G., Fairclough, S., Solovey, E.T.: Physiological computing. Computer **48**, 12–16 (2015)
26. Vourvopoulos, A., Faria, A.L., Cameirão, M.S., Bermudez i Badia, S.: RehabNet: a distributed architecture for motor and cognitive neuro-rehabilitation. In: 2013 IEEE 15th International Conference on e-Health Networking, Applications Services (Healthcom), pp. 454–459 (2013)
27. Fisher, J.G., Hatch, J.P., Rugh, J.D.: Biofeedback: Studies in Clinical Efficacy. Springer, Boston (2013)
28. Johnson, B.R.: Crucial Elements of Police Firearms Training. Looseleaf Law Publications (2007)
29. Muñoz, J.E., Gouveia, E.R., Cameirão, M.S., i Badia, S.B.: PhysioLab-a multivariate physiological computing toolbox for ECG, EMG and EDA signals: a case of study of cardiorespiratory fitness assessment in the elderly population. Multimed. Tools Appl., 1–26 (2017)
30. Plews, D.J., Scott, B., Altini, M., Wood, M., Kilding, A.E., Laursen, P.B.: Comparison of heart-rate-variability recording with smartphone photoplethysmography, Polar H7 chest strap, and electrocardiography. Int. J. Sport. Physiol. Perform. **12**, 1324–1328 (2017)
31. Sanei, S., Chambers, J.A.: EEG Signal Processing. Wiley, Hoboken (2013)
32. McMahan, T., Parberry, I., Parsons, T.D.: Evaluating electroencephalography engagement indices during video game Play. In: FDG (2015)
33. Kamzanova, A.T., Matthews, G., Kustubayeva, A.M., Jakupov, S.M.: EEG indices to time-on-task effects and to a workload manipulation (cueing). World Acad. Sci. Eng. Technol. **80**, 19–22 (2011)
34. Fairclough, S., Gilleade, K.: Construction of the biocybernetic loop: a case study. In: Proceedings of the 14th ACM International Conference on Multimodal Interaction, p. 578. ACM, New York (2012)
35. Kennedy, R.S., Lane, N.E., Berbaum, K.S., Lilienthal, M.G.: Simulator sickness questionnaire: an enhanced method for quantifying simulator sickness. Int. J. Aviat. Psychol. **3**, 203–220 (1993)
36. Teasdale, N., Lavallière, M., Tremblay, M., Laurendeau, D., Simoneau, M.: Multiple exposition to a driving simulator reduces simulator symptoms for elderly drivers (2009)
37. Csikszentmihalyi, M.: Toward a psychology of optimal experience. Flow and the Foundations of Positive Psychology, pp. 209–226. Springer, Dordrecht (2014). https://doi.org/10.1007/978-94-017-9088-8_14
38. Peifer, C.: Psychophysiological correlates of flow-experience. In: Engeser, S. (ed.) Advances in Flow Research, pp. 139–164. Springer, New York (2012). https://doi.org/10.1007/978-1-4614-2359-1_8
39. Sandweiss, J.H.: Biofeedback and sports science. In: Sandweiss, J.H., Wolf, S.L. (eds.) Biofeedback and sports science, pp. 1–31. Springer, Boston (1985). https://doi.org/10.1007/978-1-4757-9465-6_1
40. Grossman, D.: On Killing: The Psychological Cost of Learning to Kill in War and Society. Open Road Media, New York (2014)

41. Dey, A., Piumsomboon, T., Lee, Y., Billinghurst, M.: Effects of sharing physiological states of players in a collaborative virtual reality gameplay. In: Proceedings of the 2017 CHI Conference on Human Factors in Computing Systems, pp. 4045–4056. ACM (2017)
42. Cacioppo, J.T., Tassinary, L.G., Berntson, G.: Handbook of Psychophysiology. Cambridge University Press, Cambridge (2007)
43. Bombeke, K., et al.: Do not disturb: psychophysiological correlates of boredom, flow and frustration during VR gaming. In: Schmorrow, D.D., Fidopiastis, C.M. (eds.) AC 2018. LNCS (LNAI), vol. 10915, pp. 101–119. Springer, Cham (2018). https://doi.org/10.1007/978-3-319-91470-1_10
44. Pugnetti, L., Meehan, M., Mendozzi, L.: Psychophysiological correlates of virtual reality: a review. Presence Teleoperators Virtual Environ. **10**, 384–400 (2001)
45. Wiederhold, B.K.: Virtual reality and applied psychophysiology. Appl. Psychophysiol. Biofeedback **30**, 183–185 (2005)
46. Stephens, C., et al.: Biocybernetic adaptation strategies: machine awareness of human engagement for improved operational performance. In: Schmorrow, Dylan D., Fidopiastis, Cali M. (eds.) AC 2018. LNCS (LNAI), vol. 10915, pp. 89–98. Springer, Cham (2018). https://doi.org/10.1007/978-3-319-91470-1_9
47. Fuchs, S., Schwarz, J.: Towards a dynamic selection and configuration of adaptation strategies in augmented cognition. In: Schmorrow, D.D., Fidopiastis, C.M. (eds.) AC 2017. LNCS (LNAI), vol. 10285, pp. 101–115. Springer, Cham (2017). https://doi.org/10.1007/978-3-319-58625-0_7
48. Pereira, M., Argelaguet, F., Millán, J. del R., Lécuyer, A.: Novice shooters with lower pre-shooting alpha power have better performance during competition in a virtual reality scenario. Front. Psychol. **9**, 527 (2018)
49. Pugnetti, L., Mendozzi, L., Barberi, E., Rose, F.D., Attree, E.A.: Nervous system correlates of virtual reality experience. In: European Conference on Disability, Virtual Reality and Associated Technology (1996)
50. Friedman, D.: Brain-computer interfacing and virtual reality. In: Nakatsu, R., Rauterberg, M., Ciancarini, P. (eds.) Handbook of Digital Games and Entertainment Technologies, pp. 1–22. Springer, Singapore (2015). https://doi.org/10.1007/978-981-4560-52-8_2-1
51. Malińska, M., Zużewicz, K., Bugajska, J., Grabowski, A.: Heart rate variability (HRV) during virtual reality immersion. Int. J. Occup. Saf. Ergon. **21**, 47–54 (2015)
52. Mason, P.H.: Recovering from the War: A Guide for All Veterans, Family Members. Friends and Therapists. Patience Press, High Springs (1998)
53. Muñoz, J.E., Rubio, E., Cameirao, M.S., Bermúdez i Badia, S.: Closing the loop in exergaming - health benefits of biocybernetic adaptation in senior adults. In: Proceedings of the 2018 Annual Symposium on Computer-Human Interaction in Play (2018)

Author Index

Printed in the United States
By Bookmasters